Ethical Implications of Reshaping Healthcare With Emerging Technologies

Thomas Heinrich Musiolik
Berlin University of the Arts, Germany

Alexiei Dingli
University of Malta, Malta

A volume in the Advances in Medical Technologies and Clinical Practice (AMTCP) Book Series

IGI Global
PUBLISHER of TIMELY KNOWLEDGE

Published in the United States of America by
IGI Global
Medical Information Science Reference (an imprint of IGI Global)
701 E. Chocolate Avenue
Hershey PA, USA 17033
Tel: 717-533-8845
Fax: 717-533-8661
E-mail: cust@igi-global.com
Web site: http://www.igi-global.com

Library of Congress Cataloging-in-Publication Data

Names: Musiolik, Thomas Heinrich, 1980- editor. | Dingli, Alexiei, editor.
Title: Ethical implications of reshaping healthcare with emerging technologies / Thomas Heinrich Musiolik and Alexiei Dingli, editors.
Description: Hershey, PA : Medical Information Science Reference, [2021] | Includes bibliographical references and index. | Summary: "This book shows the current state of research in the fields of health care and medicine, how the new technologies can be used for patient communication, health monitoring or for the treatment of patients"-- Provided by publisher.
Identifiers: LCCN 2020057923 (print) | LCCN 2020057924 (ebook) | ISBN 9781799878889 (hardcover) | ISBN 9781799878889 (ebook)
Subjects: MESH: Biomedical Technology--ethics | Bioethical Issues | Health Services--trends
Classification: LCC R724 (print) | LCC R724 (ebook) | NLM W 82 | DDC 174.2--dc23
LC record available at https://lccn.loc.gov/2020057923
LC ebook record available at https://lccn.loc.gov/2020057924

This book is published in the IGI Global book series Advances in Medical Technologies and Clinical Practice (AMTCP) (ISSN: 2327-9354; eISSN: 2327-9370)

British Cataloguing in Publication Data
A Cataloguing in Publication record for this book is available from the British Library.

All work contributed to this book is new, previously-unpublished material.
The views expressed in this book are those of the authors, but not necessarily of the publisher.

For electronic access to this publication, please contact: eresources@igi-global.com.

Advances in Medical Technologies and Clinical Practice (AMTCP) Book Series

ISSN:2327-9354
EISSN:2327-9370

MISSION

Medical technological innovation continues to provide avenues of research for faster and safer diagnosis and treatments for patients. Practitioners must stay up to date with these latest advancements to provide the best care for nursing and clinical practices.

The **Advances in Medical Technologies and Clinical Practice (AMTCP) Book Series** brings together the most recent research on the latest technology used in areas of nursing informatics, clinical technology, biomedicine, diagnostic technologies, and more. Researchers, students, and practitioners in this field will benefit from this fundamental coverage on the use of technology in clinical practices.

COVERAGE

- Diagnostic Technologies
- Biomechanics
- Biometrics
- Clinical Nutrition
- Patient-Centered Care
- Clinical High-Performance Computing
- Medical Informatics
- Telemedicine
- Nursing Informatics
- Nutrition

IGI Global is currently accepting manuscripts for publication within this series. To submit a proposal for a volume in this series, please contact our Acquisition Editors at Acquisitions@igi-global.com or visit: http://www.igi-global.com/publish/.

The Advances in Medical Technologies and Clinical Practice (AMTCP) Book Series (ISSN 2327-9354) is published by IGI Global, 701 E. Chocolate Avenue, Hershey, PA 17033-1240, USA, www.igi-global.com. This series is composed of titles available for purchase individually; each title is edited to be contextually exclusive from any other title within the series. For pricing and ordering information please visit http://www.igi-global.com/book-series/advances-medical-technologies-clinical-practice/73682. Postmaster: Send all address changes to above address.

Titles in this Series

For a list of additional titles in this series, please visit:
http://www.igi-global.com/book-series/advances-medical-technologies-clinical-practice/73682

Machine Learning and Data Analytics for Predicting, Managing, and Monitoring Disease
Manikant Roy (Lovely Professional University, India) and Lovi Raj Gupta (Lovely Professional University, India)
Medical Information Science Reference • © 2021 • 241pp • H/C (ISBN: 9781799871880) • US $395.00

Advancing the Investigation and Treatment of Sleep Disorders Using AI
M. Rajesh Kumar (Vellore Institute of Technology, Vellore, India) Ranjeet Kumar (Vellore Institute of Technology, Chennai, India) and D. Vaithiyanathan (National Institute of Technology, Delhi, India)
Medical Information Science Reference • © 2021 • 291pp • H/C (ISBN: 9781799880189) • US $345.00

Machine Learning in Cancer Research With Applications in Colon Cancer and Big Data Analysis
Zhongyu Lu (University of Huddersfield, UK) Qiang Xu (University of Huddersfield, UK) Murad Al-Rajab (University of Huddersfield, UK & Abu Dhabi University, UAE) and Lamogha Chiazor (University of Huddersfield, UK)
Medical Information Science Reference • © 2021 • 263pp • H/C (ISBN: 9781799873167) • US $345.00

Handbook of Research on Nano-Strategies for Combatting Antimicrobial Resistance and Cancer
Muthupandian Saravanan (Mekelle University, Ethiopia & Saveetha Dental College, Saveetha Institute of Medical and Technical Sciences (SIMATS), India) Venkatraman Gopinath (University of Malaya, Malaysia) and Karthik Deekonda (Monash University, Malaysia)
Medical Information Science Reference • © 2021 • 559pp • H/C (ISBN: 9781799850496) • US $375.00

Handbook of Research on Solving Modern Healthcare Challenges With Gamification
Ricardo Alexandre Peixoto de Queirós (uniMAD, Escola Superior de Media Artes e Design, Portugal) and António José Marques (LabRP, School of Health, Polytechnic of Porto, Portugal)
Medical Information Science Reference • © 2021 • 382pp • H/C (ISBN: 9781799874720) • US $425.00

IGI Global
PUBLISHER of TIMELY KNOWLEDGE

701 East Chocolate Avenue, Hershey, PA 17033, USA
Tel: 717-533-8845 x100 • Fax: 717-533-8661
E-Mail: cust@igi-global.com • www.igi-global.com

Table of Contents

Detailed Table of Contents

One of the conversations that emerged forcefully during the past year, in the context of the COVID-19 pandemic, is linked to the use of artificial intelligence (AI) in healthcare, and it touches both its effectiveness and its ethics. The chapter starts with three examples of using automated systems in healthcare and continues by proposing an understanding of the ethics from the perspective of the meaning assigned to optimisation. The argument is that we need to deeply explore the aim of optimisation in order to shed a different and perhaps more revealing light on ethical questions related to AI use in general, and in healthcare in particular. The chapter ends with a few propositions on how to approach optimisation and reconsider the way in which automation is both adopted and adapted.

The importance of robotics and assistive technologies for healthcare is increasing. For their introduction into practical application, the continuous integration of the user perspective is crucial to ensure acceptance and usability. This can be achieved by the user-centered design approach. In an earlier publication, several problems with its functional implementation within research and development (R&D) projects were pointed out. This chapter discusses possible solutions to promote an effective integration of the user perspective in R&D projects based on six interviews with experts from Germany. The results can be summarized in three main requirements: first, the generation of a common understanding of the target group; second, a scientific research approach considering the context of technology usage; third, projectification, with a focus on efficient resource planning, the development of generic technologies, and technology evaluations with the user group. Leaders of innovative projects can benefit from implementing these strategies in the development process.

Modern advanced tools of artificial intelligence assist healthcare professionals in a variety of complex tasks related to medical care. Digitalization and automation accelerate the development and deployment of innovative artificial intelligence tools tailor-made for clinical applications; decision support systems represent an important example of such tools. This chapter is devoted to discussing the role of artificial intelligence in current and prospective medical care and ethical aspects of their deployment. As developed countries currently go through remarkable transforms of medical care involving informatization and centering around medical information and knowledge, this chapter also discusses future ideals of medical care characterized by the concept of information-based medicine. Ethical and patient safety implications of using artificial intelligence within information-based medicine are overviewed here. Specific attention is paid to mental healthcare and ethical aspects of using artificial intelligence in its context.

Artificial intelligence has a huge array of current and potential applications in healthcare and medicine. Ethical issues arising due to algorithmic biases are one of the greatest challenges faced in the generalizability of AI models today. The authors address safety and regulatory barriers that impede data sharing in medicine as well as potential changes to existing techniques and frameworks that might allow ethical data sharing for machine learning. With these developments in view, they also present different algorithmic models that are being used to develop machine learning-based medical systems that will potentially evolve to be free of the sample, annotator, and temporal bias. These AI-based medical imaging models will then be completely implemented in healthcare facilities and institutions all around the world, even in the remotest areas, making diagnosis and patient care both cheaper and freely accessible.

For a long time, the primary approach to control pain in patients involved the use of specially designed drugs. While these drugs have proved to be sufficient to reduce the perception of pain in patients of all ages, they do not come without any potential side effects. The prolonged use of such drugs can have adverse effects on the health of a patient. This research proposes a shift away from such practices and proposes the use of technology as an adjunct tool to help patients cope with pain. Through the adoption of affective computing, this research presents Morpheus results obtained at the time of writing confirm that the approach presented by this research is indeed useful and can achieve results that are in line with the set out as part of this study. The authors firmly believe that the approach presented in this research can lay the foundations for the research and development of similar applications in pain reduction scenarios.

Mental health students, who are still undergoing training, might find it challenging to visualise and fully understand what their patients experience. For this reason, the authors created a virtual reality simulator which mimics the symptoms of a person suffering from schizophrenia at a virtual workplace. The simulation is managed by an artificial intelligence system which asks the user to attempt simple tasks, while simultaneously facing both visual and auditory hallucinations. The AI also adapts the storyline and character behaviour dynamically to increase the immersiveness of the experience. A pilot study was carried out, and the initial results were very encouraging. In fact, the absolute majority of the users stated that the simulation has helped increase their understanding of schizophrenia. In this chapter, the authors evaluate this experiment but from a different perspective. They focus mainly on the use of emerging technologies such as AI and VR and discuss the ethical considerations of their use within the field of mental health.

This chapter introduces the field of advanced technology within the orthotics and prosthetics profession, a healthcare profession that combines technology and engineering science with medical and health science to produce medical devices (orthoses and prostheses) to treat medical conditions that cause physical dysfunction. The chapter sets the background to the ethical dilemmas that are encountered within the field, which technologically advanced devices cause such dilemmas and why, and then discusses the ethical dilemmas as encountered by the three stakeholders within the profession, namely the manufacturers/innovators, the prosthetic and orthotic practitioners, and the users of the devices themselves, the patients. In conclusion, the chapter looks at some solutions and recommendations to overcome or at least reduce these dilemmas.

Skin disease rates have been increasing over the past few decades. It has led to both fatal and non-fatal disabilities all around the world, especially in those areas where medical resources are not good enough. Early diagnosis of skin diseases increases the chances of cure significantly. Therefore, this work is comparing six machine learning algorithms, namely KNN, random forest, neural network, naïve bayes, logistic regression, and SVM, for the prediction of the skin diseases. The information gain, gain ratio, gini decrease, chi-square, and relieff are used to rank the features. This work comprises the introduction, literature review, and proposed methodology parts. In this research paper, a new method of analyzing skin disease has been proposed in which six different data mining techniques are used to develop an ensemble method that integrates all the six data mining techniques as a single one. The ensemble method used on the dermatology dataset gives improved result with 94% accuracy in comparison to other classifier algorithms and hence is more effective in this area.

Foreword

Like many obsessions, my journey into telling stories with data started at an early age. I can still remember as a 9-year-old drawing maps overlaid with the different time zones so that I could, at a glance, see what time it was around the world and dream of exotic locations.

Since then, I have been fascinated not only with telling my own stories, but also how others can understand data and tell their own stories, uncover things previously unknown and identify new insights.

And so, when I was asked to write a foreword to this book, I was pleased to discover that the ethical issues of Artificial Intelligence (AI) within healthcare was being discussed with serious consideration. My own journey into AI has always focused on data and how, as with any algorithm, it can only perform as well as the data that is fed into it. Issues of fairness and more broadly ethics when it comes to technology needs more attention than it is currently receiving, not only to highlight the effects of bias, but more practically, what needs to be done to mitigate bias.

Healthcare is also somewhat unique in that it is a regulated industry that is undergoing a huge transformation effort in part due to the emergence of AI. In the US alone, the FDA has already approved 161 AI powered products since 2017 and is set to be more than 600 by 2025 – a huge rate of growth! However, a recent investigation by STAT discovered that of those 161, only 73 have publicly disclosed how much data was used to validate their models (Ross, 2021). Of the ones that have, the numbers of items in the validation sets ranged between 100 and 15,000 patient records and only 13 included a gender breakdown. What this really highlights that there is not a standardised approach to how these algorithms are validated or how they are reported.

It is worth stating up front that building AI is hard and unlike traditional software development it can be difficult to put together a clear specification for how it should behave and perform. Issues of bias, fairness and explainability continue to challenge even experienced data scientists and researchers. While (hopefully!) no one intentionally sets out to create biased AI, like any endeavour there are always constraints to manage, and quality (read error rate) is always at odds with budget and time. There needs to be balance between all of these and one must continually question what the acceptable level of quality and scope for any project is.

The tasks of creating, validating, and deploying AI still presents daily challenges to companies looking to take advantage of this technology. Much of what is involved is still very manual and significant amounts of time is spent sourcing, preparing, and cleaning data.

On the surface it looks easy enough to cobble together some data and train a model – there are plenty of open-source data sets, articles and competitions online doing just that. But the reality is that these generally are not suitable for much more than to determine basic feasibility.

Most resort to building their own bespoke in-house tooling and data processing pipelines to help manage all this, but these turn out to be not only expensive to maintain but fragile - constantly breaking or taking time away from higher value activities.

When it comes to machine learning, bias is typically a data issue. Machine learning models feed on data as they are *trained*. By its very nature variability is inescapable when it comes to data, and AI is only as good as the data that was used to train it – as they say, garbage in, garbage out. Not only that, once you have trained a model it is even more difficult to ensure that they are robust and are free of bias when running in the real world. Explainability, or being able to understand how an AI product was able to come up with a result is key to addressing issues of ethics and fairness, especially in regulated environments.

Bias in datasets is an issue that can lead to significant consequences in healthcare. Recent publications have reinforced the fact that medical AI solutions, when trained on biased data, are biased themselves and may exacerbate societal inequalities by limiting access to care, advising inadequate care, and leading to poorer patient outcomes for underrepresented groups or those with rare conditions.

The point here is that if you do not know how an AI system was trained and tested, you can't evaluate the risk of concept or data drift as real-world conditions and distributions change. What does "data drift" mean? It means that changes in the real-world data that cause a model to perform differently than expected or tested when it was initially deployed.

The best way to get started is to fully understand the data that has been used to train an AI system through exploratory data analysis, coupled with visualisation. The aim of which is to know the distributions across each dimension, the outliers and areas that are underrepresented. It is not an easy task, especially when dealing with unstructured data like text and images. By visualising your data, trends can appear that are not immediately obvious just by looking at individual data points, you need to be able to sort, group, pivot and graph the data.

The other key is to provide as much access to the data to others as possible. By only looking at the data yourself, it only confirms assumptions from a singular perspective. By collaborating with others, you can gain insight from a wider, more diverse group of individuals and backgrounds that can help to uncover broader issues of unfairness and bias that we individually can be unaware of. Having the right tools and infrastructure to make this as easy as possible is key, with the goal of transparency and explainability in mind and not relying on aggregated values like sensitivity and specificity as these can hide the edge cases.

While the media likes to portray AI with the lens of a dystopian future, I firmly believe AI has huge potential to save lives and reduce the burden of repetitive tasks. As a technologist it's easy to get wrapped up in the mechanics of solving a problem with a new approach, and I need to be constantly reminded that it is right and correct to first ask – yes, but at what cost?

Roger Noble
Zegami, UK

REFERENCES

Ross, C. (2021). *Explore STAT's database of FDA-cleared AI tools*. https://www.statnews.com/2021/02/03/fda-artificial-intelligence-clearance-products/

Preface

We are constantly striving to improve people's quality of life, especially those who are the most vulnerable in our society. Irrespective of all the wealth one possesses, the single significant problem that everyone faces is always related to health. There is nothing one can do apart from hoping to gain access to the latest medical solutions. Because of this, we believe that by marrying emerging technologies with medicine, we can manage to speed up the innovations in our healthcare system, which ultimately reach the people. Of course, to do that, we have to consider the various ethical implications that surface when we introduce new approaches. Let's not forget that in such cases, the end does not necessarily justify the means since we are ultimately talking of human lives and their dignity.

Every day, new technologies are revolutionising medicine and opening up new opportunities for patients, doctors, clinics and hospitals. Artificial Intelligence (AI), Blockchain, Internet of Medical Things, Augmented Reality, Virtual Reality (VR), Robotics, 3D Printing and many others disrupt the work of health professionals. Autonomous systems constantly monitor the patient's well-being using smartphones, wearable devices, and other sensors connected to the ambient assisted systems permeating our homes. The data-rich medical records generated from these systems, augmented with AI, simplify the everyday tasks of clinical workers. When professionals are not available on location, robots can take over in the operating room, controlled remotely by professionals using VR. It is very clear from the previous list of examples that innovations in healthcare will change the quality of the treatment the patients receive and will change the work of doctors, clinics, and hospitals forever.

This book contains a list of the most up-to-date state-of-the-art solutions in healthcare and medicine worldwide, thus highlighting novel forms of treatment that are already available today and shines over the future possibilities currently under research. While tackling these issues, it also examines the ethical implications in healthcare and medicine associated with the rapid development of these technologies.

All the topics mentioned in this book should be of interest to both medical doctors and technology specialists seeking ideas on how to combine the two areas of study. By showcasing the current state of the art research in these two fields, we can illustrate how new technologies can ultimately enhance patient communication, health monitoring and medical treatment. At the same time, it proves that the integration of emerging technologies is available from today. Long gone are the days where innovation stays secluded in a lab. The critical aspect is to bring it to market as quickly as possible whilst always guaranteeing the safety of the users. Hence why the ethical implications should be considered and given due importance. Furthermore, the book can be used as part of lectures, seminars or workshops since it offers a concise set of case studies within the medical domain.

The chapters in this book are varied and far-reaching, touching different areas such as:

- **Ethics, Health, and AI in a COVID-19 World.** One of the conversations that emerged forcefully during the past year, in the context of the COVID-19 pandemic, is linked to the use of Artificial Intelligence (AI) in healthcare, and it touches both its effectiveness, and its ethics. The article starts with three examples of using automated systems in healthcare, and continues with proposing an understanding of the ethics from the perspective of the meaning assigned to optimisation. The argument is that we need to deeply explore the aim of optimisation in order to shed a different and perhaps more revealing light on ethical questions related to AI use in general, and în healthcare în particular. The article ends with a few propositions on how to approach optimisation and reconsider the way in which automation is both adopted and adapted.
- **Managing User Integration: Insights From the Field of Publicly Funded Research and Development Projects in Germany.** The importance of robotics and assistive technologies for healthcare is increasing. For their introduction into practical application, the continuous integration of the user perspective is crucial to ensure acceptance and usability. This can be achieved by the User-Centered Design approach. In an earlier publication, several problems with its functional implementation within research and development (R&D) projects were pointed out. This article discusses possible solutions to promote an effective integration of the user perspective in R&D projects, based on six interviews with experts from Germany. The results can be summarized in three main requirements: first, the generation of a common understanding of the target group; second, a scientific research approach considering the context of technology usage; third, projectification, with a focus on efficient resource planning, the development of generic technologies, and technology evaluations with the user group. Leaders of

innovative projects can benefit from implementing these strategies in the development process.

- **Ethical Aspects of Information-Based Medicine (With a Focus on Mental Health).** Modern advanced tools of artificial intelligence allow to assist healthcare professionals in a variety of complex tasks related to medical care. Digitalization and automation accelerate the development and deployment of innovative artificial intelligence tools tailor-made for clinical applications; decision support systems represent an important example of such tools. This chapter is devoted to discussing the role of artificial intelligence in current and prospective medical care and ethical aspects of their deployment. As developed countries currently go through remarkable transforms of medical care involving informatization and centering around medical information and knowledge, this chapter also discusses future ideals of medical care characterized by the concept of information-based medicine. Ethical and patient safety implications of using artificial intelligence within information-based medicine are overviewed here. Specific attention is paid to mental healthcare and ethical aspects of using artificial intelligence in its context.
- **Artificial Intelligence in Medical Care: Ethical Aspects of Information-Based Medicine.** Already before the outbreak of the COVID-19 pandemic, modern advanced tools of artificial intelligence have been introduced to assist in a variety of complex tasks related to medical care. Digitalization and automation accelerate the development and deployment of innovative artificial intelligence tools tailor-made for clinical applications. This chapter is devoted to discussing the role of artificial intelligence in current and prospective medical care. A survey of selected inspiring examples of artificial intelligence applications in health-related tasks is presented here. As developed countries currently go through remarkable transforms of medical care, involving informatization and centering around medical information and knowledge, this chapter also discusses future ideals of medical care characterized by the concept of information-based medicine. Ethical and patient safety implications of information-based medicine are overviewed. Specific attention is paid to psychiatry, which may greatly benefit from promising recent results of neuroscience research.
- **Reducing Pain Through Affective Computing.** For long, the primary approach to control pain in patients involved the use of specially designed drugs. While these drugs have for long proved most cases proved to be sufficient to reduce the perception of pain in patients of all ages, they do not come without any potential side effects. The prolonged use of such drugs can have adverse effects on the health of a patient. This research proposes a shift away from such practices and proposes the use of technology as an adjunct

tool to help patients cope with pain. Through the adoption of Affective Computing, this research presents Morpheus Results obtained at the time of writing confirm that the approach presented by this research is indeed useful and can achieve results that are in line with the set out as part of this study. We firmly believe that the approach presented in this research can lay the foundations for the research and development of similar applications in pain reduction scenarios.

- **Assistive Technologies.** The field of robotics is becoming extremely important in the use of assistive technologies for health systems. Thus, the user's roles and interactions with the mechanical component are crucial to ensure successful adoption. A high degree of usability is essential to achieve user acceptance through the entire development process. Because of this, this chapter focuses on the User-Centered Design approach. This approach is also associated with a variety of challenges when bridging the gap between conceptualisation and realisation. This chapter discusses possible solutions to close the gap.
- **Ethical Considerations of Using VR in Mental Health Training**. Mental Health students, who are still undergoing training, might find it challenging to visualise and fully understand what their patients experience. For this reason, we created a Virtual Reality simulator which mimics the symptoms of a person suffering from schizophrenia at a virtual workplace. The simulation is managed by an Artificial Intelligence system which asks the user to attempt simple tasks, while simultaneously facing both visual and auditory hallucinations. The AI also adapts the storyline and character behaviour dynamically to increase the immersiveness of the experience. A pilot study was carried out and the initial results were very encouraging. In fact, the absolute majority of the users stated that the simulation has helped increase their understanding of Schizophrenia. In this paper, we will evaluate this experiment but from a different perspective. We will focus mainly on the use of emerging technologies such as AI and VR and discuss the ethical considerations of their use within the field of Mental Health.
- **Ethical Considerations in Prosthetics and Orthotics.** This chapter introduces the field of advanced technology within the orthotics and prosthetics profession, a healthcare profession that combines technology and engineering science with medical and health science to produce medical devices (orthoses and prostheses) to treat medical conditions that cause physical dysfunction. The chapter sets the background to the ethical dilemmas that are encountered within the field, which technologically advanced devices cause such dilemmas and why, and then discusses the ethical dilemmas as encountered by the three stakeholders within the profession, namely the

manufacturers/innovators, the prosthetic and orthotic practitioners, and the users of the devices themselves, the patients. In conclusion, the chapter looks at some solutions and recommendations to overcome or at least reduce these dilemmas.

- **Prediction of Skin Diseases Using the Machine Learning.** Skin diseases rate has been increasing since past few decades. It led to both fatal and non-fatal disabilities all around the world, especially in those areas where medical resources are not good enough. Early diagnosis of skin diseases, increases the chances of cure significantly. Therefore this work is comparing six machine learning algorithm namely KNN, Random forest, Neural Network, Naïve Bayes, Logistic Regression and SVM for the prediction of the skin diseases. The information gain, gain ratio, gini decrease, chi-square and relieff are used to rank the features. This work comprises the introduction, literature review and proposed methodology part. In this research paper, a new method of analyzing skin disease has been proposed in which six different data mining techniques are used and then developed an ensemble way, that integrates all the six above mentioned data mining techniques as a single one. The ensemble method used on the dermatology dataset gives improved result with 94% accuracy in comparison to other classifier algorithms and hence is more effective in this area.

As can be seen from the wide selection of topics mentioned above, the book gives a very comprehensive overview of the different technologies which are currently affecting modern medical practices. Each chapter also gives a peep into the future, thus sowing inside the brains of professionals ideas which they can build upon in the coming years. Notwithstanding this we hope that through this collection of paper, we can manage to make an impact by keeping people informed about these developments and help them get in touch with researchers worldwide that are creating state-of-the-art innovations. Of course, is always framed within ethical parameters thus allowing patients to get the best treatment possible while ensuring that their rights are being protected. Only if we do so can we hope to create a better future for everyone, one where the most needy, get the most out of the emerging technologies that are reshaping healthcare.

Acknowledgment

Thomas Heinrich Musiolik aka Prof. Brain would like to acknowledge his mentors and heroes, Professor Dr. David Adrian Cheok, Dr. David Levy, Albert Einstein (RIP) and Abū Alī al-Husain ibn Abd Allāh ibn Sīnā (RIP). Furthermore, he would like to acknowledge his two supervisors Professor Dr. Christian Blümelhuber and Professor Dr. Stephan Porombka for the trust and the freedom to be able to grow professionally, yet also humanely. He wishes to acknowledge his enchanting wife Sophie, daughter Emilia Viktoria and son Leon Vincent aka. Mr. Lion for being happiness and magic in his life and to express his gratitude and love to them forever.

Prof. Dr. Alexiei Dingli would like to thank the almighty for creating such an incredible Universe which serves as a daily source of inspiration for researchers worldwide to achieve amazing feats. He would also like to thank his personal source of inspiration; his wife Anna, his three kids Ben, Jake and tiny Faye, together with his dear parents who are always there to support all of his endeavors.

Chapter 1
Ethics, Health, and AI in a COVID-19 World:
Why Contextual Dynamics Matter and Culture Beats Algorithms

Alec Balasescu
Royal Roads University, Canada

ABSTRACT

One of the conversations that emerged forcefully during the past year, in the context of the COVID-19 pandemic, is linked to the use of artificial intelligence (AI) in healthcare, and it touches both its effectiveness and its ethics. The chapter starts with three examples of using automated systems in healthcare and continues by proposing an understanding of the ethics from the perspective of the meaning assigned to optimisation. The argument is that we need to deeply explore the aim of optimisation in order to shed a different and perhaps more revealing light on ethical questions related to AI use in general, and in healthcare in particular. The chapter ends with a few propositions on how to approach optimisation and reconsider the way in which automation is both adopted and adapted.

INTRODUCTION

One of the conversations that emerged forcefully during the past year, in the context of the COVID-19 pandemic, is linked to the use of Artificial Intelligence (AI) in healthcare, and it touches both its effectiveness, and its ethics. Based on the author's experience in healthcare and on the current examples of the adoption and adaptation

DOI: 10.4018/978-1-7998-7888-9.ch001

of automating systems, this article will discuss the impact of the possible use of AI as decision support for allocation of medical resources in emergency situations. The main question of the article is: How is optimisation understood and used in healthcare in relation to AI, what are possible pitfalls of adopting automated systems, and how can they be possibly avoided?

Exploring possible answers to this question will lead us to analyse the impact of the dynamic socio-cultural environment on the predictive capacities of algorithm-based AI models. The article will emphasize the importance of integrating culturally specific dimensions in AI development and deployment, and to approach ethics as applied to AI in a culturally aware manner.

The article starts with three examples of using automated systems in healthcare, and continues with proposing an understanding of the ethics from the perspective of the meaning assigned to optimisation. The argument is that we need to deeply explore the aim of optimisation in order to shed a different and perhaps more revealing light on ethical questions related to AI use in general, and healthcare in particular. The article ends with a few propositions on how to approach optimisation and reconsider the way in which automation is both adopted and adapted.

DECISIONS, DECISIONS, DECISIONS

Optimisation is a major selling point of Artificial Intelligence (AI)-based automation systems. It consists of clear and obvious applications — such as optimising the image-based diagnosis in healthcare. All the same, it bears promises of a perfectly optimised lifestyle for those who embrace total monitoring of their lives, from food intake to daily activities — a hallucination of a perfectly optimised life that is.

The ethics of decision making applied to AI gave birth to an entire field, AI ethics, with specialized journals, publications, and books that cover the most diverse domains, from justice and policing application to cultural variance of AI applications. While some authors approach the structural determinants that influence the very design of automated systems (Noble, 2018; D'Ignazio et al.,2020), others look at the ways in which these designs reinforce the current inequalities instead of addressing them (Hong, 2020; Eubanks, 2019; Hicks, 2018). Healthcare, AI and ethics constitute a special subfield, in which decision making is analyzed from ethical, human-machine interaction, and efficiency lenses (Perreira, 2019; Musen el al., 2014; Park et al., 2019; Pontefract el al., 2018; Kohli et al., 2018). While the field is ripe with theoretical and practical approaches, this paper proposes a perspective on the question of AI ethics in healthcare that is both philosophical and practical. Philosophically it asks the question of the limits of optimisation, it concretely shows how ethics is highly dependent on the material and cultural context, and it emphasizes the practicality of the method in approaching these particularities in order to avoid formulaic answers.

Some would say that life is a sum of decisions. When we make decisions that influence others lives as directly as they do in healthcare, we want to make sure we actually take the right decision. Automated systems using evidence-based AI algorithms promise an *a priori hindsight* in our decision making and that's why they are so seductive. They can also be misleading.

Users and beneficiaries of AI come from a variety of cultural spaces with different representations of health, body, privacy, wellbeing, and ethics. Patients and health providers may experience healthcare in the same institutional context, but in intellectually and emotionally different manners. For instance, the mere use of a device for electronic medical data recording for example can generate two contradictory feelings and attitudes.

On the one hand a patient can feel neglected, while the health worker is absorbed behind the screen. The health worker, in turn, may feel pressed by the natural urgency of giving care, but completely absorbed by the mandatory computing routine, at only arm's reach from the patient.

In even more dramatical ways, automation systems may be used in informing on, or even taking decisions about, how the limited care unit resources are allocated in ways that literally may end lives. At the same time, the algorithms involved in these decisions are often inscrutable, not only for the health workers but even for IT specialists themselves. However, they are designed on principles that may not be as universal as we like to believe, but highly dependent on cultural biases.

Healthcare has different domains in which decision making needs to be rapid and accurate. The examples below illustrate three separated and interrelated instances: medication, diagnosis, and triage or resource allocation. Discussing them together will point to the intricate web of relations formed at the intersection of technology, healthcare, biology and culture. It will also reemphasize the importance of human centered systemic approaches and analysis in case of adoption of automated systems in clinical settings and elsewhere.

Automating Medication - What can go Wrong?

For two years the author was part of a team that designed, prepared, implemented and evaluated the introduction of an electronic healthcare system in a Canadian province. Currently used all over the world, the electronic healthcare systems combine the patients records, also known as patient charts, with the automation of certain operations, data extraction and storage, in order to facilitate and enhance the quality of decision making based on evidence, subsequent healthcare, and medical research. The system itself embeds a series of decision support features, under the form of alerts - i.e. alerts in case of the risk of sepsis or for the possible wrong dosage administration The system user has the option to ignore, override, or follow the instructions attached to any type of message, however the system will register the option, sometimes with unexpected consequences (I will return to this in a moment).

The automated system the author worked with entails a specific medication workflow that combines the medication in itself with scanning both the medication labels and the patients' Wristbands. This requires the manipulation of a computer on wheels with a scanner attached that displays the patient's record, occasional alerts, and standardized warnings based on real time analysis of the medical data input. Medication itself is part of the real time data input in patient's records. The computer on wheels (aka COW) is rather clumsy—with a rather large display on which all the complex patient medical history must be exposed at once. Not to mention the weight of the COW. So much for AI immateriality...

To optimise medication meant to follow precisely the workflow briefly described above in order to scan as many instances of medication as possible. The operation itself consists in the following steps: access the medication from storage, bring it together with the COW wherever the patient is, scan the patient's wristband, scan the medication, check the patient's identification, ask verbal identification from the patient (if the patient's state allows for it), and administer the medication as prescribed. Each vial or pill needs to be scanned. If in any of the instances above the machine gives out an alert, such as wrong medication, wrong patient, or wrong dosis, the healthcare worker (usually a nurse) has the option to override the system or to insert data manually. Nevertheless, the new standardized workflow emphasizes the scanning over the manual insertion.

In the view of the Quality Insurance (QI) department, the measure of efficiency of work is the rate of medication scanning per distributed dose of medication in each department. Thus, the new workflow is supposed to have a twofold utility: to record real time accurate data, and to ensure the accuracy of the records. This is why the QI department considers the manual insertion of the information post-medication a failure in the correct procedure, and thus in healthcare practice. Moreover, scanning is raised to the rank of efficiency measure and work ethics in this environment.

QI narrowly defined efficiency independent of context, and of the complexity of the process involved in work. This soon proved to be the Achile's heel of the system.

First, the system was designed in the United States, where medical doctors are not allowed to write subscriptions for medication in variable doses. On the contrary, in Canada variable doses subscriptions are rather common, leaving to the caregiver the decision regarding the appropriate dose in function of the state of the patient. Because the system could not be twitched to accept variable doses, the alerts were set to fire up as "wrong dose" for any medication administered in lower doses than the maximum prescribed, and the nurses were instructed to override them manually.

Therefore the system generated statistics that showed an increased percentage of "wrong doses", without the ability to differentiate between genuine wrong doses and legitimate overriding. The intersection between design and practice proved to be the generator of an error, that may aliment error in judgments regarding the efficiency of the healthcare workers on the floor, and about the quality of the service.

Second, in the first couple of weeks the system generated statistics showed that the rate of completed medication scanning workflow had decreased drastically in the Emergency department. The QI department promptly concluded that there was a problem, edging on outright blaming the floor personnel for "not doing their job", as data "showed". Now, data usually points out where there might be a problem, but it does not precisely indicate what the problem is (this is frequent confusion at the basis of many decisions taken while using what "data says"). In consultation with the hospital management, the author did a "rapid ethnography" (Palinkas, 2019) adapted to the context, meant to understand where the personnel experienced impediments in the medication administration workflow.

The findings were telling regarding the importance of understanding context—including physical context—when we decide to implement any technology, and particularly AI-based technology. As mentioned before, although AI systems function in a perceived virtual space, they comprise a great deal of materiality (Deibert, 2020). The COWs, to begin with, seemed, at the first glance, rather slick, with ergonomic design, variable geometry that could be adapted to sitting or standing positions, nicely rolling wheels, and big screens that could accommodate the simultaneous display of all the patient chart's information. They may seem close to perfection. And they were, if it wasn't for the context. In an ideal healthcare site, rendered on a computer, they probably looked like the peak of hospital technology. In the physical reality of this emergency department, designed in the late 1970s, with narrow corridors, even narrower doors, and multifunctional spaces, the COWs looked clumsy, almost encumbering, and somehow out of place. The author observed that both the computers and their charging station had names, written on stickers and attached to them. When asked why, a nurse prompted the author to think about what happens in case of a blackout. It would be much easier, she said, to tell your colleagues "Nemo is working", and eventually rapidly find him, instead of "LC32450X4 is working"—a great example of human-machine interaction effects, and the importance of integrating technology in the pre-existent cultural forms If for industrial designers form still follows function, for new virtualised technology its function must follow cultural forms once it leaves the lab conditions.

Let's return to, and review, the medication workflow. In the ideal case, it implies that the nurse first checks the patient system using a barcode reader attached to the COWs, does the verbal identification by asking the patient their name and DOB, scans the patient's barcode on the bracelet attached at admission, scans the medication label, and finally administers the medication. After the first medication is administered the nurse will only repeat the scanning for vials and packages. The entire operation must happen with the patient in sight, at their bedside, which means that the nurse needs to manoeuvre the COW to wherever the patient is. This workflow may work well when patients are hospitalized already, and are waiting patiently to receive their doses. However, this is not always the case.

First of all, some patients arrive in a critical state and all the operations listed above take time. Minutes, even seconds, may be crucial in an emergency situation. In many cases, the first life saving medication must be administered even before the patient is registered in the system, that is before having a wristband to scan, or an electronic chart for the nurse to refer to.

Second, leaving aside the life threatening situations, patients arriving at the emergency ward are assigned a priority rank based on a first rapid consultation and assessment. In the hospital the author am referring to, a 5 tier system is in place, with the first two receiving immediate assistance, while the last three needed to wait longer. The procedure of assigning ranks is called triage. Due to lack of space, the waiting room for the patients already triaged is the same with those who have just entered the department. The place can get really crowded at times, and manoeuvering the COW between the waiting chairs rows proves sometimes unnerving. Medication is administered either by using manual input, or by overriding altogether the system.

Third, there are cases in which a patient state may rapidly deteriorate. And here an interesting design feature comes into play. The COWs work with an usb antenna, and the antena is inserted by design in the lateral of the large screen. Many times, while running along the corridors and entering the narrow doors to reach the patient, the antena would hit the threshold and breaks inside. There is obviously no time to search for another available COW.

Fourth, some barcodes on vials and packages may not work. It is frustrating, particularly in emergency situations. Also, due to the design factor explained above, range doses and constantly popping alerts distract the personnel and need to be overridden regularly. These instances are recorded by the system as "wrong dose" or "override", and may be interpreted by the QI department in many different ways.

This relationship between humans and machines mediated is further complicated by newly standardized workflows. Sometimes healthcare personnel identified workarounds that would allow feeding the machine with required data, while responding to their own definition of efficiency informed directly by the workfloor experience. This happened beyond the emergency department floor. In order to avoid the cumbersome and often frankly impossible maneuvering of the COWs in patient's narrow salons, nurses found an alternative solution for the medication administration. They would bring the medication and the COW at the entry of the room (usually populated by one or two patients); print duplicates of the wristbands;

scan the duplicate and each medication outside the salon; and they take them to the patient inside, without bringing in the COW. They would come out and repeat the procedure for the subsequent patient. This procedure would not meet the standards of the workflow designed for the use of the new system, but it would nonetheless register in the system as the correct procedure.

As a result of the rapid ethnography in the Emergency department, an agreement has been reached: unless major modifications in the system will be operated, medication in the emergency department would not necessarily need to follow the scanning workflow.In order to reach a happy ending like this one, the stakeholders involved must agree/be opened enough to reconsider the meaning of optimization and adapt it to the context. Unfortunately, this is not the case everywhere, everytime. Also it certainly did not address all other instances of workarounds, or the series of unintended consequences that the standardization of the procedure led by the automatic system adoption had on the healthcare processes.

Systems and the City

One of the important aspects of any systemic analysis is deciding on the limits of the system. In the case of the automatic system discussed, does the system comprise the entire hospital or only the department in focus? Does it include the pharmacy that prepares the daily medication according to the system's records? Does it include the relationship with other hospitals and care centers that adopt the same interlinked system? What about the urban setting? Should it also be included? The answer to all of the above is, well, yes. In fact, the best approach is in terms of *nested systems*—in which each system is part of a bigger one—, and to identify their intricate web of relations.

The automated system promises a so-called "closed medication loop". This means that the medication prescribed by the medical doctor is introduced into the electronic system that can be accessed instantly by the hospital pharmacy where medication is verified, prepared, and readied for delivery daily. Any modifications to an individual's patient doses, or medications are registered automatically in the system and actualised daily. This saves a lot of work for the night shift nurses. Prior to the electronic system, they had to insert manually the new subscriptions in special folders or check if there are modifications for already registered patients, and then send these folders to the pharmacy, every night at 3 am. Based on these folders, the pharmacy technicians prepared the required medications everyday. In the particular hospital the author worked with, prior to the introduction of the automated system, the cut-off hour for the morning medications to be ready was set at 7:30 am. This meant that the technicians would start their working day at 6:30 am.

The introduction of the automated system imposed a region wide standardization: it required the medications to be ready at 7:00 am, as opposed to 7:30 am, in order to harmonize the hour of the first medication for all the patients included in the new system. In consequence, the technicians in charge of preparing the medication needed to start their working day at 6:00 am instead of 6:30 am.

Let us take a look at the bigger system that nests the hospital: the city. This particular hospital is located in a prime real estate region, where house and rental prices are prohibitive for many people, including our nurses and technicians. Most of them commute to work using public transport which is a fairly good option and, pricewise, a much better alternative to owning a car. The commute is long, and the first buses only arrive in the vicinity of the hospital at 6:20 am giving no option for the technicians to show up before 6:30 am. Hence the unexpected happened: all technicians from the hospital's pharmacy resigned. The hospital's quick and the only possible fix was to hire pharmacists at the beginning of their career - who most likely owned cars or could afford one - and offer them entry salaries that were automatically higher than those of experienced technicians. This, in turn, created a certain professional tension and disillusionment among the new hires: although pharmacists, they were required to perform technicians' duties and, despite their limited experience,, the frustration was understandable. Where would the experience come from, if not nurtured from the beginning of the career?

In this example we can count at least 6 nested systems: the medication closed loop nested in the electronic health records system, nested in the hospital system, nested in the network of hospitals adopting the same electronic health records system, nested in the urban setting with its real estate and transport peculiarities, nested in the system of labour and social inequalities reflecting back on the entire ensemble. Each modification in one of the systems reverberates with unforeseen consequences at every level of the others.

In the previous example the electronic system settings and automated responses intersected with workflow designs, and interior layout and organization of the emergency department. In this case the standardization of procedures meant to adapt to the need of consistency in the networked medical system reverberated with urban settings and labour conditions, and created a perfect storm that destabilised the financial and HR managerial resources of the hospital in unforeseen ways.

They both point out the need of human centred approaches in any attempt to adopt automated systems and standardization, particularly in healthcare. They also reveal the importance of understanding automated systems, AI included, in their entirety, that is including the materiality that accompanies them.

Imag(in)ed Diagnosis

Image based diagnosis is one healthcare domain in which AI using Machine Learning (ML) and Deep Learning (DL) for image recognition proved highly efficient. That high the efficiency that many radiologists fear their profession is soon to disappear (Ford, 2015). However, despite the hype around image-based diagnosis using AI, up until now, the most efficient and accurate diagnosis process proved to be the one that combines a human supervised with machine diagnosis. In other words, when a specialist double checks the algorithm results. We are talking rather about a symbiotic relationship (Russell, 2019), and not of an outright replacement. However, human-machine symbiosis does not always work as designed in the lab.

The study of the use of DL in diagnosing retina damage done by Google in Thailand (Beede et al., 2020) is pioneering in the field of human-centered research and evaluation in healthcare. While human centered, and patient centered approaches are becoming more and more the norm in healthcare related research, this study is perhaps the first that looks systematically at how algorithms, technology, and human expectations intersect the reality of caregiving in the industry. The study took place between 2018 and 2019 and a first article was published in 2020.

The article rightfully observes the disadvantage, and even the danger of the lack of formal requirement, in the adoption of automated systems in healthcare with human centered observational evaluation. The research revealed both the necessity and the urgency for these types of studies and evaluations, in order to make sure that the implemented automated system works not as designed, but as intended in relationship with the users and beneficiaries. In this case, the expectation of efficiency was met by the reality of real physical conditions when the system was implemented.

In the workflow of diagnosing retina damage using DL, a key step is taking of retina photos. This step is fulfilled by nurses, who later fed the images into the image recognition machine. The variable quality of light, the use or absence of pupil dilating solutions, and the impossibility to take more than two shots per patient (otherwise the retina risked to be damaged) sometimes produced images unusable by the machine, but perfectly readable by a human interpreter. In many cases two lower quality shots from different angles could be read together by a human, and give a complete image of the retina state. However, the machine only accepted one shot per patient. According to the workflow, in case of the system's refusal of the image, the patient should be automatically referred—even if a human could have read the image accurately. For the purpose of the study and for the implementation of the system, the decision to further refer the patient to a specialist had to be based solely on the machine reading.

However, nurses were attuned to the patients' difficulties in their attempts to reach the specialists, which could imply a full day of travel using public transport, or the necessity that the patient their children owning cars to drive them, upsetting their work schedule. In many cases, nurses considered that patients' comfort was an integral part of caregiving. Therefore, if the image was refused by the machine but readable by humans, they would "workaround" the workflow and choose to not further refer the patient.

The results of this study point out to similar issues and challenges as those described above, regarding the Canadian clinical setting. The nested systems of care, algorithms, family ties, work relationships, interior design and public transport act interdependently and create a new reality that is unforeseeable in the lab conditions in which any system is designed. Culture as embedded in both relationships and materiality, different understanding of what giving care means, particular and particularly diverse arrangements in healthcare settings that do offer the same services speak to the necessity to understand the context, understanding that can be acquired only through observational, human-centred methods of research and evaluation.

Adoption and adaptation of automated systems together with the hype created around them continue to reveal complex and rather problematic interactions between AI models and the reality on which they are deployed, as well as the conflict between competing AI ethical principles. Let's turn for the moment towards the latter, and discuss it in the context of the current pandemic.

Ethics - Principles versus Practices

Former UN Secretary-General Kofi Annan said in his lecture at Tübingen University: "One thing that should be clear is that the validity of universal values does not depend on their being universally obeyed or applied. Ethical codes are always the expression of an ideal and an aspiration, a standard by which moral failings can be judged rather than a prescription for ensuring that they never occur." (Annan, 2003)

This is a powerful statement, touching at the heart of the ethical challenges of leadership. It may also contain a major flaw: while ethical codes can be framed as an expression of universal aspirations, the standards by which we could judge moral failings cannot equally be universal. Whether we like it or not, morality is culturally dependent - and, in many cases,moral failings fall into a cultural blind-spot. This does not mean that, in the name of "cultural particularities", we can abdicate from universal ethical codes (although this is a current practice among authoritarian figures, particularly regarding the respect of human rights). It merely means that we need to be aware of how these aspirational universal codes are expressed in daily practices, and how the transformation of these practices can (and does) generate new moral norms that, in their turn, shed light on those very cultural blind-spots.

Valuing human life is a universal ethical code. But what type of human life is more "valued" than others in different societies? And how do these societies make decisions based on that? Is a young life more valuable than an old one? How is this valuing expressed in daily practices? Is life at any cost more valuable than the individual choice to "not resuscitate" or dignity in dying? Is it possible to have an "equally valuable" approach to human life even in moments of scarcity? Is collective survival more important than individual well-being—and can they be separated after all?

These types of questions emerged forcefully during our current COVID-19 pandemic crisis, and scientists, ethicists, and politicians are tackling the answers (or act as if they know them already).

Two major conversations have dominated the public sphere lately: the use of data tracking systems for forecasting viral spread, and the possible use of AI as decision support for the allocation of medical resources in emergency situations. By analyzing the conversations and practices around this topic, this text will advocate a bottom-up approach on AI governance. We will see how, sometimes, ethical codes may compete with one another. We will also catch sight of how the attempt to codify them in universally applicable AI algorithms can lead to the emergence of new types of biases instead of eliminating the existing ones. Thus, both deciding on the instances of using AI, and designing and relying on AI to make decisions need to have as starting points the practices that embody moral norms, and not universal ethical codes and their presumed possible codification in AI algorithms. The immateriality of AI models received a reality check, and so are about to experience the AI ethics themselves.

A Material World

At a higher level of analysis the pandemic in fact seems to be an eloquent reminder of the fact our world is material, despite a discourse of virtualisation of everything, from markets to life itself. All of a sudden COVID-19 forced us to experience at least three major types of materialisations:

Materialisation of borders - while borders are not always easy to cross, and some are more material than others, in the past pandemic year, the transfrontalier movement has almost come to a stop. Most countries in the world have become inaccessible to others other than their citizens or residents. While writing this text many countries around the world remain closed to foreigners.

In parallel, extraordinary forms of collaboration at regional and global levels showed that only an open approach may offer long term solutions - for example, the German hospitals uptaking French patients at frontier regions in order to relieve the over-stretched French hospitals. At the same time, displays of solidarity were also suspiciously received, raising questions about using solidarity as mechanisms of soft power, particularly in China's case.

(De-)Materialisation of movement - Movement has become materialized and virtual, both at the same time. During lockdown, it has entered a controlled phase at all levels, with much of the workforce passing through a sort of mass experiment: work from home. Many of those for whom the ability to move was as natural as breathing experienced it for the first time as a privilege. Movement was dis-placed to online platforms, and dematerialized into bytes and pieces of data (more on this in a bit).

Materialisation of our bodies - most important we are called upon to acknowledge the importance of our bodies. We, individually and collectively, have realised in a dramatic way that our lives are very real and unequivocally linked to our material bodies. The variations of the abstract indicators of the economy showed that the entire global complex system is not separated from, but heavily dependent on our human bodies, their health and their movement (see above). This will contribute to the gradual dismantling of the illusion that we live in a virtual world in which the body is merely an instrument among others, a tool to be refined in gyms and yoga sessions, or a resource to be overstretched during long, caffeine fueled working hours. Somehow our bodies became ourselves again.

Tracking

The data tracking systems (DTS) are not a novelty - the US police, for example, use it at large scale, nor is their use by marketing companies that rely on the individual users' data to push products through targeted advertising. The question of online data tracking was brought to the public's attention as early as 2012 (Madrigal, 2012), but the generalised use of smartphones made possible the extension of tracking from virtual movement to material movement in space and time. Apps that use the phone GPS (many times as a default option) track, store, and sell movement data to third parties for targeted marketing purposes. The same data can be used in instances by police in order to "prevent crime" - a practice that is both contested and not yet fully understood, let alone regulated (Friedersdorf, 2019).

The European Union (EU) enacted a data protection act that obliges developers to design, pseudonymisation and/or anonymisation of users' data, and to fully inform, and to obtain consent from the consumers regarding their use of data (General Data Protection Regulation 2016/679, implemented starting May 2018). This regulation impacts the use of data tracking systems, and makes it more difficult to apply it indiscriminately, or sell it to third parties (like US based corporations tend to do). More recently the EU adopted a series of policy papers regarding the more general use of AI.

What DTSs actually do is to combine borders, movements, and bodies and recreate them in the immaterial world of algorithms, while juxtaposing them to pre-designed models, assigning the individual user to typologies within the models. It does not matter if the models are of consumer habits, potential delinquency, or the likelihood to pay one's mortgage. The trouble with the AI models is largely discussed in the specialty literature (O'Neil, 2019, Broussard, 2018, Galison, 2019), and it emerges from a few major sources:

1. Models are based on previous behaviour and aggregated data, and have a probability rate of correct identification. They are not 100% accurate! This may not be a major problem in cases in which we have models of success for an athlete's performance, but what happens when they are used to decide upon the finance or the justice delivery for individuals? Another drawback is that models function as long as the reality matches the conditions of the data collection, and they are highly dependent on the data quality and accuracy. Under normal circumstances (read *long periods of status quo*) the models more or less function as designed (emphasis on *as designed*). But, as the COVID-19 crisis showed, a sudden disruption can cause a "model drifting" - that is, models do not correspond anymore to reality, and they need to be redesigned. This drifting was first signaled in the Amazon use of AI, and then spotted in all major industries that use Artificial Intelligence. (Castellanos, 2020, Heaven, 2020)
2. The use of proxy measurements in order to decide how values are attributed within a typology. For example, such a model may use the students' exams performance in order to determine the value of an educator, disregarding the whole series of other factors that impact on the exam results, apart from the educator's qualities and qualifications. At the same time, an educator who feels his livelihood threatened may be compelled to polish his students' results - giving birth to further distortions (see O'Neil).
3. Models are designed by humans and more often than not they embed the biases held by designers and developers. This is also a topic highly discussed in AI ethics. The solutions offered range from increasing the diversity in designer and product development teams to renouncing the use of the tool itself altogether.

With the COVID-19 pandemic, eyes turned towards the possibility to use DTS in order to predict and prevent the rapid spread of the virus by creating early warning mechanisms. The idea is relatively simple: once downloaded, DTS Apps track the user's movements using their phones, and identify if the user is in the vicinity of someone who has already been registered as COVID-19 positive. The App would then alert the user and also create an anonymous map of possible viral spread.

AI ethicists raised first concerns, particularly regarding the tension between two AI major ethical principles: the user's autonomy (including rights to privacy) and usage for common good. First, the DTS cannot ensure 100% autonomy, especially when the GPS system is used for tracking. When movement data becomes health data (as in this case), anonymity is all the more important. Individual health data are highly sensitive. They are stored in highly secure environments, anonymized and used exclusively by specialists in healthcare. But what if the movement becomes a predictor for health? What if movement data are sold to third parties, interested in evaluating it through approximate models, in order to anticipate the individuals' health risks? Based on this data, can we decide who can and who cannot return to work, travel, or even visit friends? Or who receives scarce treatment if those who need it are too numerous?

Up to now, the ethical solution for the dilemma concerning movement data is a greater degree of anonymization. The design solutions proposed for the app gravitate are twofold: use the bluetooth systems of the device instead of the GPS to signal proximity only (and not location), and store all the relevant data on the device (not on third parties servers). Downloading and using the app is voluntary. A diversity of Apps featuring these solutions are being currently deployed.

The US had a fragmented approach, they granted the companies with the decisions on the design and the deployment of tracing apps, as well as with the subsequent ethical decisions.. European countries, on the other hand, have a more centralized approach, in that the government is more involved in financing and developing the Apps, with features that need to meet the European standard of privacy. At the time of writing, Germany only started the deployment of their 20 millions Euro App, and reassures its users that the data is not accessible to the platform provider they use (Android or Apple), but only to public healthcare specialists in the country. At the same time Norway decided to pull its own off use because the reliability was questionable at least. Being based on voluntary download and reporting, and built on the assumption that people always carry their smartphones with them, the Norwegian government concluded that the App models do not necessarily correspond to human behaviour.

For an external observer the situation seems to be completely different in countries that appear to have a centralized, all powerful system of data tracking and AI use, such as China. While an European observer may conclude easily that the balance between common good versus individual anonymity is already tilted towards the first in China's case, and that China already can use the Social Credit System in order to track and prevent COVID-19 spread, the reality is not precisely this. The approach in China seems to be more fragmented than in some European countries. Some provinces developed their own DTS, some of the Apps use GPS while others are based on voluntary input of location by the user. Regional governments and cities may use different apps that may result in different "health scores" assigned to the same person. (Ye, Josh, et al. 2020). As Ding (2018) observes in his analysis of China's

AI strategy, the Western perception is that AI deployment in China is top down and monolithic, hyper centralized and controlled, with no room for ethics. Far from the truth, as Ding shows in his work. In parentheses, this perception is a common trope of the depiction of "the East" in Western popular thinking. The doctrine of social peace and its attainment does guide the actions in China, however, ethical debates are present and lead by private enterprises, such as the Tencent's Research Institute.

In conclusion, the use of DTS poses ethical dilemmas because they reveal the opposition between individual autonomy and common good. They also raise practical issues regarding accuracy and efficiency because of the way in which data is collected, stored, and used (Canca, 2020).

DTS also raises an interesting issue about healthcare and data generation and usage: any data about a person can arguably be used as healthcare data, or as marketing as convenient. Lifestyle can indicate stages of life and states of health. This raises the question of interchangeability of data. Individuals as data generators become themselves interchangeable between the systems of knowledge interested in their lives, healthcare being one of them. How are we to relate to the vast amount of data potentially available about an individual when a decision of life and death is made?

Back to Triage

The COVID-19 spread put an important strain on healthcare systems all over the world, and each country has approached the crisis in different ways. From avoiding testing and sending patients that were not in a critical state home—as it happened in the UK at the beginning of the pandemic to carefully planning the lockdown and the bed allocations in places like Germany, we have witnessed countless examples of uplifting solidarity action.

The insufficient resources, such as hospital beds and respiratory units, and the necessity to allocate them to an increasing number of patients in critical states put a lot of pressure on the medical personnel. Ideally, all health systems should have guidelines for extreme situations such as pandemics, indicating how to triage the patient and allocate scarce resources. The guidelines contain more often than not a set of recommendations about triaging the patients and allocating scarce resources, but they do not necessarily contain the practical ways in which the recommendation can be implemented - so nurses and doctors are left scrambling to create their own procedures in this type of emergency.

The particularity of this pandemic puts strain on the Intensive Care Units (ICUs) rather than on Emergency (ER). The ERs around the world currently use a diversity of triage systems, and there usually one decides what type of treatment a patient needs, and in what order of emergency. This is different from the pandemic situation in overstretched ICUs, where the treatment may not be available for everyone who needs it, and access to it has to be selective. This is an important distinction, and this is what happens today in many ICUs around the world. ER triage procedures do not apply to this situation. So what do the healthcare providers around the world do? They are trying to follow the recommendations and to devise their own procedures in order not only to best serve patients and the common good, but also to reduce their own enormous emotional stress.

There are few criteria they may use, and as Philip Rosoff, ethicist and MD at Duke University explained[1], we know how **not** to take a decision of this kind: not in a rush, not at the bedside, and not using judgment based on privilege. In his words, in healthcare at least in the US, there are ordinary situations in which there is a distinction made between VIPs and VUPs (Very Unfortunate Persons). In the case of the COVID-19 pandemic this distinction is eliminated, and so is the question of age. Age is not a decisive factor in providing treatment in case of scarcity (contrary to what an AI ethicist argued in a conversation on this very topic).

The only criteria that should play a role, Rosoff explained, is the clinical chances of survival that the patient has. This can be assessed by healthcare professionals based on the healthcare records of the respective patient and on the current clinical state displayed. Here, one can see that artificial intelligence powered tools may come forcefully into play. Electronic Health Records (EHR) facilitate the preservation of patients' medical history, and combined with the data of the current chart of a patient they could, theoretically, match the patient's history and current state with a recommendation regarding a triage decision. This may provide a certain relief in the high stress situations, and the decision may be supported by this type of evidence based approach.

However there are two important factors that need to be taken into consideration here:

1. The AI models embedded that pass a judgment on the state of health of the patients may be themselves flawed: the use of proxy measures in order to establish the health state of a patient (such as money spent in the past x years in health related issues) can be very misleading: for example, such an AI powered tool kept showing that black patients' health is much better than white ones, and as a result they may receive less medical attention. The fact that less resources were spent on patients identified as black was considered by the AI system to be a sign of health. This was in fact due to the reversed type of causation: blacks in the US received less medical attention due to financial hardships and systemic racism, resulting in less money spent on health. If a subsequent decision is taken based on this, in fact it will continue the spiralling of inequality (Obermeyer et al., 2019).

2. The risk of errors induced by the way in which the humans interact with the machines. One important aspect in AI as a decision support tool, particularly in healthcare, is that the system should remain a tool for support, and not be transformed in the decision maker. However, the high emotional stress amplified by the workload experienced by health workers may generate the so-called "suspension of clinical thinking"—that is taking the AI recommendation as the ultimate authoritative decision. In other words, under a variety of circumstances, particularly high stress, humans may be tempted to evacuate the weight of the decision to the machine. While this may be possible in a driverless car, it may prove disastrous in medical settings. Ironically, it seems (although it is not) easier to create an algorithm advising doctors (because everything happens between the screen and the health worker) than an integrated AI system that drives a car.

In conclusion, although AI may provide assistance in patients triage for resource allocation in a pandemic situation, it should not be transformed into an automated decision making instrument, precisely because, as we have seen, biases and model dysfunctionalities may create irremediable medical errors. As with the case of retina scanning,the use of DL algorithms to decide on referrals, or in the case of ER medication administration, we need to develop workflows that integrate the human-machine interaction and avoid overreliance on the standardized answers of the machines. And of course, there is the question of accountability...

AI Ethics and Models

Both instances analysed above (DTS and possible AI use in triage for medical resource allocation in ICU) have in common the question of ethics.

When we try to make an ethical decision based on allegedly universal principles (such as „Life is the most valuable asset"), we should always be aware of the ethical codes that unavoidably vary from a context to another (between different social classes, working contexts and so forth). What we practically (and many times unconsciously) do when we take a decision (or allow AI to take in an automated manner) is to hierarchize those principles or codes and to put them in a particular sequence. This is why an ethical decision taken in a certain context may look unethical if we apply it to another context.

According to ethical decision making theory, there are five major methods to arrive to an ethical decision: the utilitarian approach (to make the most good and the least harm), the rights based approach (to best protect the moral rights of those affected), the fairness and justice approach (to insure that the decision fair), the common good approach, and the virtue approach (to decide in accordance with the decision maker values).These methods are present and expressed as AI ethical codes in most of the approaches.

Currently a series of organisms are stating principles for ethical AI that ought to be taken into consideration when designing and using AI. The EU put forth 7 principles for trustworthy AI: Human agency and oversight, Technical Robustness and safety, Privacy and data governance, Transparency, Diversity, Non-discrimination and fairness, Societal and environmental well-being, Accountability. Each of these principles comes with a list of recommendations meant to explain what they mean. Under privacy and data governance we may find anonymity, respect for individual rights. Under Societal and environmental well-being we may find concerns for common good. As argued above, these principles may compete in different cases. They are also highly abstract, and they may be interpreted differently in different socio-cultural contexts. (European Commission 2019)

However, AI models interact with institutional, social and cultural contexts and may fail if they are not designed for the context. This happens in fact in most of the cases in which AI works directly with humans, as shown in this article.

Ethical models do the same, so in order to avoid their drifting, we should develop them by firstly observing practices. The ethical codes themselves do not exist in theory, despite the fact that some ethicists generate them first theoretically. In fact they are first expressed in different practices. Their very meaning is translated through practices, but practices vary in time and space. Different practices show the crack in models—as in the AI deployment cases. We should look at practices and their variations first in order to make our way back to judgments on values and ethics. Returning to the question of rights and valuing life - how is this expressed in various practices? How can we design decision making mechanisms (automated or not) that correspond to the variability of practices and their dynamic transformations?

Matter Matters

The major lesson for AI, and for Ethics that COVID-19 brings is that **adoption means adaptation** in a world in which matter matters. Therefore:

1. AI is a tool—it does not have to **be ethical** (it's absurd)—it should be designed in accordance with ethical principles understood contextually, leading to it **acting ethically within the context.** Therefore, we first need to understand the context - ask an anthropologist.
2. Always set off having in mind that models are always wrong. Models do not drift because people behave weird. They drift because they are... models.Their accuracy is limited in time, and the faster we change, the faster they drift. Carrying them across contexts will implicitly make them drift. That's why we

first need to study the cultural context (regional, institutional, professional) and to work our way back from here into the design of AI systems.

3. The design process should start in the field, not in labs. We need to design AI for specific cultural contexts, building models starting from reality, not trying to model reality according to abstract lab-designed models—and this applies to ethical models as well. Sooner or later, lab-made models will "drift", and ethics is one of the most important domains where they fail.
4. We need to create constant evaluation feedback loops. Remember: AI is material. It has a material support and it interacts with the material world which means it is not going to flow smoothly. Be prepared to reassess and adjust it based on how its adoption develops.

What does the Pandemic Teach us?

The rippling effects of the current pandemic will be felt in economy, culture, and politics. In terms of AI, this means both a great opportunity to see where it is really helpful, and a wake up call to demystify some of the hype around it. One major lesson is that AI not only interacts with a material world in continuous transformation, but its functioning depends on this very materiality (and material culture). The crisis also re-emphasizes the importance of understanding socio-cultural variations—geographical or institutional—when approaching ethics. Moreover, it urges us to be more aware of the fact that AI design, deployment, and adoption has ethical implications. One major question that was overlooked till recently would be: what domains and instances need the deployment of AI? Is decision making based on AI appropriate for all the domains where we stubbornly try to implement it? Should we optimize everything just because we can? As Rosoff observed in his dialogue with David Remnick, the US healthcare is a multibillion-dollar business, so in this particular context, the AI optimization may not always be in the best interest of the patient. Let's be patient and better ponder on where AI is really useful, and where it has the potential of becoming a "weapon of math destruction".

CONCLUSION

Artificial Intelligence could Optimise Every Aspect of our Lives, but Should we Allow it?

In 2019 at the Unfinished festival, the author organised and mediated a conversation between Angelica Dass, a Madrid based artist born in Brazil, who is most famous for her project Humanae, and Moran Cerf, an Istraeli neuroscientist now based in the

US, specialised in human machine interaction at the brain level. He explores the ways in which technology may hack into consciousness. The question the author posed was how would a life perfectly optimized by technology look. More specifically, the author asked them to imagine how life would be if most of our decisions were to be taken by an algorithm that had access to all our data, from genetic make-up to neural mapping, to every bit and byte of lifestyle choices made up to the present. What would they themselves do if the machines indicated a kale and salmon sandwich on oat crackers, perfect for the health improvement, over the butter croissant they crave? While Angelica chose the croissant, Moran argued that he would prefer to use his cognitive power for things more important than trifling choices, and would go for the sandwich. He also hoped for a prolonged healthy productive life.

So, what does optimisation mean in this example? **What is it that we optimise, and where do we leave space to suspend our decisions and follow the algorithmic ones?** This is a fundamental ethical problem to be added to current AI debates.

Ethics may look like "universal laws" but, put into practice, they are decodified according to a series of very different societal, religious, lawful hierarchies. We will need to deeply understand the effect of this fact in our rush to automatize. The hierarchies are furthermore interiorized by individuals into unconscious biases, and further down these biases are embedded in algorithms. Identifying this variance has been in focus of many mental and physical experiments, from the trolley dilemma to the moral machine (Awad, 2018) - the latter being essentially a gamification of the former. No easy answer is at hand. But in this context my questions are: how are we to optimise these types of decisions? Should we optimise them? And **how precisely are we optimising them?**

And this brings us back to the initial observation in ER, in which following indiscriminately the optimized workflow for medication in order to feed the automated system, the supposedly correct data in a standardized manner would jeopardize the caregiving process and even render difficult to save lives. More often than not efficiency is defined independent of context, and fails to account for the complexity of the process involved in any work environment. The view from the finance department, for example, of what efficiency means can be at times at odds with the perspective of quality assurance, and the way quality is understood in the latter may be completely different from what persons on the work floor strive for. The third major question is brought to mind: **What do we optimise (for)?**

In conclusion,the authorwould suggest that we spend more time thinking about these three questions before implementing automated decision making systems, before designing algorithms, and before considering the parameters of that design:

1. Why do we optimize? In other words, what does optimization mean? Reducing costs or increasing well-being and happiness? Answers to these questions may

be found into a better care given to the definitions of metrics and measurements when deciding on the usefulness of an automated system.

2. How do we optimise? Did we take into account as many variables as possible, including the socio-cultural context and the type of activity we'd like to optimise? It is possible, probable, and even desirable to explore the array of unforeseen effects before designing and implementing an automated system in context?
3. What do we optimise (for)? Perhaps there are domains in which a certain type of optimisation should be kept at bay, or should be rethought for the domain itself.

Answers to these questions can be found only through observational, human-centered research and evaluation techniques that integrate ethnographic methods with institutional analysis, and design thinking.

After understanding the context, we should approach optimisation as a tool for a well-defined scope, and not as the scope itself while usually using a very narrowly defined optimisation definition.

More often than not, in the case of AI algorithms and automated systems, the latter seems to be the case. Perhaps it is high time to ponder on the variance of optimization and AI in function of context by redefining optimisation in the first place. And perhaps not every domain of life needs to be optimized in an algorithmic manner.

REFERENCES

Annan, K. (2003). *Universal Values - Peace, Freedom, Social Progress, Equal Rights, HUman Dignity - Acutely Needed.* SG/SM 9076. https://www.un.org/press/en/2003/sgsm9076.doc.htm

Awad, E., Dsouza, S., Kim, R., Schulz, J., Henrich, J., Shariff, A., Bonnefon, J.-F., & Rahwan, I. (2018). The Moral Machine experiment. *Nature*, *563*(7729), 59–64. doi:10.103841586-018-0637-6 PMID:30356211

Broussard, M. (2018). *Artificial Unintelligence. How Computers Misunderstand the World.* The MIT Press. doi:10.7551/mitpress/11022.001.0001

Canca, C. (2020). *Why 'Mandatory Privacy-Preserving Digital Contact Tracing' is the Ethical Measure against COVID-19.* https://medium.com/@cansucanca/why-mandatory-privacy-preserving-digital-contact-tracing-is-the-ethical-measure-against-covid-19-a0d143b7c3b6

Castellanos, S. (2020). Pandemic-Related Disruptions Hurt Reliability of Some AI Models. *Wall Street Journal*. https://www.wsj.com/articles/pandemic-related-disruptions-hurt-reliability-of-some-ai-models-11591781402

D'Ignazio, C., & Klein, L. F. (2020). *Data Feminism*. The MIT Press. doi:10.7551/mitpress/11805.001.0001

Deibert, R. (2020). *Burning Data*. CBC Massey Lecture #5. https://www.cbc.ca/radio/ideas/reset-reclaiming-the-internet-for-civil-society-1.5795345

Ding, J. (2018). Deciphering China's AI Dream The context, components, capabilities, and consequences of China's strategy to lead the world in AI. Centre for the Governance of AI, Future of Humanity Institute, University of Oxford.

Emma, B., Baylor, E., Hersch, F., Iurchenko, A., Wilcox, L., Ruamviboonsuk, P., & Vardoulakis L. (2020). A Human-Centered Evaluation of a Deep Learning System Deployed in Clinics for the Detection of Diabetic Retinopathy. *CHI '20: Proceedings of the 2020 CHI Conference on Human Factors in Computing Systems*. 10.1145/3313831.3376718

Eubanks, V. (2019). *Automating Inequality. How High-Tech Tools Profile, Police, and Punish the Poor.* Picador Editions.

European Commission. (2019). *Shaping Europe's digital future - Ethics guidelines for trustworthy AI*. https://ec.europa.eu/digital-single-market/en/news/ethics-guidelines-trustworthy-ai

Ford, M. (2015). *Rise of the Robots. Technology and the Threat of a Jobless Future*. Basic Books.

Friedersdorf, C. (2019). Mass Surveillance Is Coming to a City Near You. A tech entrepreneur wants to track the residents of a high-crime American community. *The Atlantic*. https://www.theatlantic.com/ideas/archive/2019/06/mass-surveillance-tech/592117/

Galison, P. (2019). Algorists Dream of Objectivity. In Possible Minds. 25 Ways of Looking at AI. New York: Penguin Press.

Heaven. (2020). Our weird behavior during the pandemic is messing with AI models. *MIT Technology Review*. https://www.technologyreview.com/2020/05/11/1001563/covid-pandemic-broken-ai-machine-learning-amazon-retail-fraud-humans-in-the-loop/

Hicks, M. (2018). *Programmed Inequality. How Britain Discarded Women Technologists and Lost Its Edge on Computing*. MIT Press.

Hong, S.-H. (2020). *Technologies of Speculation. The Limits of Knowledge in a Data-Driven Society*. New York University Press. doi:10.18574/nyu/9781479860234.001.0001

Kohli, A., & Jha, S. (2018). Why CAD failed in mammography. *Journal of the American College of Radiology*, *15*(3), 535–537. doi:10.1016/j.jacr.2017.12.029 PMID:29398499

Madrigal, A. C. (2012). I'm Being Followed: How Google—and 104 Other Companies—Are Tracking Me on the Web. *The Atlantic*. https://www.theatlantic.com/technology/archive/2012/02/im-being-followed-how-google-151-and-104-other-companies-151-are-tracking-me-on-the-web/253758/

Musen, M. A., Middleton, B., & Greenes, R. A. (2014). Clinical Decision-Support Systems. In *Biomedical Informatics* (pp. 643–674). Springer. doi:10.1007/978-1-4471-4474-8_22

Noble, S. U. (2018). *Algorithms of Oppression. How Search Engines Reinforce Racism*. New York University Press. doi:10.2307/j.ctt1pwt9w5

O'Neil, C. (2019). *Weapons of Math Destruction. How Big Data Increase Inequality and Threatens Democracy*. Broadway Books.

Obermeyer, Powers, Vogeli, & Mullainathan. (2019). Dissecting racial bias in an algorithm used to manage the health of populations. *Science, 366*(6464), 447-453. doi:10.1126/science.aax2342

Palinkas, L. A., & Zatzick, D. (2019). Rapid Assessment Procedure Informed Clinical Ethnography (RAPICE) in Pragmatic Clinical Trials of Mental Health Services Implementation: Methods and Applied Case Study. *Administration and Policy in Mental Health*, *46*(2), 255–270. doi:10.100710488-018-0909-3 PMID:30488143

Park, Kuo, Barbarin, Kaziunas, Chow, Singh, Wilcox, & Lasecki. (2019). *Identifying Challenges and Opportunities in Human-AI Collaboration in Healthcare*. Academic Press.

Perreira, C. (2019). Consumed by Disease. Medical Archives, Latino Fictions, and Carceral Health Imaginaries. In Captivating Technology. Race, Carceral Technoscience, and Liberatory Imagination in Everyday Life (pp. 50-66). Duke University Press

Pontefract, Coleman, Vallance, Hirsch, Shah, Marriot, & Redwood. (2018). The impact of computerized physician order entry and clinical decision support on pharmacist-physician communication in the hospital setting: A qualitative study. *PloS One, 13*(11), e0207450.

The Shock Wave of COVID-19. (2020). In *The New Yorker Radio Hour* [podcast]. https://www.newyorker.com/podcast/the-new-yorker-radio-hour/the-shock-wave-of-covid-19

Waterson. (1990). "Calvin and Hobbes", January 9, 10, 11. In *The Complete Calvin and Hobbes, Book Three 1990-1992*. Adrew McMeel Publishing.

Wittenberg-Cox, A. (2020). What Do Countries With The Best Coronavirus Responses Have In Common? Women Leaders. *Forbes*. https://www.forbes.com/sites/avivahwittenbergcox/2020/04/13/what-do-countries-with-the-best-coronavirus-reponses-have-in-common-women-leaders/#36f031293dec

Ye, J., Feng, C., & Xue, Y. (2020). *Contact tracing – the privacy vs urgency dilemma for governments in the fight against Covid-19*. South China Morning Press. https://www.scmp.com/tech/big-tech/article/3087325/contact-tracing-privacy-versus-urgency-dilemma-governments-fight

ENDNOTE

1 Philip Rosoff in dialogue with David Remnick, the New Yorker Radio Hour "The Shock Wave of COVID-19"

Chapter 2
Managing User Integration:
Insights From the Field of Publicly-Funded Research and Development Projects in Germany

Cornelia Eicher
Charité – Universitätsmedizin Berlin, Germany

Robert Klebbe
Charité – Universitätsmedizin Berlin, Germany

ABSTRACT

The importance of robotics and assistive technologies for healthcare is increasing. For their introduction into practical application, the continuous integration of the user perspective is crucial to ensure acceptance and usability. This can be achieved by the user-centered design approach. In an earlier publication, several problems with its functional implementation within research and development (R&D) projects were pointed out. This chapter discusses possible solutions to promote an effective integration of the user perspective in R&D projects based on six interviews with experts from Germany. The results can be summarized in three main requirements: first, the generation of a common understanding of the target group; second, a scientific research approach considering the context of technology usage; third, projectification, with a focus on efficient resource planning, the development of generic technologies, and technology evaluations with the user group. Leaders of innovative projects can benefit from implementing these strategies in the development process.

DOI: 10.4018/978-1-7998-7888-9.ch002

INTRODUCTION

Publicly funded research and development (R&D) projects typically serve to develop and investigate socially, economically, and technologically risky developments, such as innovative products or processes (Fellbaum, 1982, p. 88). Within the framework of interdisciplinary collaborative projects, manufacturers, and industry (e.g., hardware and software developers), scientific institutions (e.g., research institutions), and social and healthcare institutions closely work together on innovative solutions. By contributing and sharing their expertise, collaborative project partners can enhance their own knowledge and test early-stage developments or methods. Due to third-party funding, financial risks are limited, and failure has no impact on the partners' credibility or success outside the project's framework.

Particularly, innovation-driven projects with societal significance are often the focus of R&D projects. Due to the crucial impact of worldwide demographic change on various areas of society, such as the working world, social security systems, and the healthcare sector, robotics for assistance and care are at the center of global discussion. In the healthcare sector, those discussions affect patients, healthcare stakeholders, policy makers, and industrial players, and are therefore the object of many R&D projects (Dolic et al., 2019). While robotic systems are generally used for various tasks in healthcare, such as surgery or logistics (Acosta Calderon et al. 2015; Peters et al., 2018), a vast amount of development is invested into the care of older adults (Graf, 2020). Reasons are the increasing number of the elderly, a shortage of professional caregivers and related to that, an increased burden for social security systems. Furthermore, elderly are a highly heterogeneous group characterized by different health conditions, disease patterns, coping strategies and therefore have individual care requirements. In this context, care robots are being attributed great potential to support persons with physical and/or mental impairments and disburden formal and informal caregivers (Law et al., 2019). Potential fields of robot application include support for activities of daily living, e.g., eating, toileting, mobility, household management, and social participation as well as the cognitive and physical relief of formal and informal caregivers (Becker 2013, p. 21 ff.; Kehl 2018, p. 59 ff.).

Despite the wide range of possible applications, it must currently be stated that the developed systems often do not go beyond the project status (Bedaf et al., 2015, p. 80). Furthermore, robotics research in the field of care and nursing is still in its infancy, so that there is little evidence of the solutions developed compared to existing forms of care and nursing. Barriers of the implementation of care robots comprise socioeconomic, user acceptability and ethical issues related to the care-receiving individual in particular as well as the care provision as a whole (Johansson et al., 2014; Servaty et al., 2020). Finally, it must also be critically noted that existing user concepts, especially regarding older people, do not adequately consider the individual backgrounds, prerequisites, needs and institutional embedding (Flandorfer, 2012, pp. 1–13).

The User-Centered Design (UCD) approach aims to counteract this phenomenon. The objective of UCD is to achieve high usability levels and the best possible user experience of a product or service by placing the user in the center of the development process. The UCD consists of several components (Rubin & Chisnell, 2008, pp. 12–13). Starting with a requirements analysis, which identifies the requirements, needs, and barriers of the user group, the approach continues to prioritize and transform them into an adequate concept for the subsequent project development process. Followed by several iterative user tests, the prototype can be adapted during the development process to pursue a user-oriented design. The UCD also considers the integration and implementation of the final product version through a comprehensive evaluation with the user group, regarding usability, acceptability, and efficacy.

However, there seem to be various challenges in managing the user-centered design approach in R&D projects, especially those with a focus on innovative technologies such as robotics. In a prior article, we critically examined the role of user perspectives within R&D projects on innovative assistive technology and robotic solutions in healthcare, and identified consequences for health and robotic technologies with regard to usability and user acceptability (Klebbe & Eicher, 2020, pp. 220–252). We held interviews with six experts from the fields of R&D, health technology industry and application partners and determined conditions and consequences of current user integration for different phases of R&D projects. The results will be presented as a short summary in the following section, serving as a basic understanding of the gap between conceptualization and implementation of user needs.

Background

In addition to technical, economic, and normative aspects, the integration of the user perspective plays a decisive role in the development of assistive technologies. Our previous article examined the consideration of user perspectives in R&D projects (Klebbe & Eicher, 2020, pp. 220–252). The findings regarding challenges and obstacles of user-centered research in publicly funded R&D projects form the background of this article. In the following, we will summarize these on the five levels of *user-centered research, conceptualization, development, demonstrator (pre-prototype), and continuation of the project results.*

User-Centered Research

The integration of the user perspective takes place primarily at the level of accompanying scientific research at different points during the project. The project usually starts with a requirements analysis followed by the realization of the identified requirements and interim evaluations of the development status. Each project closes with a thorough evaluation of the overall developed system. We identified access to the target group, sample size and structure, evaluation duration, consideration of the situational and natural environment of the target group, and limited project resources as key factors in adequately capturing user-centered design and development principles.

Conceptualization

Another area of possible challenges and obstacles concerns the concept phase. The identified prerequisites from the requirements analysis are gradually transformed into practicable solutions, considering the available resources and competencies. Limitations of the methodological approach of the requirements analysis, as mentioned above, can affect the conception phase, and impede the successful user-oriented development approach. A further influencing factor consists in the allocation of financial, material, and personnel means, which can limit the project goals if estimated too short.

Development

Regarding the development process, the focus on a technological problem-solving approach was highlighted as a decisive influencing factor. If a technical problem forms the conceptual starting point, a de-contextualization of the user is presumable, resulting in partial solutions for singular problems. From the point of view of technical development, it was also critically emphasized that due to limited resources often no generic development can take place. Instead, the use of proprietary technical solutions leads to additional restrictions for user-centered development.

Demonstrator

A demonstrator is a version of the device or system still in the early technology phase and designed to demonstrate feasibility and applicability. Demonstrator projects thus facilitate the development of high-risk innovative solutions and make it possible to pursue research questions that could otherwise not be considered. At the same time, there are three key challenges. First, such experimental models are difficult to evaluate in terms of efficiency and effectiveness. Second, the flexibility of the project outcome has an impact on its transferability. Third, there are few incentives for application partners to participate in such high-risk, innovative technologies projects.

Exploitation of the Project Results

A final essential field for the integration of the user perspective is the transfer of research results to politics, science, and industry. Usually, this takes place at the level of economic utilization by the technology and industry partners as well as the level of scientific utilization in the form of publications or conference contributions. Regarding economic utilization, often merely individual solutions pursued by the respective project partners are reused in the context of their own product portfolio. The further development of the overall solution often fails due to unclear right of use or the lack of resources to enter the market. In the area of scientific utilization, key influencing factors are the availability (open source), the access restrictions to the respective scientific community, and the publication characteristics of the different disciplines. Finally, a fundamental limitation consists in the predominantly research-proposal-oriented approach. Thus, transferability is only possible with restrictions due to object, time, and context limitations.

Overall, it became evident that although user-centered development plays an important role in the design, usability, and acceptability of robot solutions, it can also be subject to many restrictions. The challenges and obstacles to appropriate user integration, summarized here, are discussed in the results section of this article, supported by further literature. Based on these findings, solutions are presented that may also be relevant for areas other than publicly funded R&D projects.

Methodology

For a detailed insight into the practice of publicly funded R&D projects, six experts with long-standing experience in R&D projects focusing on robotics and/or assistive technologies were interviewed. The participants were recruited as a conscious case selection (Akremi, 2014, p. 272) based on the interdisciplinary cooperation structure within R&D projects as described at the beginning. In this respect, two experts each with project experience in the fields of health and nursing science research, engineering science research and development, and health management and care were included. All participants demonstrated a high level of experience in R&D projects with the target group of geriatric people and people in need of long-term care. The central subject of the guided interviews was the role and inclusion of the user perspective in the research and development process as well as associated difficulties and barriers. In addition, the experts were asked about their role as well as their focus and goals within R&D projects. Finally, the experts were asked to evaluate the current state of development of robotics in care and the associated application possibilities. The interviews were conducted as telephone interviews in four cases and as face-to-face interviews in two cases. All interviews were recorded as digital audio files and written transcripts. Following the interviews, the transcripts were reviewed for consistency using the digital recordings. The resulting text material was analyzed by two trained researchers according to the principles of systematic structured content analysis according to Mayring (cf. 2015, p. 98). In an inductive coding procedure, each of the two researchers first coded the interview transcripts independently. The codes were then compared, and a common code system was developed, based on which a new run of material was conducted. After final paraphrasing, generalization, and reduction, the codes were categorized to generate the requirements. To reduce errors in the evaluation process, the two researchers worked according to the "four-eyes principle", coding and evaluation were controlled alternately. The interviews revealed three central fields of requirements for future R&D projects with a focus on assistive and robotic health systems: a common understanding of the user group, the user-centered accompanying research, and projectification.

RESULTS: RECOMMENDATIONS FOR EFFECTIVE USER INVOLVEMENT

In the following, we will discuss the three central requirement areas for future R&D projects on the basis of further literature. In addition, we provide recommendations to promote effective integration of the user perspective.

Creating a Shared Understanding of the Target Group

According to the interviewees, a common understanding of the project partners regarding the needs, skills and living conditions of the target group is essential for the successful integration of the user perspective into the project development process. Various factors were identified that counteracted this common understanding. For example, the consideration and integration of the user perspective became less important once the project partners started to pursue different partial interests. This was the case, if the focus within a project was to overcome technical challenges instead of the development of one user-centered solution. In addition to diverting objectives, the involved project partners were characterized by different patterns of perception and interpretation, according to their respective institutional field of practice (e.g., science or industry). In this context, the project partner responsible for user involvement faced certain challenges, such as mediation work between the different partners. This involved both raising awareness of user concerns and translating them into task-oriented development and construction concepts. Thus, according to the experts, technology manufacturers must be able to empathize with the position and role of the users. Often, however, they only had an inaccurate idea of the target group. A compounding factor can result from abstract or even contradictory outcomes of the scientific requirements analyses, for example, due to methodological limitations. Additionally, outcomes were sometimes provided at a late stage within the development process and could not be considered adequately.

Overall, the experts recommended establishing a common communication level for the successful integration of the user perspective within the R&D process. According to them, this could be attained for example by a comprehensive target group analysis, as already carried out in commercial and industrial enterprises. Different methods are used that reflect the characteristics, specific needs, prerequisites, skills and living conditions of the target group to generate a precise picture of the targeted user group (Maguire & Bevan, 2002, p. 135). One method, which is being increasingly applied in R&D projects, is the use of personas and scenarios, involving the contribution of all project partners. By working together closely, technological, ethical, legal, social, and user-specific requirements can be considered, comprehension gaps can be closed directly between the partners, and a common objective for the development process can be created (Nielsen, 2013, pp. 91–92). Ideally, this process should take place as early as possible in the project—preferably during the project initiation phase—and the outcomes should be used during the project to monitor and reflect on internal processes. Furthermore, a holistic user understanding includes the institutional context in which the potential user group is embedded (Peter & Olson, 2010, p. 251). Approaches should be pursued that examine the target group in its natural environment (e.g., at home or in inpatient facilities), focusing on the user, his/her socio-demographic background, and his/her (socio-) psychological factors. On the other hand, a holistic approach also considers the patterns of acceptability and use of caregiving and care service networks. As they are highly involved in the consultation with and implementation of assistive technology for those in need, caregivers can have a decisive impact on the target group's perception and acceptability of technology (Frennert & Östlund, 2014, p. 302; Vollmer Dahlke et al., 2021).

Although R&D projects increasingly consider the role of older technology users and users in need of care, it must be noted that stereotypes continue to influence the development processes. With reference to Neven (2010), Flandorfer (2012, p.2) points out that older people are portrayed as frail, dependent, and ill, as well as incapable or anxious about the use of technological aids in the context of the discourse on aging and innovation. Frennert and Östlund (2014) describe this aspect as a "lack of mutual inspiration in the development of robotics for older people." These kinds of stereotypes neglect the fact that older people constitute a very heterogeneous group, which is largely cognitively and physically healthy and creatively adapts technology to their individual needs (Frennert & Östlund, 2014, p. 303). The same applies to other groups who need care and support. By focusing on technological requirements and by developing the robotic system before having it (pre-) evaluated with the potential target group in a lab setting, the user is assigned a passive role. Thus, a predefined artefact is the result at the end of the development phase, which is being evaluated regarding usability and acceptability to no purpose (Flandorfer, 2012, p. 6). About acceptability and usage patterns, studies also show the importance of positive experience with innovative technologies, especially for user groups characterized by their low self-efficacy and greater restraint in the use of technology (Flandorfer, 2012, p. 3).

Another important aspect is the user representation. Stereotypes conveyed by technology and its status in society can have a negative impact on the self-perception of older people. Since the aging process is being constituted as a social problem associated with demographic change, target groups might show a low acceptability towards technological solutions, despite their potential benefits. Reasons for this may lie in both the rejection of the underlying role models and the disappointment towards the expectations generated by political and scientific discourses (Flandorfer, 2012, p. 6).

Closely linked to a potential stigmatization by technology, ethical, social and legal implications (ELSI) also play a crucial role. With reference to Sharkey and Sharkey (2012), Frennert and Östlund (2014) cite six main ethical concerns about the use of robots in care: the loss of interpersonal contacts, the loss of privacy, deception and infantilization, the loss of control and self-determination, and liability aspects. Other ethical concerns include the potential impact of long-term robot use on user behavior and the possibility of emotional dependence.

Requirements for the Scientific Research Approach

Regarding the integration of the user perspective within the framework of accompanying scientific research, it became apparent that central challenges existed, particularly in the fields of recruitment or access to the target group, sample size and composition, generalizability and comparability of study results, frequency and duration of user-centered tests, and consideration of the user context.

Regarding access to the target group and the recruitment of study participants, both the expertise of the project partner responsible for user involvement and regional conditions played an important role. These resulted in limitations in access to the target group, for example, if the target group is small and regionally diffuse, and/or if the study participants themselves are not capable of giving their consent. According to the interviewed experts, it is necessary to enter the field at an early stage to determine both the framework conditions for the inclusion of the test persons and the evaluation setting. At the same time, this procedure could offer the possibility of determining different moderating factors influencing the use and acceptability of technology at an early stage, and to include them in the conception of the study design. In this context, Flandorfer (2012, p.3) emphasizes the importance of socio-demographic factors and their interactions for the acceptability of robotic systems. These include age, gender, education, cultural background, marital status, income, living conditions, social environment, religious background, occupation, and socio-economic status. At the same time, Flandorfer (2012) underlines the special role of moderating factors, such as previous experiences with technology in general, which can have a mediating effect against the influence of age- and gender-specific differences. With reference to Heerink (2011), Flandorfer (2012, p. 9) also emphasizes the importance of a complete inventory of various influencing factors for future research, stating, "The assumption is that, in addition to sociodemographic variables, there is a plethora of moderating factors (e.g., physical and mental condition, self-directed use, living conditions, decline of cognitive skills, and depressed mood) or such short-term factors as tiredness."

Although there is a common awareness about the importance of these factors, current research does not yet sufficiently consider them. This is mainly because the sample sizes in most studies is too small to draw reliable conclusions (Flandorfer, 2012, p. 9). Furthermore, it is also critically emphasized that some studies attempt to achieve statistically significant results based on small sample sizes (Bemelmans et al., 2012; Broekens et al., 2009). At the same time, it is not possible to reflect heterogeneity within the population based on small sample sizes, so specific groups may be represented disproportionately, and results therefore are biased.

The period of evaluation studies was pointed out as a further aspect affecting the generalizability of the study results. Various factors during the project led to a shortening of the evaluation periods, which on the one hand reduced the possibility of system adaptations to user needs and on the other hand influenced the collection of reliable study results regarding applicability, usability, and acceptability. Furthermore, effects such as a temporary change in natural behavior in response to the participation in a scientific study (Hawthorne effect) and the tendency towards increased use of a new technology due to its novelty (Novelty effect) could not be ruled out. According to Kachouie et al. (2014), these effects still receive insufficient attention in current research, although they can negatively influence external validity.

In addition, an inadequate description of the study design, applied analyses, and evaluation methods, as well as an unclear description of the study results, were identified as further limitations. Overall, these limitations have far-reaching consequences for the reproducibility of studies and their results, which, however, are required to counteract low proof of efficacy.

Another bias for the generalizability and comparability of the study results may lie in the focus on application-oriented research. There is no consistent methodological procedure available for the evaluation of developed assistive robotic systems. Instead, many different research approaches are used, which are methodologically strongly oriented towards these robotic systems (Flandorfer, 2012, p. 9). Missing or inadequate control conditions within evaluation studies are also critically discussed. In this context, Kachouie et al. (2014) criticize the lack of (randomized) control groups, which are necessary to credit observed effects on the actual intervention.

Finally, the results of the expert interviews reported an insufficient consideration of the target group's caregiving and health service networks within the accompanying user-centered research. The aim of the project, to prove the technological feasibility of specific user requirements and unforeseen expenses during the project, often led to the de-contextualization of the development process. Often only partial solutions were developed and evaluated, which could eventually not be integrated into an existing (healthcare) infrastructure. In particular, the required technological complexity had a limiting effect: due to the dynamic and highly variable environments, only a small part of the studies was carried out in the home of people in need of care. Accordingly, most studies took place under laboratory conditions or in the inpatient sector, which raises the question of the transferability of the observed effects. Bemelmans et al. (2012) also stated that the robotic systems they examined were often not clearly embedded in a nursing intervention.

In the context of these different limitations, the interviewed experts suggested various recommendations for an effective integration of the user perspective within the framework of accompanying research. The first is to get an early impression of the identified problem through an inspection of the field. Ideally, at least one representative of each project partner should take part. Especially, but not limited to, design and development partners can thus increase their awareness of the specific needs of the target group. Depending on the study design and the pursued knowledge generation, the experts recommended keeping the requirements analysis relatively short, if only highly abstract requirements can be generated. In this context, they suggested a triangulation of qualitative and quantitative approaches. Thus, qualitative, explorative pilot studies could contribute to gaining deeper insights into the different needs, perceptions, acceptability, and usage patterns of people in need of care. Subsequent quantitative results could be used to determine generalizability, potential correlations, and interaction effects. Overall, when evaluating user needs for system conceptualization, the focus should be on a quick and detailed generation of requirements. In this context, the experts reported positive experiences with user-centered tests using prototypes that convey the shape or function of the future system early, from the project start. Especially for robotics research, the use of image and video material to determine acceptability and usage patterns was not sufficient compared to demonstrations or tests with real robotic systems. Furthermore, the experts stressed the urgent need for generic evaluation methods to ensure comparability of the results. A further requirement lies in the need for detailed descriptions of the study design and the results obtained, to ensure their reproducibility. Finally, sufficient funds and resources for an evaluation should be ensured—ideally randomized trials with large sample sizes, control groups, and long evaluation periods.

In summary, the presented challenges for an adequate user integration and user representation as well as the restrictions to a specific research item have far-reaching consequences for a target-oriented ELSI research. On the one hand, this consists in the scientific access to the object. Thus, different disciplines are involved in the ethical, legal, social and economic evaluation of robotic solutions based on heterogeneous theoretical models and associated methodological procedures (Spindler et al., 2020). In this context, the described limitations may hinder the process of forming unified and general research methods, both at the level of a single scientific discipline and across different disciplines. Furthermore, the question arises to what extent the produced findings can capture societal needs, potential barriers to acceptability, and the disruptive potential of innovative technologies beyond the local scope of the project (Bellon & Nähr-Wagener, 2020) and be reflected in the development and introduction process. Finally, from a transdisciplinary perspective, another question is to what extent research results are made accessible to a larger audience and to what extent civil society actors are included in the innovation discourse as required as a dimension of the EU's Responsible Research and Innovation approach (Röß & Warnke, 2020).

Tackling Projectification

Another key factor influencing user integration was how R&D projects were structured and organized. In this context, the way a technical or scientific issue was projectified and the duration of the project, which is usually set at three years, were of central significance. The experts confirmed the statement by (Fellbaum, 1982, p. 88) that the focus of R&D projects is the development and research of socially, economically, and technologically risky developments (products, processes, technologies) with an associated high risk of failure. At the same time, the objectives of the projects set during the project application process and the subsequent work plan were often regarded as too ambitious. Another problem constituted the fact that necessary expenses for the planning of resources and development could not be estimated adequately. Unforeseen additional expenses emerging during the project had several negative impacts on the project results. First, only partial aspects of the original project idea were implemented, and phases of user integration had to be reduced or abandoned. Furthermore, due to limited resources, proprietary systems had to be used instead of developing a generic technology for a specific problem. Barriers in their operability resulted in further limitations. However, according to the experts, a generic development approach that produces technologies compatible with existing technological infrastructures and workflows could prevent a variety of limitations in implementation and, at the same time, support sustainable use.

In addition to partially unclear framework conditions of the development prerequisites and environment, the linear and, in separate development work packages structured, work plan formed another relevant, influencing factor on user integration. Although it is possible to test the progress of single work packages at different stages in the development process, the respective development stages are integrated relatively late during the project. Once again, development problems of all participating project partners negatively affected the entire course of the project and the associated possibilities of user evaluation of the overall system. During the interviews, a central requirement in this context were both a stronger parallelization of processes and an agile development process, to test intermediate development results by users early in the project and in several loops. This will allow the findings to be used immediately for the ongoing development and design process. Another central requirement was the realization of a long-term evaluation of the overall system to achieve reliable results.

Another requirement in the promotion of innovative health technologies is to abandon the construction of a technical or economic understanding of innovation and instead consider a societal perspective based on different reference systems (Rammert, 2010).

Although the collaborative structure of R&D projects implies an interdisciplinary composition, the individual opportunities for each project partner to act are often structured around the demonstrator (pre-prototype) concept, which is primarily focused on technical feasibility. Although the demonstrator status prevents the pressure to succeed in technological development (Stubbe 2020), there are far-reaching limitations for science and practitioners (health care institutions) in terms of the connectivity of their communication and action possibilities in their own social subsystems. For an effective transfer of project knowledge, it therefore seems necessary to consider the different user groups within their institutional embedding as well as the associated social framework conditions of diffusion and integration (especially regarding ELSI implications). On the other hand, the challenge is to better distribute and coordinate the resulting research desiderata within the framework of different funding guidelines. In this context, the establishment of independent committees for the evaluation and review of project plans, progress, and results could be a further approach.

Finally, the question arises as to whether the duration of R&D projects should be linked more closely to the complexity of the development objective. After a basic project period, research projects should be able to apply for an extension of the project, providing a certain technological complexity as well as social, economic, and technological risks. To counteract the phenomenon of describing an overambitious project objective within research applications, the established practice of reporting to the project-managing agency could be expanded by a monitoring system. In addition, independent committees could also be involved in the research evaluation process. Since research with robotics for the health care sector is still at an early stage, the R&D sector has to take equal account of the complexity of the systems, their current social diffusion, and their integration prerequisites, as well as the potential social consequences.

Limitations

Our methodological approach is associated with different limitations, which we will reflect in the following.

A first lies in the criteria-based case selection (Akremi, 2014, p. 272). Despite the fundamental consideration of the three core perspectives of research, industry, and practice within the sample, the results are subject to a certain bias. This bias especially concerns the logic of practice of the experts' organizations/institutions as this influences their perceptions, goals, and actions. A second limitation is that the interviewed experts were predominantly involved in national application-oriented R&D projects. Although most of the experts had additional experience, for example, in European R&D projects, projects funded by the Federal Ministry of Education and Research (Bundesministerium für Bildung und Forschung, BMBF), in particular, were the focus in the interviews. The transfer of the results to an international level is therefore limited. Finally, to be able to assess the effects of various identified influencing factors adequately, it would be necessary to include other actors into the analysis. These include representatives from the fields of research funding (project management agencies, ministries), patients and family associations, medical staff, the health industry, and health policy.

CONCLUSION

This work presented requirements for the successful integration of user needs into R&D projects with a focus on innovative health technologies. Furthermore, recommendations were provided to close the gap between user-centered design and its realization to achieve users' expectations on the efficacy, effectiveness, and usability regarding everyday-life activities. These recommendations concerned the collaboration and motivation of all collaborative partners, who are responsible to contribute fully to a common goal. However, project sponsors are also in demand to adapt both preliminary work on project funding applications, including adequate research objectives, and R&D process structures to the research purpose. Furthermore, they should closely monitor the processes and interim results to intervene, if necessary. Finally, it must be acknowledged that the interdisciplinary nature of R&D projects creates an environment to consider different ethical, social, legal, and technological perspectives, whose realization is a key driver of innovative technology and user acceptability. Although our results are predominantly connected to R&D practices within publicly funded projects, we believe that various outcomes are transferable to the industrial area. Therefore, leaders and managers of innovative development projects can benefit from implementing the presented strategies into the process of user integration to create products that are highly accepted by their user groups.

ACKNOWLEDGMENT

The authors express their special thanks of gratitude to all those who contributed to this publication.

This research received no specific grant from any funding agency in the public, commercial, or not-for-profit sectors.

REFERENCES

Acosta Calderon, C. A., Mohan, E. R., & Ng, B. S. (2015). Development of a hospital mobile platform for logistics tasks. *Digital Communications and Networks*, *1*(2), 102–111. doi:10.1016/j.dcan.2015.03.001

Akremi, L. (2014). Stichprobenziehung in der qualitativen Sozialforschung [Sampling in qualitative social research]. In N. Baur & J. Blasius (Eds.), *Handbuch Methoden der empirischen Sozialforschung*. Springer Fachmedien Wiesbaden. doi:10.1007/978-3-531-18939-0_17

Becker, H. (Ed.). (2013). Robotik in Betreuung und Gesundheitsversorgung. Zürich: vdf Hochschulverl. doi:10.14512/tatup.22.1.62

Bedaf, S., Gelderblom, G. J., & de Witte, L. (2015). Overview and categorization of robots supporting independent living of elderly people: What activities do they support and how far have they developed. *Assistive Technology*, *27*(2), 88–100. doi:10.1080/10400435.2014.978916 PMID:26132353

Bellon, J., & Nähr-Wagener, S. (2020). Interdisziplinarität, ELSI und Integrierte Forschung – aus Einem Vieles und aus Vielem Eines? In B. Gransche & A. Manzeschke (Eds.), *Das geteilte Ganze* (pp. 37–52). Springer Fachmedien Wiesbaden. doi:10.1007/978-3-658-26342-3_2

Bemelmans, R., Gelderblom, G. J., Jonker, P., & de Witte, L. (2012). Socially assistive robots in elderly care: A systematic review into effects and effectiveness. *Journal of the American Medical Directors Association, 13*(2), 114–120.e1. doi:10.1016/j.jamda.2010.10.002 PMID:21450215

Broekens, J., Heerink, M., & Rosendal, H. (2009). Assistive social robots in elderly care: A review. *Gerontechnology (Valkenswaard), 8*(2), 94–103. doi:10.4017/gt.2009.08.02.002.00

Dolic, Z., Castro, R., & Moarcas, A. (2019). *Robots in healthcare: A solution or a problem? Workshop proceedings.* Brussels. https://www.europarl.europa.eu/RegData/etudes/IDAN/2019/638391/IPOL_IDA(2019)638391_EN.pdf

Fellbaum, K.-R. (1982). *Telekommunikation von A – Z* [Telecommunication from A to Z]. VDE-Verl.

Flandorfer, P. (2012). Population ageing and socially assistive robots for elderly persons: The importance of sociodemographic factors for user acceptance. *International Journal of Population Research, 2012*, 1–13. doi:10.1155/2012/829835

Frennert, S., & Östlund, B. (2014). Review: Seven matters of concern of social robots and older people. *International Journal of Social Robotics, 6*(2), 299–310. doi:10.100712369-013-0225-8

Graf, B. (2020). Assistenzroboter für die Pflege: Verfügbare Produkte und Forschungsfelder. *Zeitschrift für Gerontologie und Geriatrie, 53*(7), 608–614. doi:10.100700391-020-01782-7 PMID:32986162

Johansson-Pajala, R.-M., & Gustafsson, C. (2020). Significant challenges when introducing care robots in Swedish elder care. *Disability and Rehabilitation. Assistive Technology*, 1–11. doi:10.1080/17483107.2020.1773549 PMID:32538206

Kachouie, R., Sedighadeli, S., Khosla, R., & Chu, M.-T. (2014). Socially assistive robots in elderly care: A mixed-method systematic literature review. *International Journal of Human-Computer Interaction, 30*(5), 369–393. doi:10.1080/10447318.2013.873278

Kehl, C. (2018). *Robotik und assistive Neurotechnologien in der Pflege - gesellschaftliche Herausforderungen*, Berlin: Büro für Technikfolgen-Abschätzung beim Deutschen Bundestag (TAB). https://www.tab-beim-bundestag.de/de/pdf/publikationen/berichte/TAB-Arbeitsbericht-ab177.pdf

Klebbe, R., & Eicher, C. (2020). Wer sind eigentlich diese Nutzer? Zur Rolle älterer und pflegebedürftiger Erwachsener in der Entwicklung robotischer Assistenzsysteme [Who are exactly these users? The role of older adults and people in need of care in the development of robotic systems]. In J. Hergesell, A. Maibaum, & M. Meister (Eds.), *Genese und Folgen der Pflegerobotik - Die Konstitution eines interdisziplinären Forschungsfeldes* (1st ed.). Beltz Juventa in der Verlagsgruppe Beltz.

Law, M., Sutherland, C., Ahn, H. S., MacDonald, B. A., Peri, K., Johanson, D. L., Vajsakovic, D.-S., Kerse, N., & Broadbent, E. (2019). Developing assistive robots for people with mild cognitive impairment and mild dementia: A qualitative study with older adults and experts in aged care. *BMJ Open*, *9*(9), 1–9. doi:10.1136/bmjopen-2019-031937 PMID:31551392

Maguire, M., & Bevan, N. (2002). User requirements analysis. In J. Hammond, T. Gross, & J. Wesson (Eds.), Usability: Gaining a competitive edge. Springer US. doi:10.1007/978-0-387-35610-5_9

Mayring, P. (2015). *Qualitative Inhaltsanalyse: Grundlagen und Techniken (Qualitative content analysis: Principles and techniques)* (12 überarbeitete Auflage). Beltz Verlag.

Nielsen, L. (2013). *Personas - User Focused Design*. Springer London. doi:10.1007/978-1-4471-4084-9

Peter, J. P., & Olson, J. C. (2010). *Consumer behavior & marketing strategy* (9th ed.). McGraw-Hill Irwin.

Peters, B. S., Armijo, P. R., Krause, C., Choudhury, S. A., & Oleynikov, D. (2018). Review of emerging surgical robotic technology. *Surgical Endoscopy*, *32*(4), 1636–1655. doi:10.100700464-018-6079-2 PMID:29442240

Rammert, W. (2010). Die Innovationen der Gesellschaft [The innovations of society]. In J. Howaldt & H. Jacobsen (Eds.), *Soziale Innovation: Auf dem Weg zu einem postindustriellen Innovationsparadigma*. VS Verlag für Sozialwissenschaften. doi:10.1007/978-3-531-92469-4_2

Röß., A., & Warnke, P. (2020). Organisationale Rahmenbedingungen für Integrierte Forschung: Perspektiven aus einer angewandten Forschungsorganisation. In B. Gransche & A. Manzeschke (Eds.), *Das geteilte Ganze* (pp. 119–132). Springer Fachmedien Wiesbaden. doi:10.1007/978-3-658-26342-3_6

Rubin, J., & Chisnell, D. (2008). *Handbook of usability testing: How to plan, design, and conduct effective tests* (2nd ed.). Wiley Pub.

Servaty, R., Kersten, A., Brukamp, K., Möhler, R., & Mueller, M. (2020). Implementation of robotic devices in nursing care. Barriers and facilitators: An integrative review. *BMJ Open*, *10*(9), e038650. doi:10.1136/bmjopen-2020-038650 PMID:32958491

Spindler, M., Booz, S., Gieseler, H., Runschke, S., Wydra, S., & Zinsmaier, J. (2020). How to achieve integration?: Methodological concepts and challenges for the integration of ethical, legal, social and economic aspects into technological development. In B. Gransche & A. Manzeschke (Eds.), *Das geteilte Ganze* (pp. 213–239). Springer Fachmedien Wiesbaden. doi:10.1007/978-3-658-26342-3_11

Stubbe, J. (2020). Sechs Thesen für gelingende Integrierte Forschung. In B. Gransche & A. Manzeschke (Eds.), *Das geteilte Ganze* (pp. 197–211). Springer Fachmedien Wiesbaden. doi:10.1007/978-3-658-26342-3_10

Vollmer Dahlke, D., Lee, S., Smith, M. L., Shubert, T., Popovich, S., & Ory, M. G. (2021). Attitudes Toward Technology and Use of Fall Alert Wearables in Caregiving: Survey Study. *JMIR Aging*, *4*(1), e23381. doi:10.2196/23381 PMID:33502320

Chapter 3
Ethical Aspects of Information-Based Medicine (With a Focus on Mental Health)

Jan Kalina
https://orcid.org/0000-0002-8491-0364
ICS CAS, Prague, Czech Republic

Nicole Tobišková
ICS CAS, Prague, Czech Republic

ABSTRACT

Modern advanced tools of artificial intelligence assist healthcare professionals in a variety of complex tasks related to medical care. Digitalization and automation accelerate the development and deployment of innovative artificial intelligence tools tailor-made for clinical applications; decision support systems represent an important example of such tools. This chapter is devoted to discussing the role of artificial intelligence in current and prospective medical care and ethical aspects of their deployment. As developed countries currently go through remarkable transforms of medical care involving informatization and centering around medical information and knowledge, this chapter also discusses future ideals of medical care characterized by the concept of information-based medicine. Ethical and patient safety implications of using artificial intelligence within information-based medicine are overviewed here. Specific attention is paid to mental healthcare and ethical aspects of using artificial intelligence in its context.

DOI: 10.4018/978-1-7998-7888-9.ch003

INTRODUCTION

The whole society worldwide is affected by the COVID-19 pandemic and seems to undergo the most dramatic progress in the history of humankind. Naturally, medical care can hardly remain untouched by the negative impact of the pandemic but may at the same time benefit from new perspectives and opportunities (Alimadadi et al., 2020). Indeed, after the outbreak of the COVID-19 pandemic in 2019 caused by the SARS-CoV-2 coronavirus, medical care has experienced complex transforms basically in all countries around the world (Sigurdsson et al., 2020).

The digitalization and automation contribute to an increasing availability of big medical data (Lin & Hou, 2020). Innovative tools of artificial intelligence (often abbreviated as AI) allow to obtain new medical knowledge from the available big medical data (Tripathi, 2021). The digitalization and automation (including deployment of robots) have enabled development and deployment of modern telemedicine tools such as clinical decision support systems. The information technology contributes to a paradigm shift from medical care approaches formulated for an average patient towards personalized approaches based on specific medical knowledge obtained for a particular individual patient. Further, artificial intelligence has a potential to interconnect very particular medical specialties and to overcome the granulation (or fractalization) of current medicine by offering a holistic approach to clinical care for an individual patient. This chapter is devoted to ethical aspects related to deployment of artificial intelligence in medical care, with a focus on the transforms of medicine from evidence-based medicine towards prospective ideals denoted here as information-based medicine. An array of issues related to the use of artificial intelligence in medical care is presented here with a particular focus on the field of mental health.

On one hand, we currently experience the boom of artificial intelligence tools for healthcare applications. On the other hand, ethical issues of using artificial intelligence in healthcare are often reduced to technical (software engineering) problems of data privacy, anonymization, confidentiality, and sharing, without paying attention to a broad spectrum of other ethical issues. A more complex overview of ethical aspects of artificial intelligence in healthcare in general and particularly in specific fields of clinical care thus remain to represent a hot interdisciplinary topic connecting the worlds of ethics, medicine, medical informatics, or computer science. This paper fills the gap of a missing broad discussion of diverse topics of using artificial intelligence in general, with a focus on mental healthcare, where the ethical debates still have not come to generally acknowledged conclusions.

The chapter has the following structure. The next section introduces basic concepts of artificial intelligence and machine learning. An overview of selected inspiring health-related artificial intelligence applications follows, documenting the recent ability of artificial intelligence to reshape medical care. Then, it is discussed how medical care is centered around the key concepts of medical information and machine learning. A vision of ideals of information-based medicine is then presented. A number of ethical aspects of information-based medicine are discussed. A separate section on specific ethical aspects for the field of mental healthcare follows, which shows that a specific field of healthcare has to face its very specific ethical issues, not relevant for other clinical fields. Apart from finding new connections among particular ethical aspects, the chapter comes to the main conclusion that ethical considerations cannot be successfully solved as an appendix (additional extra component) of medical care relying on artificial intelligence, but have to pervade all clinical decision making tasks of the medical care as their integral part.

ARTIFICIAL INTELLIGENCE AND MACHINE LEARNING

Artifical intelligence tools can be introduced as software devices with diverse abilities, which are nowadays able e.g. to analyze (possibly big) medical data and to perform advanced clinical decision making by solving complex machine learning tasks. Artificial intelligence tools in medical care include clinical decision support systems, sensors or chatbots, tools for diagnostic imaging or gene expression analysis, tools for natural language processing (for analyzing unstructured medical reports) etc.; the potential and at the same challenges and limitations of artificial intelligence in healthcare were extensively described in an overview by Jiang et al. (2017). Analyzing medical data combines established methods for exploratory data analysis (EDA), descriptive modelling, predictive machine learning with heuristic principles; numerous computational techniques commonly used in current healthcare were overviewed in Kalina (2015).

Methods of machine learning (including modern tools of neurocomputing such as deep neural networks) as well as multivariate statistics may be exploited for the analysis of numerical data (in the form of numbers) and also for extracting features from medical images and signals. Their implementation in freely available software packages can be nowadays considered as highly reliable. The classification (supervised learning) task has the aim to learn a rule allowing to assign a new measurement (i.e. an independent individual) to one of several given groups. Solving the classification task within a clinical decision support system requires to capture the multivariate structure (correlation structure) of biomedical data, but at the cost of (sometimes quite strong) assumptions. Machine learning tools may obtain knowledge from data with a large dimensionality or complexity, possibly encompassing an intrinsic dimensionality reduction (variable selection) so that the resulting solution is sparse, i.e. trimming away some of the available features or parameters such as in the classification method of Kalina & Matonoha (2020).

Deep learning, a class of machine learning algorithms, represents a promising field with an enormous potential for a suitable automatic analysis of massive datasets. Deep learning is particularly suitable for analyzing multimodal data, i.e. data available in various forms acquired from various sources. An example of multimodal data is a combination of functional magnetic resonance images (fMRI) and gene expression measurements allowing to bring unique knowledge related to genetic predispositions for schizophrenia. Deep learning methods are understood as universally valid, i.e. they do not require a specific probabilistic distribution of the data; still, they commonly require some assumptions, which are in practice rarely validated. Testing the assumptions together with the transparency of the algorithms thus belongs to the ethical issues related to using deep learning tools (Piano, 2020).

SELECTED APPLICATIONS OF ARTIFICIAL INTELLIGENCE IN HEALTHCARE

In this section, selected inspiring recent artificial intelligence tools successful in health-related applications are overviewed, which document the recent ability of artificial intelligence to reshape current medical care.

Brain Sciences and Mental Health

Artificial intelligence has been repeatedly applied to analyze electroencephalography (EEG) signals or fMRI measurements (Bučková et al., 2020), which have a potential to reveal e.g. an early onset of Alzheimer's disease. In the near future, the promising results of artificial intelligence may lead to an increasing recommendation of preventive brain examinations by primary physicians, and thus to an improved diagnostics of brain disorders.

Artificial intelligence has allowed a complex modelling of the human brain as a whole. Earlier models of the brain had a static (fixed) point of view according to the organization of the central nervous system, exploiting the knowledge of specific functions of individual parts of the brain. Nevertheless, dynamical models of the brain are currently acknowledged as more appropriate, which are based on large-scale distributed and interactive networks. While different parts of the brain are already known to be responsible for specific functions, principles of spontaneous brain activity (in a resting state) and especially connections between pairs of brain parts in the resting state represent an important open problem in current neuroscience. Their discovery requires to capture the brain processes at various activities or to find a method for an effective monitoring of the brain. It has been conjectured that certain modifications of the resting-state brain networks are characteristic for schizophrenic patients (Hlinka et al., 2011). Because neuroimaging is known to be highly sensitive to outliers due to measurement errors and complicated structure of acquiring the images, a robust (resistant) analysis of fMRI images is highly desirable.

Let us describe a particular study of fMRI data of spontaneous brain activity of various parts of the brain. In this study of Kalina & Hlinka (2017), the brain activity of 24 probands was measured by means of fMRI under 7 different situations. One of them can be characterized as a resting state, without any stimulus. Besides, the probands were observing each of 6 different movies while measuring the brain activity in the same way. The data have the form of 4005 correlation coefficients among fMRI measurements in three-dimensional regions of the brain measured on 24 probands. Each of the correlation measures evaluates the connectivity between two parts of the brain. The basic task is to classify (separate) the resting state from a movie on the high-dimensional data with 24 probands and 4005 variables. Because the measurements are contaminated by outlying values (outliers), robust methods (i.e. resistant with respect to the presence of outliers in the data) were applied. Such robust tools (cf. Kalina (2012)) turned out to be reliable in the particular task to analyze brain measurements. Particularly, the model based on a robust linear discriminant analysis, based only on 81 selected (most relevant) variables, yields the 100% classification accuracy here. Thus, the study reveals the benefits of robust algorithms within artificial intelligence tools.

Naturally, understanding the human brain may contribute to understanding mental health disorders (Kalina, 2021). Indeed, the current (i.e. rather limited) understanding of mental health disorders may become largely improved with the help of artificial intelligence applied to the study of human brain. The number of mental health disorders started to increase rapidly after the outbreak of the COVID-19 pandemic, so there arguably arises an increasing need for digital psychiatry (Ćosić et al., 2020). So far, however, decision support systems have not become extensively used in mental healthcare, as various attempts for decision support systems for a distant diagnosis or therapy have led to frustrations. In spite of their currently rare applications, telepsychiatry tools (i.e. tools of telemedicine in psychiatry) have a potential to offer the mental healthcare also to patients who would otherwise stay reluctant to seeking a classical therapy, e.g. to patients with substance abuse problems.

Fetology

Recent examples of artificial intelligence tools in fetology, i.e. the field related to diagnosis and care of fetal (prenatal) patients before birth, include an advanced method of Hynek et al. (2018) for assessment fetal size (and thus of gestational age) by means of linear models tailor-made for data, which are clustered (in different groups) and longitudinal (i.e. observed sequentially from the same probands over time). Such modelling considers not only the time development of the mean values but also the time series of variances. Another application is a method for quality evaluation of nuchal translucency measurements by means of statistical control charts proposed by Hynek et al. (2021). Their real-time monitoring of the quality of the measurements by means of exponentially weighted moving average charts turned out to outperform traditional methods for sequential quality control.

Nursing

Nursing informatics is currently acknowledged as a self-standing discipline aiming at supporting nurses with their decisions regarding the nursing care tailor-made for an individual patient or for family-centered care. Artificial intelligence tools including decision support systems have recently penetrated also to nursing. In numerous hospitals, nursing information systems represent autonomous parts of the hospital information systems. Available evidence-based nursing tools use specific nursing nomenclatures (classification systems), which however complicate the communication between nurses and physicians. Nurses throughout the world have become more self-governing and have obtained an increasing authority but are at the same time expected to demonstrate an improved responsibility, education, and health literacy.

As evidence-based nursing uses statistical evidence again recommended for the average patient, statistical literacy represents an important expectation from qualified nurses. This is true also for artificial intelligence tools developed for the care of patients infected with COVID-19; such a system by Keim-Malpass & Moorman (2021) was developed for early selection of patients under a higher risk with a potential need for cardiovascular decompensation. The need for statistically literate nurses is not a novelty; the founder of modern nursing, Florence Nightingale (1820-1910), namely contributed to the development of statistics and was able to promote social reforms in the United Kingdom in the fields of hygiene and public health.

Biometric Authentication

An application for biometric authentication, i.e. the task to identify an individual based on biometric characteristic, invented to meet specific needs within a large university hospital was presented by Kalina & Schlenker (2018). The implemented software procedure based on typing on a keyboard captures the keystroke dynamics of a given user when entering a username and a fixed password; the data are collected directly from the operation system of the computer. The application allows to record the code of every key, its name, time of pressing, and time of releasing the key automatically without any delay.

A particular study of the results of the application will be now presented. The data were acquired from 32 probands, who were demanded to write a fixed password ("kladruby") 5-times slowly and 5-times at the habitual speed. Thus, 15 variables including 8 keystroke durations (pressing each of the keys) and 7 keystroke latencies (pauses between pressing two keys) were measured, all in milliseconds. The biometric authentication represents a classification task to 32 groups, where each group corresponds to one of the individuals in the study. Although the number of variables is small, it exceeds the number of measurements (the number of repeated typing the password), which severely complicates the analysis of the data, together with the fact that they are highly contaminated by outlying values. Robust versions of linear discriminant analysis turn out to perform better on the noisy data for classification to a small number of groups, but lose their performance because there are as many as 32 groups. On the other hand, a support vector machine classifier turns out to be the most suitable among the available classification methods. However, the method is sensitive to the presence of outlying values (outliers) and improved results were obtained if outliers were manually discarded prior to learning the classification rule. This study, which has been tested within a university hospital, shows (again) the need for robust statistical procedures if artificial intelligence tools should analyze data contaminated by outlying values.

FROM INFORMATION TO MEDICAL KNOWLEDGE

Before we describe the future ideals of information-based medicine, we explain our understanding of medical information and knowledge, the harmful role of misinformation, and the focus of current healthcare on the average patient.

Medical Information and Knowledge

To make a clear distinction between information and knowledge, information in the form of raw available data can be hardly used for the particular decision making task. Only knowledge in the form of relevant and useful facts obtained (extracted) from the raw data may be useful for a particular decision making task. Medical knowledge has three components: electronic, economic, and environmental (Zvárová & Zvára, 2011); naturally, clinical decision making should take all these three knowledge components into account. Medical care exploits the knowledge from a clinical trial within a clinical task for an individual patient. As medical information (and the knowledge derived from it) starts to play a prominent role in medical care, it will be necessary to adopt processes allowing the knowledge (instead of patients) to circulate among physicians or care providers naturally under given rules of data privacy and protection. It can be distinguished between two dimensions of medical knowledge:

- Knowledge relevant for a particular patient;
- General knowledge, typically acquired within clinical trials by averaging the results over a group of patients. Such averaged knowledge is however relevant and reliable only for a fictitious average patient (as discussed below).

Trustworthy Information Contribute to Public Trust

Healthcare systems in individual countries may be effective only in the atmosphere of a public trust (Gopichandran et al., 2020). A major unethical phenomenon endangering public trust is the spread of misinformation, such as the boom of misinformation contradicting all available scientific evidence about the COVID-19 pandemic. This boom started soon after the outbreak of the pandemic throughout the world (Mian & Khan, 2020) and scientists worldwide have been constantly demanding to fight against misinformation. Misinformation, in spite of being false and useless, reduces the uncertainty of the recipient and in this way fulfils the formal definition of information, generally acknowledged within information theory. Still, because unreliable information cannot be transformed to useful medical knowledge, data quality represents an ethical issue (as discussed later).

Let us describe the situation during the COVID-19 pandemic in the Czech Republic, where the state has been intensively criticized for insufficient popularization of the vaccination against the disease. Shortly after the beginning of the pandemic situation, there were presented conspiracy theories, pseudoscientific opinions about the pandemic, or evident lies in media. In emotional debates, scientists have revealed their contradictory opinions and lack of unity, which naturally led to the loss of their own credibility, but also to a general loss of public trust in science or in medical care as such. The public was puzzled and a general reluctance to the vaccination turns out to be a natural consequence. In reaction to the low quality of data related to the pandemic development or unavailability of detailed data related to the vaccination, the Czech Statistical Society launched an expert group focusing on epidemiological modelling of the COVID-19 pandemic in January 2021. The current authors consider the activity of the expert group to be praiseworthy and agrees with their demands for providing the data about the pandemic to the public, because making the data publicly available would contribute to improving the public trust in the healthcare system. At the same time, the Czech Academy of Sciences started to promote the idea to establish its new Institute of Virology. However, the authors hold the opinion that decision making related to medical care as well as epidemiological and political steps against the pandemic has to take into account not only biological knowledge, but also delicate sociological, demographic, or economic aspects.

Focus on Average Patient

Traditionally, medical care is directed at an average patient. The medical knowledge within biomedical research is typically obtained by averaging (aggregating) the results over selected groups of probands. In other words, the methodology of biomedical research leads to conclusions, which are naturally formulated for an average human; such concept was in fact introduced already by the Belgian polyhistor Adolphe Quetelet (1796–1874). Also current clinical trials, which remain to be the main source of medical knowledge, use biostatistical methods to yield averaged results for averaged (virtual, imaginary) patient, without reflecting the individual situation of a real patient at the point of care. However, medical care would be very different if aiming at e.g. a median patient, or if using a trimmed mean for aggregating the results of clinical trials; the trimmed mean is obtained as the mean after trimming away a given percentage of outlying (atypical, anomalous) values from the given data and is thus more suitable for data contaminated by outliers. On the other hand, such analysis of the entire dataset observed within a clinical trial would not allow to draw more precise conclusions for a possibly atypical (anomalous, outlying, statistically extreme) individual patient.

FROM EVIDENCE-BASED MEDICINE TOWARDS INFORMATION-BASED MEDICINE

As the COVID-19 pandemic accelerated a development of advanced artificial intelligence tools allowing to extract medical knowledge from available information, the most developed countries can anticipate further permanent transforms of medical care. Currently, evidence-based medicine (EBM) has been widely accepted as a unifying concept describing perfect or optimal practices of medicine. The clinical practice is gradually undergoing improvements towards more advanced ideals which are denoted in this section as the ideals of information-based medicine (Kalina, 2021).

The pioneering approach to EBM proposed in the 1990s was primarily focused on the best available evidence in making decisions related to care for individual patients. Later, EBM was refined (and redefined) as a thorough, unique, and critical use of the best objective and most topical proofs in the process of decision making about the diagnosis, therapy, and prognosis for individual patients (Straus et al., 2018). Such proofs cannot be however understood as rigorous proofs but have only the form of statistical evidence. The practice of evidence-based medicine integrates clinical expertise of individual physicians with clinical evidence acquired within systematically performed clinical research. The cornerstones of EBM require that physicians are able to use up-to-date research results and exploit them in their everyday clinical practice. This includes e.g. searching and systematic critical evaluation of clinical research publications, analysis of activities, risk analysis, or analysis of ethical and legal consequences of using a given approach. By considering economic analysis of costs, EBM contributes also to healthcare effectiveness.

The knowledge used within EBM is typically obtained within clinical research, i.e. within **clinical trials**. The current practice of clinical trials is still criticized for the usually low quality of data collection or for (unintentional but common) avoiding of some important variables (James et al., 2015). Besides, proponents of personalized medical care promote clinical trials with small sample sizes, i.e. performed on several very specific patients with the same risk factors. In reality, there apparently emerges a tendency for clinical trials to become bigger and more expensive. In addition, the response to therapy is known to be influenced by the sole presence of the patients in a clinical trial, naturally only if the patient is aware of taking part in the trial. Decision support systems may also help to decide whether a new clinical study should be performed. While each clinical study must undergo an ethical review process, many of current clinical studies seem superfluous, i.e. the same studies are carried out repeatedly. It is also highly ethically sensitive that clinical trials often have an inappropriate design without a possibility to generalize the results to modified conditions, which are different than the laboratory (artificial) conditions of the original clinical trial.

Next to clinical trials, the importance of **basic research** relevant for medical care quickly increases thanks to the development of artificial intelligence. We expect the knowledge obtained within basic (nonclinical) research to become dominant, so that the medical care is shifted beyond the ideas of EBM towards an ideal state characterized by the model of information-based medicine (Borangíu & Purcarea, 2008), connecting basic biomedical research with patient-specific information. The potential of artificial intelligence tools is to perform the integration of knowledge from various sources, primarily from basic research (i.e. understanding diseases on a molecular level), epidemiological studies, and examinations of an individual patient. At the same time, basic research together with information technology and big data analysis extend the possibilities for a targeted medical care solution beyond the current concept of EBM and allow to overcome its limitations.

Information-based medicine requires much deeper transforms of the best practices (gold standard of the medical care) beyond technical improvements of tools of information technology. The future medical care will require a paradigm shift from approaches formulated for an average patient towards personalized approaches based on specific medical knowledge obtained for a particular individual patient.

The concept of information-based medicine as a recent and perspective medicine paradigm describes the effort to transform the statistical evidence for an averaged patient towards a real participative patient based on individual data with clinical as well genetic or metabolic parameters. The concept of information-based medicine starts to find first applications, such as in the study of Senders et al. (2018) exploiting artificial intelligence in clinical decision making; particularly, the study exploited deep learning to analyze massive brain imaging data and to personalize treatment decisions for patients with a brain tumor.

Information-based medicine will profit from using clinical decision support systems together with other electronic health (e-health) tools and with results of the basic research (e.g. in neuroscience or molecular genetics). All these sources of medical knowledge will contribute to bringing the decision making process closer to an individual patient, improving the effectiveness of therapy and patient safety. The availability of big data together with a new biomedical knowledge may allow to make the therapy efficient, compared to the current state; it is not uncommon e.g. in current mental healthcare that the therapy aims only at easing the suffering of patients. As a by-product, the transform of healthcare will be accompanied by the transform of nursing towards principles of information-based nursing.

From the data analysis point of view, the personalized medical care within information-based medicine will consider clusters (homogeneous subgroups) of patients or a set of several quantiles instead of averaging the results, where e.g. a typical patient with a high risk of a given disease, an average patient, and a typical patient with a low risk are considered. Such considerations require new concepts of machine learning, although we have to expect physicians to prefer a unified and much simpler approach for groups of patients even further, without following the trends of personalized care. It should be stressed that the progress consists mainly in the methodology and not in statistical software, which represents only a tool for acquiring knowledge from the data.

Information-based medicine, aiming at committing to ethical standards, will have to refuse misinformation. Thus, in contrary to the current experience with a plethora of misinformation, future medical care needs to be more open to the public. Its democratization and renewal of trust of the public will need an intensive popularization and publicizing.

One might have the feeling that physicians remain limited or constrained by narrow perspectives of artificial intelligence. While medical specialists become overspecialized with an increase of medical knowledge (Moreau, 2020), they are less able to solve more general problems or to change to a new subspecialty. It is however exactly the information technology, which offers to capture human body and/or healthcare in a holistic approach, because it has the capacity (if correctly organized) to store all available data (including big data) and information, to analyze them, and search for associations. In this way, information-based medicine will perform a holistic approach to information encompassing the subjective data (so useful e.g. in mental healthcare), and will capture the full bio-psycho-socio-spiritual model of health. Information-based medicine also has the potential to incorporate a high quality of diagnostics with principles of patient safety.

The ideas of information-based medicine promoted in this chapter were influenced by the personality of prof. Jana Zvárová, the founder of medical informatics in the Czech Republic, who built an interdisciplinary team around international projects, promoted health literacy, was involved in education for medical faculties, or cooperate with university hospitals already after 1990, as documented in the monograph on history of medical informatics by Masic & Mihalas (2014).

ETHICAL ISSUES OF INFORMATION-BASED MEDICINE

Information-based medical care, intensively relying on artificial intelligence tools, will have to solve serious ethical dilemmas and to anticipate potential ethical pitfalls. On a very general level, artificial intelligence must be always used according to ethical standards and ethical risks of implementation of artificial intelligence in medical care have to be minimized. Still, the majority of available papers on the topic is either very short or very theoretical, without any practical solutions (Rigby, 2019). Thus, there still remains a big potential for research of artificial intelligence ethics in medical care (Guan, 2019). Philosophical discussions about ethical aspects often focus only on the future development of the technology. However, ethical issues exist and need to be solved at the current moment. It has been debated whether artificial intelligence may become empathic (Montemayor et al., 2021); at any case, current artificial intelligence cannot solve the ethical issues automatically. Often, attention is paid to ethical algorithm design and biases within the algorithms, but the following list of ethical aspects of using artificial intelligence contains a much broader spectrum of topics related far beyond purely technical problems.

Data production quality. As only data with a sufficient quality can lead to reliable results, a high-level quality of medical data represents an ethical requirement (Firmani et al., 2019). Collecting the data in accordance with ethical principles requires to follow principles of fairness (defined as lack of bias), transparency (explainability of the data collection processes), and diversity (in order to avoid collecting too specific non-representative data). Health information quality may be evaluated by means of available criteria (metrics), e.g. for the context of reliability of publicly available data from the internet (or other unregulated sources) related to public health (Al-Jefri et al., 2018). In order to enhance data sharing and transfer, principles of data democratization have been widely discussed. Such principles require the data to be accessible for an average end user, i.e. the focus is on accessibility of health data as such, while the data should be available in an uncomplicated and easily portable format.

Data protection, safety, and privacy. Often, ethical issues are reduced to technical (software engineering) problems of health data privacy, anonymization, confidentiality, and sharing, as overviewed e.g. in the work by Ahmad et al. (2020). Physicians, nurses, other healthcare professionals, and also software systems or robots have to follow principles of data protection including ensuring privacy (or preventing from its loss), anonymization of personally identifiable data, and safety against unauthorized access to the data (Bertino et al., 2019). In each country, regulatory authorities are responsible for the policies related to regulatory affairs related to processing (protection and safety) of personal data within the given legal framework. In the European Union, technical ethical issues of data protection and privacy remain to be discussed after the General Data Protection Regulation (GDPR) became enforceable; Alaya (2020) warned that the tough privacy and security law requirements of the GDPR bring a threat of a downward spiral of risk obsession in European healthcare and lead the medical systems away from the aim of the best evidence-based care. Data protection requirements have led to the development of federated learning (collaborative learning), which allow to analyze health-related data without a need for sharing or transfer; the data remain better protected if locally analyzed by means of such machine learning techniques, which allow decentralized computations at the point of their collection.

Patient autonomy. The patients should have the possibility to give (or refuse to give) an informed consent allowing artificial intelligence to exploit their personal data (McKernan et al., 2018); such consents are more likely to be obtained in an atmosphere of a public trust in the healthcare system (as discussed above). It is natural to require that the personal data are not used for further analysis without consent of the patients, or that the clinical data are not sold to other parties.

Algorithms. The performance of artificial intelligence algorithms in healthcare may be subject to bias of diverse sources, including

- Sampling bias (also data bias, resulting in a non-representative sample so that the results cannot be generalized to the entire population);
- Selection bias (non-random sampling again resulting in a non-representative sample, but regarding mainly internal validity, i.e. the ability to obtain significant results);
- Bias due to rare cases or other extreme events (Safdar et al., 2020);
- Algorithmic bias, while the main ethical concerns discussed within the ethics of algorithms include inconclusive evidence, inscrutable evidence,

misguided evidence, unfair outcomes, transformative effects, and traceability (Tsamados et al., 2021);

- Implicit bias (unconscious bias of healthcare professionals).

The (perhaps severe) influence of two other sources of bias seems to be neglected in current discussion on ethics of algorithms:

- Bias due to violated assumptions;
- Bias of standard (non-robust) machine learning algorithms due to data contamination e.g. by outliers. To reduce the bias, robust machine learning tools should be applied (see e.g. Kalina et al., 2021).

Ethics of algorithms is also connected to the fact that any model used for artificial intelligence only approximates the reality.

Comprehensibility of algorithms. Interpretable algorithms are generally considered as preferable to black box techniques (Starke et al., 2020). Ethical discussions were devoted to possible interpretation (comprehensibility) of methods, understanding the (statistical) reasons why the software yields a particular recommendation related to medical care, or verifying if the methods are meaningful at all. Usually, however, a deep understanding why artificial intelligence recommends a particular decision cannot be achieved and remains to represent an ethical challenge. A current research trend denoted as explainable artificial intelligence attempts to propose methods for interpreting results obtained by machine learning algorithms.

Legal framework. Guan (2019) discussed possible legal ways for ensuring available artificial intelligence applications to be trustworthy and proposed administrative steps driven by governments, which would contribute to ethical governance by formulating governance concepts and principles; the administrative tasks also include formulating additional ethical guidelines beyond currently established guidelines of biomedical ethics.

Symbiosis of artificial intelligence and healthcare professionals. Because human decision making is known to be irrational, the authors hold the opinion that there remains an irreplaceable role of the tacit knowledge in a mutual communication (synergy, symbiosis, coupling) of artificial intelligence with the physician. The tacit knowledge is generally agreed to be defined as context-dependent practical knowledge of the physician within the given medical context. As artificial intelligence shapes human behavior, this will naturally affect also the relationship of physicians (or other healthcare professional) to the patient (Currie et al., 2020). Such relationship (partnership, cooperation) is also a subject of ethical debates (Nagao, 2019) and it has been proposed to construct networks connecting human and artificial intelligence inspired by biological swarms; in a particular example of Patel et al. (2019), a combination of artificial intelligence with human experts turned out to outperform each of the groups alone in diagnostics of chest radiographs.

Liability. The liability (legal responsibility) of the physician for the decisions related to medical care should be retained even if artificial intelligence participates in the decision making, as discussed by Ho (2019). Also for this reason, the physician should not over-rely on artificial intelligence.

Financial costs. Economic aspects of medical care will become more important, as the expenditures on medical care are increasing worldwide and also as the average life expectancy increases. Recommending an additional examination of a given patient, which is not expected to bring new information related to the care for the given patient, should not be regarded as ethical. In addition, artificial intelligence has already been applied to revealing unethical transactions; particularly, it turns out to be able to detect fraudulent claims, representing nowadays a costly problem for healthcare insurance companies (Dhieb et al., 2020).

Triage and population screenings represent an important ethical issue, because their algorithms are not free of human induced biases. In emergency situations, e.g. in the pandemic era, artificial intelligence may be used for resolving ethical dilemmas related to triage (prioritization of patients); Soltan et al. (2021) used an artificial intelligence procedure to order (rank) patients according to their priority of being hospitalized. As another example, software tools may be applied for the decision making task related to selecting a set of individuals who would get the vaccination.

Ethical issues related to triage in clinical scenarios were described by Herreros et al. (2020), who described the dilemmas of triage decision during the COVID-19 pandemic in Spain. In the conditions of scarce resources, physicians had to evaluate ten-year life expectancy of COVID-19 patients based on age and comorbidities, severity of their illness, expected duration of treatment, and recovery potential without a sufficient prior experience with the disease as such. Especially at the onset of the pandemic, criteria for triage decisions were not unified and recommendations were discussed overrating the importance of age or social value of patients (e.g. prioritizing healthcare professionals), which were later agreed as unsuitable criteria.

Genetic testing. With a better understanding of the genetic information, which was accelerated thanks to the analysis of the genome by artificial intelligence tools, predictive genetics (including prenatal diagnostics) becomes more complex and raises thus more ethical concerns, requiring adequate counseling of the clients and respecting their confidence. At the same time, the progress in epigenetics confirms that the genetic information encrypted in the DNA must not be necessarily manifested in a particular individual. Only the physician (but not the software) is able to fully capture that the gene may be manifested only with a certain probability. Still, the public inclines to perceiving genetics as predictive (fated, deterministic) instead of probabilistic with its conclusions formulated with some uncertainty.

Patient autonomy. An involvement of artificial intelligence in the decision making tasks may suppress the patient autonomy, i.e. participation of patients on decisions related to their medical care. On the other hand, ongoing discussions about modern medical care put an increasing emphasis on patient autonomy (Kilbride & Joffe, 2018) and are critical to replacing the patient-physician relationship by a nonhuman therapy.

Patient Safety

All artificial intelligence solutions have to be integrated within the medical practice following general principles of patient safety, so that patient safety is related to ethical aspects of using artificial intelligence in modern medical care (Currie et al., 2020). Information-based medicine should seriously focus on reducing medical malpractice (improper treatment resulting in injury or loss) and maleficence (intentional harmfulness or mischief). The focus of patient safety may be characterized as maximizing harm prevention, or in other words introducing freedom for the patient from unnecessary (real or potential) harm associated with healthcare. It is possible to distinguish between two types of errors in healthcare:

(1) Errors caused by the limitations of the current technologies or level of medical knowledge;
(2) Adverse effects of healthcare, i.e. preventable errors caused by human factors or system failures.

Patient safety as a self-standing healthcare discipline considers only the errors of the second type. An ineffective therapy of a (correctly or incorrectly diagnosed) rare disease, which has not been well investigated by biomedical researchers, is not well does not represent an issue for the area of patient safety. If however a physician fails to perform an important clinical examination of a particular patient and this leads to a wrong diagnosis and harmful therapy of a common disease, we speak about the error of the second type, which may subsequently lead to a superfluous time in the hospital or even a preventable death of the patient.

Because patient safety will never be automatically guaranteed by medical procedures corresponding to the most recent scientific knowledge, information-based medicine will have to study adverse effect of healthcare and propose ways for eliminating them. Wachter & Gupta (2018) drew the attention of experts on the alarming situation worldwide pointing at incidents, injuries and deaths as consequences of errors in medical care. It has been recently estimated that about 15% of the total hospital activity and expenditures in the OECD countries represents a direct consequence of adverse events (Slawomirski et al., 2017). This is true in spite of numerous recent efforts in place in the most developed countries, which have consequently led to an improvement in the area of patient safety. Such adverse effects remain to be intense in spite of the penetration of modern technologies (including artificial intelligence tools) to medical care. Our understanding of quality of care in information-based medicine involves the integration of a correct and effectively determined diagnosis and safety.

INFORMATION-BASED MENTAL HEALTHCARE AND ITS SPECIFIC ETHICAL ISSUES

While the specific field of psychiatry (or mental health as a more general concept) was remaining at the boundaries of interest of the society always throughout the history, the current paradigm of evidence-based medicine in the specialty field of psychiatry has been called by various synonyms in the literature, including evidence-based medicine in psychiatry, evidence-based clinical practice in psychiatry, evidence-based mental health, or evidence-based practices for mental health. This section discusses mental healthcare from the point of view of ethical aspects related to the transform of mental healthcare through emerging technologies.

Transforms of mental healthcare can be anticipated in the near future, which will be enabled by a vast number of technological tools recently introduced for mental healthcare. The fast improvement of technology and rise of big data of various types and formats from unthinkable sources have a potential to contribute to clinical usage. For all these reasons, the paradigm of evidence-based mental healthcare should be replaced by deeper ideas going more beyond and the information-based medicine can be expected to develop also in the area of mental healthcare. Thus, it is possible to introduce the concept of information-based mental healthcare. In addition, decision support systems may contribute to shared (collaborative) decision making in routine mental healthcare. A particular evidence of the drift of mental healthcare towards participative principles is the current transition of mental health services towards community-based services, applying patient-centered (client-centered) approaches in healthcare; such transforms have been taking place across many developed countries.

Information-based mental healthcare will especially benefit from new knowledge obtained in psychiatric genetics. Current research in this field, which is primarily devoted to whole-genome associations and whole-genome sequencing, reveals a very complex genetic architecture of the most of mental health disorders. Integration of molecular medicine and the already known polygenic risk scores with clinical psychiatry will be a demanding task due to a large gap between the two fields; indeed, a transform of psychiatry will be feasible only by means of a paradigm shift leaving aside the genetic determinism (pre-programming) of mental health and accepting the intricacies of mental health disorders (Demkow & Wolanczyk, 2017).

As the number of mental health disorders keeps increasing worldwide, the field of mental healthcare may strongly benefit from an advent of useful artificial intelligence tools. Starke et al. (2020) stressed that the wide range of ethical aspects of artificial intelligence in mental healthcare requires to understand the decision making processes in the particular field. Such ethical aspects were characterized as interdisciplinary topics requiring a discussion of experts on mental healthcare with experts on artificial intelligence (informaticians). The ethical issues formulated already above for a general context are valid also for the context of mental healthcare; in fact, some of the references cited above for the general context are related to mental healthcare. Let us thus pay attention to only additional specific ethical topics related to mental healthcare.

Data protection and privacy. Among all the ethical aspects in this list related to artificial intelligence, data protection and privacy issues have received the largest attention in the mental healthcare literature. The issues of guarding privacy rights, ensuring informed consent, transparency of machine learning models, should be carefully considered by regulatory agencies, physicians, patients, as well as ethicists and legal experts. Close collaboration of experts with different backgrounds was recommended e.g. by Mostert et al. (2018), which should finally agree on safeguards and improved communication about privacy protections (Rosenfeld et al., 2017). So far, the discussions continue with an ongoing need to establish consensus-based regulatory requirements and guidelines for ethics related to e-health (and particularly mobile health aka mHealth) in mental healthcare.

Algorithms. Discussion of psychiatrists about the need for interpretability of artificial intelligence algorithms came to the conclusion (see Jacobson et al., 2020) that the impossibility to explain rigorously why the algorithms yield particular results represents an important ethical issue. As big data become more available in mental health research, the decision making becomes more complex and more depending on combining massive data from various sources in various formats. Another issue is related to systematic biases of artificial intelligence tools used in mental healthcare. Algorithms designed by humans are naturally biased and biases are simply transferred, so that algorithms based on big data related to mental health may be biased just like a real psychiatrist (Fiske et al., 2019). Software itself cannot minimize human-induced biases (Walsh et al., 2020). Important examples of a systematic bias in mental healthcare decision making include sexual or racial biases; as pointed out by Starke et al. (2020), there are disproportions in the numbers of diagnoses of some mental health disorders in the United States for ethnic minorities.

Legal framework. Specific committees for (occasional or regular) auditing artificial intelligence tools for mental healthcare applications were recommended by

Mouchabac et al. (2021), who demanded that these committees should investigate new software tools in terms of their security and failures within the legal framework of psychiatric advance directives.

Suicide risk prevention. Artificial intelligence has been successfully applied to suicide prevention. Suicide risk can be predicted for patients with sleep loss, sleep disturbances, or longlife eating disorders; artificial intelligence has a potential to be active in monitoring the risk factors, prediction, and intervention. Available ethical recommendations (McKernan et al., 2018) focused on balancing between beneficence and respecting personal autonomy; false negative patients harm themselves without being identified by the software, while false positives are treated unnecessarily.

Liability. The topic of suicide risk prevention is connected to liability, which always depends on the context of legal system of a given country (Pinals, 2019). In Israel, a court sentenced a radiologist guilty for sending a radiology report directly to a psychiatric patient. The report clearly indicated lung carcinoma of this patient and the radiologist was aware that the patient was undergoing treatment against depression. The trial came to the conclusion that the physician is responsible for communicating the results of medical examinations to patients; still, the guidelines overviewed by Berlin et al. (2017) state that the patient should not obtain relevant health information if this should endanger the life or physical safety of the individual. We are not aware of any discussions about who would be liable for an analogous situation if the suicide (or suicide attempt) occurs as a direct subsequence of communication of the patient with artificial intelligence. Liability is related to patient safety issues; it must be always decided carefully whether a given patient should obtain the available medication or not, regarding possible (and serious) adversarial effects of current psychiatric medicines and patient safety considerations should be always fully integrated to mental healthcare instead of being solved separately outside of the medical care context (D'Lima et al., 2017).

Financial costs. As some brain examinations (e.g. brain imaging by fMRI) are financially very demanding, economic aspects come into play in recommending such examinations as well. To give an example, brain measurements by the fMRI technology is not always appropriate (not justified) for certain combinations of symptoms. Davis et al. (2017) formulated diagnostic tests of chronic pain based on fMRI and presented them as consensus statements, i.e. after a debate of ethical issues, subsequently led to establishing internationally recognized guidelines for pain testing based on brain imaging; naturally, the practical implementation of newly recommended guidelines has to depend on the financial possibilities of healthcare systems of individual countries.

Population screenings and genetic testing. Song et al. (2019) presented an overview of available artificial intelligence tools tailor-made for the screening of autism spectrum disorder; however, because of a lack of definite biomarkers, their paper concluded that the diagnosis must depend on behavioral observations and fully automatic diagnostics would thus not be ethical under the current state of knowledge. Epigenetics research, which brings a hope for detecting suitable epigenetic biomarkers for mental health disorders, brings a number of other ethical issues. Particularly, it is questionable whether to automatically label children with a positive test on the autism spectrum disorder (or attention deficit hyperactivity disorder, ADHD) as autists, or whether to expect people with a genetic predisposition to the major depressive disorder (based on genetic testing) to really suffer from depressions (Stein & Smoller, 2018); it is namely well known to psychiatrists that the fear from the disease or a false positive result of a diagnostic test may contribute to the development of the disease itself. Other ethical discussions were devoted to selective pregnancy interruptions recommended (and/or controlled) by artificial intelligence tools such as decision support systems (Li et al., 2021).

Dehumanization of mental healthcare. To start with an example, various wearable sensors are currently available which should help individuals to quit smoking; however, such dehumanized devices turned out not to be really effective in practice. On the other hand, McGreevey et al. (2020) described a good experience with conversational agents (robots, chatbots) in population health management (care for elderly mentally ill). Formally, dehumanization is defined as a failure to recognize the cognitive and emotional complexities of people around us (Simon & Gutsell, 2021). So far, autonomous embodied conversational agents, commonly known as chatbots, have not succeeded in creating sufficient believability in studies with mentally ill clients (Scholten et al., 2017). Because we cannot expect artificial intelligence to reach the human level of empathy, the role of psychotherapists will remain irreplaceable also because numerous mental health disorders (including addictions) are not purely biological problems. The clients may perceive dehumanized trends in mental healthcare well only if their own needs are fulfilled and if positively received jointly by the body, mind and spirit, if promoting the dignity of the patients, and if contributing to their psycho-socio-spiritual comfort.

To describe a particular case study, Heim et al. (2018) described a study of insomnia therapy exploiting avatar-based internet interventions. The patients monitored over time were repeatedly demanded to evaluate (using a 0-100 point response scale) how much they missed contact with a human therapist. This response was found to be increasing with time; such trend turned out to be statistically significant ($p<0.01$) and missing a real therapist was found as a major factor influencing the success of the therapy.

CONCLUSION

Recent transforms of medical care started already before the outbreak of the COVID-19 pandemic due to a fast digitalization, increasing availability of medical Big Data, and development of artificial intelligence tools. These tools, such as clinical decision support systems, contribute to accelerating the ongoing transforms of medical care. Instead of current practices formulated for a fictitious average patient, information-based approaches in medicine, which represent the practical fulfillment of the rather abstract concept of the knowledge society, will have the potential to be personalized and targeted to meet the needs of a real individual based on given individual medical information. Tools of artificial intelligence will enable to personalize clinical decisions related to the care for individual patients. This remains however a vision for the future; current everyday medical care practices in the developed countries still remain distant from the ideals of information-based medicine.

The transforms of the everyday medical care towards the presented vision of information-based medicine will require a democratization of medicine by increasing the participation of patients on the clinical decision making processes. The public will experience that the personalized medical care has the purpose to serve each individual patient respecting the dignity of each individual. These phenomena will renew and strengthen the public trust to the healthcare system (Burr et al., 2020). Physicians will exploit an increasing number of sophisticated artificial intelligence tools based on newly acquired biomedical knowledge. They will have to improve their statistical literacy in order to be able to better interpret (among others) the results of clinical decision support systems. At the same time, physicians are hoped to overcome the purely biological point of view and will approach the patients with empathy, respecting them as human beings. The importance of a healthy life style in accordance with epigenetic recommendations will have to be stressed; environmental factors will be acknowledged to prevent the inherited dispositions from being manifested.

As using artificial intelligence will be facing serious ethical dilemmas, the focus of information-based medicine on ethical values will hopefully not repeat the mistakes of Francis Galton (1822-1911), the father of eugenics, who conducted his anthropological research with the motivation to improve the human race by getting rid of individuals with "bad" ("undesirable") genes; his life documents that scientifically justified ideas may be vain, if not in accordance with ethical and moral values. Thus, we come to the conclusion that all recent debates on ethics or recently introduced courses on healthcare ethics would remain only toothless tools, if not accompanied by more ore less radical subsequent actions: introducing public policies reflecting the rise and expansion of artificial intelligence in healthcare. Apart from the unique overview of a number of ethical issues of artificial intelligence in healthcare presented here, the contribution of this chapter includes discovering issues much neglected in discussions about using artificial intelligence in healthcare: assumptions of machine learning methods and the need for their diagnostics, and sensitivity of machine learning to the presence of data contamination (i.e. the need to replace current machine learning tools by their robust counterparts).

Ethical considerations cannot be successfully solved as an appendix (additional extra component) of medical care relying on artificial intelligence, but healthcare performed according to ethical standards will have to be deeply pervaded by thinking about ethical values. Moral decision making has to be integrated in medical care as its integral part and considering ethical issues, which are more complex than the usually discussed topics of data protection and privacy, should find an established place at forefront of exploiting artificial intelligence in healthcare.

ACKNOWLEDGMENT

The work was supported by the grant GA19-05704S of the Czech Science Foundation and by the Ministry of Health of the Czech Republic, grant NU21-08-00432. The authors would like to thank the anonymous referees for constructive advice.

REFERENCES

Ahmad, O. F., Stoyanov, D., & Lovat, L. B. (2020). Barriers and pitfalls for artificial intelligence in gastroenterology: Ethical and regulatory issues. *Techniques and Innovations in Gastrointestinal Endoscopy*, *22*(2), 80–84. doi:10.1016/j.tgie.2019.150636

Al-Jefri, M., Evans, R., Uchyigit, G., & Ghezzi, P. (2018). What is health information quality? Ethical dimension and perception by users. *Frontiers in Medicine*, *5*, 260. doi:10.3389/fmed.2018.00260 PMID:30294599

Alaya, F. (2020). Healthcare difficulties in the post-GDPR era. *Trinity Student Medical Journal*, *20*, 8–12.

Alimadadi, A., Aryal, S., Manandhar, I., Munroe, P. B., Joe, B., & Cheng, X. (2020). Artificial intelligence and machine learning to fight COVID-19. *Physiological Genomics*, *52*(4), 200–202. doi:10.1152/physiolgenomics.00029.2020 PMID:32216577

Berlin, L., Sosna, J., & Halevy, D. (2017). Radiologist found liable for malpractice in Israel for causing a patient's suicide by sending a "bad news" report: Can this happen in the United States? *AJR. American Journal of Roentgenology*, *208*(2), 241–244. doi:10.2214/AJR.16.16804 PMID:27809563

Bertino, E., Kundu, A., & Sura, Z. (2019). Data transparency with blockchain and AI ethics. *ACM Journal of Data and Information Quality*, *11*(4), 16. doi:10.1145/3312750

Borangíu, T., & Purcarea, V. (2008). The future of healthcare-Information based medicine. *Journal of Medicine and Life*, *1*, 233–237. PMID:20108471

Bučková, B., Brunovský, M., Bareš, M., & Hlinka, J. (2020). Predicting sex from EEG: Validity and generalizability of deep-learning-based interpretable classifier. *Frontiers in Neuroscience*, *14*, 589303. doi:10.3389/fnins.2020.589303 PMID:33192274

Burr, C., Morley, J., Taddeo, M., & Floridi, L. (2020). Digital psychiatry: Risks and opportunities for public health and wellbeing. *IEEE Transactions on Technology and Society*, *1*(1), 21–33. doi:10.1109/TTS.2020.2977059

Ćosić, K., Povović, S., Šarlija, M., & Kesedžić, I. (2020). Impact of human disasters and COVID-19 pandemic on mental health: Potential of digital psychiatry. *Psychiatria Danubina*, *32*(1), 25–31. doi:10.24869/psyd.2020.25 PMID:32303026

Currie, G., Hawk, K. E., & Rohren, E. M. (2020). Ethical principles for the application of artificial intelligence (AI) in nuclear medicine. *European Journal of Nuclear Medicine and Molecular Imaging*, *47*(4), 748–752. doi:10.100700259-020-04678-1 PMID:31927637

D'Lima, D., Crawford, M. J., Darzi, A., & Archer, S. (2017). Patient safety and quality of care in mental health: A world of its own? *BJPsych Bulletin*, *41*(5), 241–243. doi:10.1192/pb.bp.116.055327 PMID:29018546

Davis, K. D., Flor, H., Greely, H. T., Iannetti, G. D., Mackey, S., Ploner, M., Pustilnik, A., Tracey, I., Treede, R. D., & Wager, T. D. (2017). Brain imaging tests for chronic pain: Medical, legal and ethical issues and recommendations. *Nature Reviews. Neurology*, *13*(10), 624–638. doi:10.1038/nrneurol.2017.122 PMID:28884750

Demkow, U., & Wolanczyk, T. (2017). Genetic tests in major psychiatric disorders—Integrating molecular medicine with clinical psychiatry—why is it so difficult? *Translational Psychiatry*, *7*(6), e1151. doi:10.1038/tp.2017.106 PMID:28608853

Dhieb, N., Ghazzai, H., Besbes, H., & Massoud, Y. (2020). A secure AI-driven architecture for automated insurance systems: Fraud detection and risk measurement. *IEEE Access: Practical Innovations, Open Solutions*, *8*, 58546–58558. doi:10.1109/ACCESS.2020.2983300

Firmani, D., Tanca, L., & Torlone, R. (2019). Ethical dimensions for data quality. *ACM Journal of Data and Information Quality*, *12*, 2.

Fiske, A., Henningsen, P., & Buyx, A. (2019). Your robot therapist will see you now: Ethical implications of embodied artificial intelligence in psychiatry, psychology, and psychotherapy. *Journal of Medical Internet Research*, *21*(5), e13216. doi:10.2196/13216 PMID:31094356

Gopichandran, V., Subramaniam, S., & Kalsingh, M. J. (2020). COVID-19 pandemic: A litmus test of trust in the health system. *Asian Bioethics Review*, *12*(2), 213–221. doi:10.100741649-020-00122-6 PMID:32837551

Guan, J. (2019). Artificial intelligence in healthcare and medicine: Promises, ethical challenges and governance. *Chinese Medical Sciences Journal*, *34*, 76–83. PMID:31315747

Heim, E., Rötger, A., Lorenz, N., & Maercker, A. (2018). Working alliance with an avatar: How far can we go with internet interventions? *Internet Interventions: the Application of Information Technology in Mental and Behavioural Health*, *11*, 41–46. doi:10.1016/j.invent.2018.01.005 PMID:30135758

Herreros, B., Gella, P., & de Asua, D. R. (2020). Triage during the COVID-19 epidemic in Spain: Better and worse ethical arguments. *Journal of Medical Ethics*, *46*(7), 455–458. doi:10.1136/medethics-2020-106352 PMID:32424063

Hlinka, J., Paluš, M., Vejmelka, M., Mantini, D., & Corbetta, M. (2011). Functional connectivity in resting-state fMRI: Is linear correlation sufficient? *NeuroImage*, *54*(3), 2218–2225. doi:10.1016/j.neuroimage.2010.08.042 PMID:20800096

Ho, A. (2019). Deep ethical learning: Taking the interplay of human and artificial intelligence seriously. *The Hastings Center Report*, *49*(1), 36–39. doi:10.1002/hast.977 PMID:30790317

Hynek, M., Kalina, J., Zvárová, J., & Long, J. D. (2018). Statistical methods for constructing gestational age-related charts for fetal size and pregnancy dating using longitudinal data. *Biocybernetics and Biomedical Engineering*, *38*(4), 992–1003. doi:10.1016/j.bbe.2018.09.001

Hynek, M., Zvárová, J., Smetanová, D., Stejskal, D., & Kalina, J. (2021). Real-time quality control of nuchal translucency measurements using the exponentially weighted moving average chart. *Taiwanese Journal of Obstetrics & Gynecology*, *60*(1), 84–89. doi:10.1016/j.tjog.2020.11.012 PMID:33495014

Jacobson, N. J., Bentley, K. H., Walton, A., Wang, S. B., Fortgang, R. G., Millner, A. J., Coombs, G. III, Rodman, A. M., & Coppersmith, D. D. L. (2020). Ethical dilemmas posed by mobile health and machine learning in psychiatry research. *Bulletin of the World Health Organization*, *98*(4), 270–276. doi:10.2471/BLT.19.237107 PMID:32284651

James, S., Rao, S. V., & Granger, C. B. (2015). Registry-based randomized clinical trials–A new clinical trial paradigm. *Nature Reviews. Cardiology*, *12*(5), 312–316. doi:10.1038/nrcardio.2015.33 PMID:25781411

Jiang, F., Jiang, Y., Zhi, H., Dong, Y., Li, H., Ma, S., Wang, Y., Dong, Q., Shen, H., & Wang, Y. (2017). Artificial intelligence in healthcare: Past, present and future. *Stroke and Vascular Neurology*, *2*(4), e000101. doi:10.1136vn-2017-000101 PMID:29507784

Kalina, J. (2012). Highly robust statistical methods in medical image analysis. *Biocybernetics and Biomedical Engineering*, *32*(2), 3–16. doi:10.1016/S0208-5216(12)70033-5

Kalina, J. (2015). Statistical challenges of Big Data analysis in medicine. *International Journal on Biomedicine and Healthcare*, *3*, 24–27.

Kalina, J. (2021). Mental health clinical decision support exploiting Big Data. In *Research Anthology on Mental Health Stigma, Education, and Treatment* (pp. 341–359). IGI Global. doi:10.4018/978-1-7998-8544-3.ch020

Kalina, J., & Hlinka, J. (2017). Implicitly weighted robust classification applied to brain activity research. In A. Fred & H. Gamboa (Eds.), *Biomedical Engineering Systems and Technologies. Communications in Computer and Information Science, 690, 87-107*. doi:10.1007/978-3-319-54717-6_6

Kalina, J., & Matonoha, C. (2020). A sparse pair-preserving centroid-based supervised learning method for high-dimensional biomedical data or images. *Biocybernetics and Biomedical Engineering*, *40*(2), 774–786. doi:10.1016/j.bbe.2020.03.008

Kalina, J., Neoral, A., & Vidnerová, P. (2021). Effective automatic method selection for nonlinear regression modeling. *International Journal of Neural Systems*. doi:10.1142/S0129065721500209

Kalina, J., & Schlenker, A. (2018). Dimensionality reduction methods for biomedical data. *Clinician and Technology*, *48*, 29–35.

Keim-Malpass, J., & Moorman, L. P. (2021). Nursing and precision predictive analytics monitoring in the acute and intensive care setting: An emerging role for responding to COVID-19 and beyond. *International Journal of Nursing Studies*, *3*, 100019. doi:10.1016/j.ijnsa.2021.100019 PMID:33426534

Kilbride, M. K., & Joffe, S. (2018). The new age of patient autonomy. Implications for the patient-physician relationship. *Journal of the American Medical Association*, *320*(19), 1973–1974. doi:10.1001/jama.2018.14382 PMID:30326026

Li, L., Li, Y., Wang, Y., & Yan, L. (2021). Intelligent medical diagnosis and misoprostol medical abortion nursing based on embedded system. *Microprocessors and Microsystems*, *81*, 103770. doi:10.1016/j.micpro.2020.103770

Lin, L. & Hou, Z. (2020). Combat COVID-19 with artificial intelligence and big data. *Journal of Travel Medicine*. doi:10.1093/jtm/taaa080

Masic, I., & Mihalas, G. (Eds.). (2014). *History of medical informatics*. Avicena.

McGreevey, J. D. III, Hanson, W. III, & Koppel, R. (2020). Clinical, legal, and ethical aspects of artificial intelligence-assisted conversational agents in health care. *Journal of the American Medical Association*, *324*(6), 552–553. doi:10.1001/jama.2020.2724 PMID:32706386

McKernan, L. C., Clayton, E. W., & Walsh, C. G. (2018). Protecting life while preserving liberty: Ethical recommendations for suicide prevention with artificial intelligence. *Frontiers in Psychiatry*, *9*, 650. doi:10.3389/fpsyt.2018.00650 PMID:30559686

Mian, A., & Khan, S. (2020). Coronavirus: The spread of misinformation. *BMC Medicine*, *18*(1), 89. doi:10.118612916-020-01556-3 PMID:32188445

Montemayor, C., Halpern, J., & Fairweather, A. (2021). In principle obstacles for empathic AI: Why we can't replace human empathy in healthcare. *AI & Society*. . doi:10.1007/s00146-021-01230-z

Moreau, N. (2020). The paradox of overspecialization: Can't see the forest for the trees. *Journal of Oral Medical Surgery*, *26*(1), E1. doi:10.1051/mbcb/2020005

Mostert, M., Koomen, B. M., van Delden, J. J. M., & Bredenoord, A. L. (2018). Privacy in Big Data psychiatric and behavioural research: A multiple-case study. *International Journal of Law and Psychiatry*, *60*, 40–44. doi:10.1016/j.ijlp.2018.07.002 PMID:30217329

Mouchabac, S., Adrien, V., Falala-Séchet, C., Bonnot, O., Maatoug, R., Millet, B., Peretti, C.-S., Bourla, A., & Ferreri, F. (2021). Psychiatric advance directives and artificial intelligence: A conceptual framework for theoretical and ethical principles. *Frontiers in Psychiatry*, *11*, 622506. doi:10.3389/fpsyt.2020.622506 PMID:33551883

Nagao, K. (2019). *Artificial intelligence accelerates human learning. Discussion data analytics*. Springer. doi:10.1007/978-981-13-6175-3

Patel, B. N., Rosenberg, L., Willcox, G., Baltaxe, D., Lyons, M., Irvin, J., Rajpurkar, P., Amrhein, T., Gupta, R., Halabi, S., Langlotz, C., Lo, E., Mammarappallil, J., Mariano, A. J., Riley, G., Seekins, J., Shen, L., Zucker, E., & Lungren, M. P. (2019). Human-machine partnership with artificial intelligence for chest radiograph diagnosis. *NPJ Digital Medicine*, *2*(1), 111. doi:10.103841746-019-0189-7 PMID:31754637

Piano, S. L. (2020). Ethical principles in machine learning and artificial intelligence: Cases from the field and possible ways forward. *Humanities and Social Sciences Communications*, *7*(1), 9. doi:10.105741599-020-0501-9

Pinals, D. A. (2019). Liability and patient suicide. *Focus (San Francisco, Calif.)*, *17*, 349–354. PMID:32047380

Rigby, M. J. (2019). Ethical dimensions of using artificial intelligence in health care. *AMA Journal of Ethics*, *21*(2), E121–E124. doi:10.1001/amajethics.2019.121

Rosenfeld, L., Torous, J., & Vahia, I. V. (2017). Data security and privacy in apps for dementia: An analysis of existing privacy policies. *The American Journal of Geriatric Psychiatry*, *25*(8), 873–877. doi:10.1016/j.jagp.2017.04.009 PMID:28645535

Safdar, N. M., Banja, J. D., & Meltzer, C. C. (2020). Ethical considerations in artificial intelligence. *European Journal of Radiology*, *122*, 108768. doi:10.1016/j.ejrad.2019.108768 PMID:31786504

Scholten, M. R., Kelders, S. M., & Van Gemert-Pijnen, J. E. W. C. (2017). Self-guided web-based interventions: Scoping review on user needs and the potential of embodied conversational agents to address them. *Journal of Medical Internet Research*, *19*(11), e383. doi:10.2196/jmir.7351 PMID:29146567

Senders, J. T., Harary, M., Stopa, B. M., Staples, P., Broekman, M. L. D., Smith, T. R., Gormley, W. B., & Arnaout, O. (2018). Information-based medicine in glioma patients: A clinical perspective. *Computational and Mathematical Methods in Medicine*, *2018*, 8572058. doi:10.1155/2018/8572058 PMID:30008798

Sigurdsson, E. L., Blondal, A. B., Jonsson, J. S., Tomasdottir, M. O., Hrafnkelsson, H., Linnet, K., & Sigurdsson, J. A. (2020). How prirmary healthcare in Iceland swiftly changed its strategy in response to the COVID-19 pandemic. *BMJ Open*, *10*(12), e043151. doi:10.1136/bmjopen-2020-043151 PMID:33293329

Simon, J. C., & Gutsell, J. N. (2021). Recognizing humanity: Dehumanization predicts neural mirroring and empathic accuracy in face-to-face interactions. *Social Cognitive and Affective Neuroscience*, *2021*(5), 463–473. doi:10.1093can/nsab014 PMID:33515023

Slawomirski, L., Auraaen, A., & Klazinga, N. (2017). *The economics of patient safety: Strengthening a value-based approach to reducing patient harm at national level*. OECD Health Working Papers, No. 96, OECD Publishing.

Soltan, A. A. S., Kouchaki, S., Zhu, T., Kiyasseh, D., Taylor, T., Hussain, Z. B., Peto, T., Brent, A. J., Eyre, D. W., & Clifton, D. A. (2021). Rapid triage for COVID-19 using routine clinical data for patients attending hospital: Development and prospective validation of an artificial intelligence screening test. *The Lancet. Digital Health*, *3*(2), 78–87. doi:10.1016/S2589-7500(20)30274-0 PMID:33509388

Song, D. Y., Kim, S. Y., Bong, G., Kim, J. M., & Yoo, H. J. (2019). The use of artificial intelligence in screening and diagnosis of autism spectrum disorder: A literature review. *Journal of the Korean Academy of Child and Adolescent Psychiatry*, *30*(4), 145–152. doi:10.5765/jkacap.190027 PMID:32595335

Starke, G., De Clercq, E., Borgwardt, S., & Elger, B. S. (2020). Computing schizophrenia: Ethical challenges for machine learning in psychiatry. *Psychological Medicine*, *1*(3), 1–7. PMID:32536358

Stein, M. B., & Smoller, J. W. (2018). Precision Psychiatry: Will genomic medicine lead the way? *JAMA Psychiatry*, *75*(7), 663–664. doi:10.1001/jamapsychiatry.2018.0375 PMID:29800947

Straus, S., Glasziou, P., Richardson, W. S., & Haynes, R. B. (2018). *Evidence-based medicine: How to practice and teach EBM* (5th ed.). Elsevier.

Tripathi, S. (2021). Artificial intelligence: A brief review. In T. H. Musiolik & A. D. Cheok (Eds.), *Analyzing future applications of AI, sensors, and robotics in society* (pp. 1–16). IGI Global. doi:10.4018/978-1-7998-3499-1.ch001

TsamadosA.AggarwalN.CowlsJ.MorleyJ.RobertsH.TaddeoM.FloridiL. (2021). The ethics of algorithms: Key problems and solutions. AI & Society. Online first. doi:10.2139/ssrn.3662302

Wachter, R. M., & Gupta, K. (2018). *Understanding patient safety* (3rd ed.). McGraw-Hill Education.

Walsh, C. G., Chaudhry, B., Dua, P., Goodman, K. W., Kaplan, B., Kavuluru, R., Solomonides, A., & Subbian, V. (2020). Stigma, biomarkers, and algorithmic bias: Recommendations for precision behavioral health with artificial intelligence. *JAMIA Open*, *3*(1), 9–15. doi:10.1093/jamiaopen/ooz054 PMID:32607482

Zvárová, J., & Zvára, K. (2011). e3Health: Three main features of modern healthcare. In E-health systems quality and reliability: Models and standards. IGI Global.

KEY TERMS AND DEFINITIONS

Artificial Intelligence: Software devices with diverse abilities, able to analyze (possibly big) data and to perform advanced clinical decision making by solving complex machine learning tasks.

Big Data: Datasets of diverse types and formats with various non-standard properties, such as large volume, enormous complexity, or heterogeneous quality.

Clinical Decision Support System: A complex software system allowing to assist physicians in decision making tasks related to diagnosis, therapy, or prognosis for a particular patient.

Evidence-Based Medicine: A thorough, unique, and critical use of the most relevant proofs (in the form of statistical evidence) in the process of decision making about the diagnosis, therapy, and prognosis for individual patients.

Information-Based Medicine: A vision describing personalized medical care of the future, exploiting advanced tools of artificial intelligence and specific medical knowledge obtained for an individual patient.

Liability: Legal responsibility for any harm or losses due to medical malpractice (improper treatment) or maleficence (intentional harmfulness or mischief).

Patient Safety: A self-standing healthcare discipline related to the study and minimization of adverse effects of healthcare.

Screening: Testing over the whole population or subpopulation, aiming at early detection of individuals under risk of a given disease.

Tacit Knowledge: In clinical decision making, it may be characterized as any context-dependent practical knowledge (domain knowledge, expert knowledge) available within the context of the given clinical task.

Chapter 4
Fairness and Ethics in Artificial Intelligence-Based Medical Imaging

Satvik Tripathi
https://orcid.org/0000-0001-6214-1464
College of Computing & Informatics, Drexel University, USA

Thomas Heinrich Musiolik
https://orcid.org/0000-0001-7749-4721
Berlin University of the Arts, Germany

ABSTRACT

Artificial intelligence has a huge array of current and potential applications in healthcare and medicine. Ethical issues arising due to algorithmic biases are one of the greatest challenges faced in the generalizability of AI models today. The authors address safety and regulatory barriers that impede data sharing in medicine as well as potential changes to existing techniques and frameworks that might allow ethical data sharing for machine learning. With these developments in view, they also present different algorithmic models that are being used to develop machine learning-based medical systems that will potentially evolve to be free of the sample, annotator, and temporal bias. These AI-based medical imaging models will then be completely implemented in healthcare facilities and institutions all around the world, even in the remotest areas, making diagnosis and patient care both cheaper and freely accessible.

DOI: 10.4018/978-1-7998-7888-9.ch004

INTRODUCTION

The word "algorithm," derived from the name of Al-Khwārizmī (Persian: خوارزمی, c. 780–850) who was a Persian mathematician. It is a step process for solving various mathematical and logical problems. In machine learning, an algorithm is a set of instructions designed to perform a specific task which may be a simple process for example multiplying two numbers, or a complex operation like playing a compressed video file. Under computer, programming algorithms are often generated as functions. A good example of an algorithm is a recipe that indicates what is to be done, step by step. In particular, deep learning algorithms promise to transform the basis for decision-making and workflow, as these types of algorithms will "learn" to perform a task by example and interpret new data. Therefore, by incorporating AI in radiology workflows, it could be possible to help health delivery organizations achieve important organizational and clinical outcomes, such as helping to increase the effectiveness of clinical workflows using imaging, helping to minimize the likelihood of "negative" clinical effects associated with delays in reading, interpreting and reporting by radiologists or empowering care teams to easily view radiology work product, accelerate clinical decision making, and streamline workflows which in turn result in a better patient experience and consequences. The intelligent workflow and clinical assistant capabilities in the sense of the radiologist himself will enable radiologists to be more efficient by automating and prioritizing tasks and data feeds, more quantitative by providing applications and resources to extract and measure information semi-automatically or automatically, and more accurate by ensuring the correct information to support the diagnosis, as well as confirming the reproducibility of any quantification procedures.

Artificial intelligence (AI) is used in medical imaging including image processing and interpretation (Lakhani et al., 2018). AI term is used when a device imitates learning and problem-solving functions (Russell & Bohannon, 2015) and presently is one of the most likely fields of the health revolution. More specifically AI refers to a computer science field committed to the development of systems that perform tasks that frequently involve human intelligence for branching off into various techniques (Chartrand et al., 2017). Machine learning (ML) is a concept introduced in 1959 by Arthur Samuel to define a subfield of AI (Samuel, 1959) that includes all those methods that enable computers to learn from information without being directly programmed and has been extensively applied to medical imaging (Lee et al., 2017). Deep learning (DL) has emerged among the techniques that come under the ML canopy as one of the most promising fields.

Figure 1. An illustration of the working of a machine learning algorithm

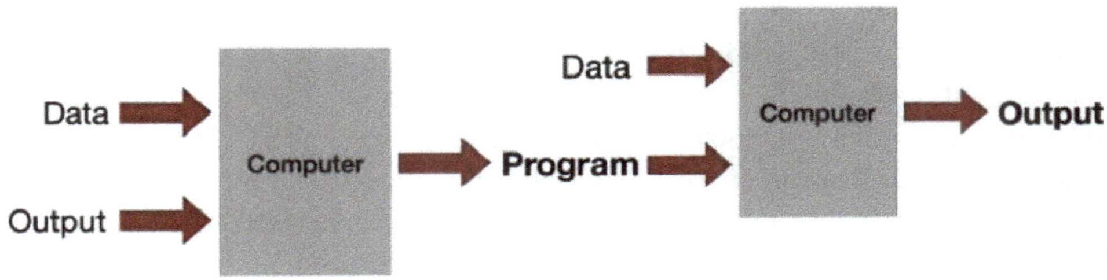

Artificial Intelligence

Artificial intelligence (AI) is the simulation of human being's intelligence processes by machines, particularly computer systems. These methods include firstly, learning which is the acquisition of information and rules for using the data, secondly, argumentation which is using rules to reach relative or definite resolutions and lastly self-correction (Tripathi, 2021).

Artificial Intelligence, a term often used interchangeably with "machine learning" – has a huge array of current and potential applications in healthcare and medicine (Rigby, 2019). Machine learning can be defined as a family of statistical and mathematical modeling techniques that can 'learn' from data to perform a diagnosis or render a treatment decision and improve the prediction, without any explicit programming. "Learning" in machine learning is the reference of the desire to create a model that can learn like a human, through experience, and achieve an objective with little to no external (human) assistance (Tripathi, 2021). Machine learning is often anthropomorphized– however, the algorithms behind the scenes use mathematical formulations to represent models and strive to learn parameters in these formulations, by tracking them back from a dataset of observations.

All computer programs consist of three basic components: an input, a function, and an output. In traditional computer programming, the programmers generally tend to knows what the input and output look like and writes a function that processes input and produces an output. The programming and potential decisions are part of a manual effort to deliberately encode the steps or knowledge needed to provide automated output, often called "rules-based systems." Whereas Machine learning relies heavily on pattern recognition and the theory that computers can learn, useful relationships in data towards an output without being explicitly programmed. Instead of relying on a computer programmer to come up with the rules of the function, we instead leverage existing input-output pairs to enable function learning, as shown in fig.1. This is called "training" the statistical model.

This has led to the development of systems that can diagnose Alzheimer's disease (Gaonkar & Davatzikos, 2013; Gaonkar et al., 2015), which can discriminate between tumor radiological images (Bakas, 2015), efficiently compute the natural history of a patient, (Attiah et al., 2019; Gaonkar et al., 2019) predict progression of cancer as well as distinguish between pseudoprogression (Macyszyn et al., 2015), and precision medicine systems that can provide personalized treatment (Davenport & Kalakota, 2019). Many healthcare applications are based on the supervised learning model– the algorithm can learn from a wide range of data recorded and images annotated by medical experts.(Sotiras, 2016).

Machine Learning is being used in many aspects of healthcare since an early time— enhancing and optimizing care delivery, improving information management, cognitive support for clinical care and prediction, early detection of diseases, and risk assessment for individuals.

There has been a huge surge in Medical AI systems, specifically due to the two most important factors:

- The availability of and access to large volumes of digital healthcare data
- The development of graphical processing units (GPUs), which enable massive parallel computation

Examples of areas in which AI could have a large impact: Automated screening and diagnosis, adaptive clinical trials, operations research, global health, precision medicine, home health and wearables, genomic analysis, drug discovery and design, robotics. (Matheny et al., 2020) With the increasing trend of ML applications, groups that will require a basic competency in both healthcare and machine learning concepts and principles are AI developers, tech companies, policy-makers and regulators, health care system leadership, pharmaceutical and device industry, frontline clinicians, ethicists, patients, and patient caregivers. (Office, 2020)

It is critically important, to begin with, an informed question. This may be from the medical literature or pressing clinical question, but you have to start with a question that includes the detailed analysis of the output of your future model and the available actions. Especially in medicine, machine learning is best understood as a means to an end that has consequences. (Schwartz, 1970)

Application of Machine Learning in Medical Imaging

The advantages of AI for radiology are multiple, according to specialists. In screening exams such as mammography, chest CT, and colonography, machine learning applications were used. Some software also assisted in deciding whether a lesion was cancerous, in addition to certain detection tasks.

"Now, AI is also helping with efficiency by automatically delineating the cardiac chambers on cardiac CT, making measurement of heart function more efficient and more reproducible," Erickson says. "AI can identify patterns in images with high reliability and may find patterns that are more complex than humans can find." By performing repetitive tasks such as segmenting frameworks, it can minimize the workload. That will then allow for more quantitative imaging, which would enhance the radiology 'output'. It can also be helpful in detecting lesions that may be subtle, which can be especially helpful if the radiologist is tired or distracted. It is proved that evidence can be found in images that humans do not interpret, such as molecular markers in tumors. (Lori, n.d.)

Artificial intelligence (AI) will make improvements to the professional lives of radiologists, just as many other areas of our lives have been changed. Since the advent of electricity, the internet, and, most recently, AI, inventions for general purposes have allowed communities to make progress and improve their quality of life. Radiologists are not the only practitioners to have their practice changed by AI, or even the first one. Therefore, other fields of medicine have been affected as well. One group of researchers recently developed mobile phone software and performed a study in which the software was shown to more reliably differentiate malignant melanomas from benign lesions than the dermatologists involved in the study.(Esteva et al., 2017)

Although the role of the dermatologist is far broader than the classification of lesions, that finding may be an initial sign that AI would also modify the labor market in that area.

In automated systems, the vast majority of laboratory samples are actually analyzed, which does not seem to concern anyone. The need to count red blood cells by trained staff has long since ceased to exist. Compared to a human study, developments in the field of computer vision have also started to produce increased sensitivity in the identification of tumors in histopathological specimens (Liu et al., 2017). The abundance of data, the development of artificial neural networks, and the increased affordability of the hardware were the primary factors that enabled such advances in artificial intelligence:

Currently, data is collected through different tools. If the new electricity is AI, the new coal is data. The development of artificial neural networks has made it possible to solve some of the problems with other techniques for machine learning. In conventional techniques, which are the basis of some auxiliary diagnostic applications, computer-aided detection, increasing the amount of knowledge to some degree improves accuracy. The accuracy appears to continue to improve with the advent of new data in the deep learning method, which uses hidden layers of artificial neural networks.

The accuracy appears to continue to improve with the advent of new data in the deep learning method, which uses hidden layers of artificial neural networks. In 2015, for instance, the output of a computer exceeded that of a person for the first time in an annual competition for object recognition in everyday images (He et al., 2017).

Increased hardware affordability, especially processing and storage equipment, has also encouraged progress in the area. A laptop with the same processing power as the most efficient supercomputer produced in 2000 can currently be purchased; the difference being that the laptop would cost around 40,000 times less than the $110 million spent on the supercomputer and will weigh far less than its 106 tonnes (Oram, 2001).

In highly lucrative fields of great global interest, developments in the field of computer vision have increased the interest of technology giants and different government sectors. Autonomous vehicles and drones with automated target recognition need image processing instantaneously, do not accept mistakes, and are not expected to rely on a human being who can easily change their operation.

Although this dispersion could apparently lead to a delay in the effect of AI on the radiology industry, developments in the automotive and space industries are typically catalysts for advances in other sectors, potentially speeding up the pace of new imaging discoveries.

There are unique obstacles to the application of AI techniques in medical imaging. Diagnoses are not always confirmed; classifications and definitions are not always unanimous and are not forever (Kohli et al., 2017). In terms of their typical dimensions and textures, the structures of the human body show considerable variety, such variation potentially masking pathological conditions.

Knowledge has spread rapidly about the automatic processing of medical images. The most recent Data Science Bowl (Kaggle Data Science Bowl, 2017), which offered a total of $1 million in awards to teams that created and made available the best-automated nodule classification algorithms for chest computed tomography, offers one example (CT). In the field of medical imaging, most participating teams had never worked, and several of them undoubtedly wanted to work in the field only because of the competitiveness.

The effect of AI on the radiologist's routine would likely occur gradually. The software can provide information that we can not extract from the scans, prioritize examination according to disease severity (Prevedello et al., 2017), and will eventually become part of the routine, among other tools. AI has already proven itself capable of producing parts of the radiological report in some areas of radiology, including a preliminary overview of the imaging results and the calculation of certain lesions.

The radiologist's key contribution, however, is not merely to provide this knowledge, but to incorporate it with the clinical data, leading to the diagnosis and individualized care of the patient in a more comprehensive way. This method of integration of information would take more time for computers to reproduce. Radiologists, however, who know how to use the technology to their benefit, would have a strong advantage over those who oppose it.

Reducing the time needed to read images will provide more time for direct patient treatment, enabling the radiologist to play a more productive diagnostic role by interpreting data from a range of sources instead of image-based data alone (Jha & Topol, 2016). Additionally, a radiologist's general training goes beyond image interpretation, covering the implementation of minimally invasive procedures, quality control, and management, as well as participating in multidisciplinary discussions and serving as a consultant so that the most appropriate imaging method be selected to address a given clinical issue.

Because of technological advancements, the demand for radiology services has already undergone extreme changes. Actually, the jobs did not cease to exist but the functions were redefined. The imaging methods that subsequently emerged, however, made it possible to broaden the radiology services market. In the current job market, radiologists who have not adapted to the modifications and have not mastered the new techniques have more difficulties. Our specialty must adjust to the numerous changes that AI will make possible, among which there will certainly be an improvement that will enhance our patients' diagnosis and treatment.

Even after numerous investments and development made, the translatability of machine learnings algorithms from laboratory to clinic isn't accomplished. Creating maximal generalization in machines is one of the key factors resulting in a delay in the development of algorithms used for diagnostics and prognostic prediction making. Algorithmic bias is one of the greatest challenges faced in generalizability. On the other side, machines do not inherently pose biases. When humans intrude on their own beliefs and ideas, whether intentionally or unconsciously, the resulting algorithm will include these human biases while discriminating two data points. As a result, ethical concerns about artificial intelligence, especially supervised machine learning, originate from human decisions incorporated during the process of development of the model.

Human feedback and model design can pass on the human bias to the model in a number of ways. The training data collection method and the surrounding process are some of the areas where various forms of bias can be taught to a model. Sample bias, annotator bias, and temporal bias are three forms of bias to discuss in regards to training data and the resulting model generalizability. Using ethical and technical aspects each of these biases can be avoided or minimized to render minimal bias. (Gaonkar et al., 2020) In the next part of the chapter, we dive deeper into ethics and biases related to machine learning algorithms.

ETHICS, BIASES, AND CHALLENGES

Sample Bias

With the exponential rise in popularity of machine learning (ML) and attempts to implement ML-based models for clinical application, to make sure that the model is not learning biases while training it is important to objectively review the training data used to train models. When an algorithm is used without appropriate training and is relied on for producing accurate predictions, in such cases it becomes unethical. In general, if any model is implemented in conditions that were not present or reflected in the training data would be considered biased. A biased ML model tends to generate inaccurate predictions because the model has not been trained on identical data resulting in the inability to make discriminate between two data points in these scenarios. Apparently, it is possible to ethically implement the same model in another population with a similar distribution to the training data population. Sample bias occurs when the reason for the model's bias is variations in the population distributions of the training and test datasets.

For developing an ML model in healthcare settings, electronic health records (EHR) are often used as the source to generate training datasets. This data source may be troublesome if any of the data is not accessible or is metadata since machine learning models can learn minute trends that could emerge in these data irregularities and discrepancies.(Gianfrancesco et al., 2018) In addition to the typical diagnostic marker functionality, researchers often use details such as drug used for medication, demographics, prognosis, and, in some cases, genomic factors in algorithms (Shivade et al., 2014; Wei et al., 2016; Wong et al., 2018).

This unstructured data necessitates manual human labor to extract and organize it in a manner that can be used to train ML models (Araujo et al., 2017; Ford et al., 2016). Perhaps this could be a tedious and time-consuming task, which means that processing a significant amount of data for training the model cost be cost-prohibitive. If the data collection process is automated, the volume of training data will be lower and the likelihood that data distribution of this smaller volume of data varies from the general population becomes significantly higher. This increases the likelihood of producing a biased and less generalizable ML model. In short, more data results in the better as well as the statistical performance of the resulting ML model.(Halevy et al., 2009).

One more great threat to generalizability that arises due to sample bias is that vulnerable groups, such as people belonging to low or marginalized socio-economic backgrounds, are much more prone to have insufficient EHR data in any provided health care system. This means that ML models trained on data generated from EHR are not reflective of, and can't be implemented ethically for, patients from these disadvantaged groups.(). This will make models trained on data from a single EHR system non-generalizable, with the risk of producing unreliable and/or biased predictions when evaluated on a group of populations not reflected in the training data (e.g., a different hospital's EHR data). A probable solution to this, as well as for creating more generalizable models at a single facility, is to practice with more external data that include a diverse group of communities.(Gianfrancesco et al., 2018).

If the training data used is too dissimilar from the population distribution on which the model would be applied, then the models' Sensitivity and Specificity would be highly jeopardized. In this world of AI-enabled technologies, data sharing by one person may help another, while a lack of such data democratization may prohibit others from receiving the best possible diagnostics as well as prognostic outcomes. This raises the fundamental ethical issue of whether data sharing ought to be compulsory to provide the best possible treatment for everyone, or A.I.-enabled healthcare should be limited to populations, mostly from the higher socio-economic backgrounds, with enough data to train the ML model on. While not forgetting the motive should be to provide the benefits of AI to everyone without violating anyone's privacy.

Annotator Bias

When two radiologists see the same scan of the same patient, they can prescribe bit distinct medications. An ML model trained on the first radiologists would,d therefore 'learn' to detect patterns and treat the patients in the same manner as the first physician. Vice versa, the model trained as per the second physician would prescribe accordingly. As a result, annotator bias is developed in the algorithmic models. It's indeed critical to distinguish annotator bias from sample bias, which arises as a result of bias in selecting training data. The objectivity of diagnosis and clinical outcomes is one of the key reasons for incorporating AI-based models into healthcare frameworks. Since annotator bias generates objective algorithms, it becomes a challenge to apply supervised machine learning (Bond et al., 2018; Goddard et al., 2012; Parasuraman et al., 1993). If a human's curation over the algorithmic decisions is not retained, any mistakes made by the initial data annotators of the training data may be propagated.

In the future, ML-based medicine and imaging will most probably be used on a massive scale in many large healthcare facilities and systems. Such models could be trained using data provided by a tiny group of annotators at a facility. The precision of these annotations would eventually determine the accuracy of the ML approach being applied, and having a limited number of annotators will most likely result in annotation bias in the trained models. Crowdsourcing annotation may be a possible alternative. In principle, crowdsourcing, which originated as a means of easily and cheaply collecting data, may have the added advantage of including a wider and much more varied group of annotators (Lease, 2011; Mason et al., 2014). It is important to note that crowdsourcing, by design, necessitates widespread data exchange, making data sharing essential to the effective growth of medical decision-making systems.

Temporal Bias

Temporal bias is a third form of bias that is seldom addressed in machine learning literature. Modern algorithms such as deep learning algorithms are essentially everlasting learning systems. A physician may practice medicine for two decades and transfer some of their knowledge to the next generation of doctors. A human physician would one day die– and would take all of the complex knowledge and experiences with them. Whereas, a machine learning algorithm is almost immortal. A computer algorithm given the power of massive computational power and memory storage will strive to 'learn' over several human generations.

As a result, a healthcare infrastructure that has deployed machine learning techniques earlier would enable:

- Training ML algorithms for a longer period.
- Collect data over a longer period of time.
- Build an ML model that can utilize this huge collected data to predict diagnosis and prognosis.
- As a result, those communities will provide their people with a "healthcare" benefit.

Temporal bias can also be regarded in the sense of an algorithm that runs over several human generations. Remember that an algorithm will keep on gathering data and training on it through various generations, while a human practitioner will ultimately decease along with their experience of serving a specific population. Since an algorithm is only constrained by computer memory and computational capacity, a population, that collects data and trains algorithms over few years before another, has a huge benefit. This sort of temporal bias is shown by ML algorithms that use genetic data or medical history to make diagnostic decisions. This benefit would most certainly extend to future generations whose ancestors' data has been already trained upon by the algorithm.

ML algorithms are prone to configuration, the volume of data used for testing, and the amount of time spent training the model. More the time spent on training the model, the better the algorithm is trained - even if using the same data for training (Goodfellow et al., 2016). Furthermore, when a group gathers data over a prolonged period of time, the amount of data gathered and annotated would keep on growing.

CONCLUSION

We conclude that the biases prevalent in algorithms are one of the most significant ethical issues that must be considered and tackled before the implementation of AI-based radiology. Even though we try to minimize the human bias in algorithms but it's very important to keep a human in the loop to have a check on the decisions made by the algorithm. A possible approach to tackle some of these ethical challenges could be by democratizing data and sharing it with institutions nationally as well as internationally. However, data sharing should be applied responsibly and not violating patient's privacy. Federated learning-, differential privacy- and homomorphic encryption-based machine learning three emerging techniques providing a solution to data sharing problems without sacrificing privacy. In brief, implementing an effective legislative and regulatory framework to allow anonymous data sharing, rethinking generalization in an algorithmic context, and developing machine learning algorithms without involving any human-generated biases are all potential solutions to implement AI-based medical imaging techniques in a modern healthcare setting.

REFERENCES

Araujo, T., Aresta, G., Castro, E., Rouco, J., Aguiar, P., Eloy, C., Polónia, A., & Campilho, A. (2017). Classification of breast cancer histology images using convolutional neural networks. *PLoS One*, *12*(6), e0177544. doi:10.1371/journal.pone.0177544 PMID:28570557

Arpey, N. C., Gaglioti, A. H., & Rosenbaum, M. E. (2017). How socioeconomic status affects patient perceptions of health care: A qualitative study. *Journal of Primary Care & Community Health*, *8*(3), 169–175. doi:10.1177/2150131917697439 PMID:28606031

Attiah, M., Gaonkar, B., Alkhalid, Y., Villaroman, D., Medina, R., Ahn, C., Niu, T., Beckett, J., Ames, C., & Macyszyn, L. (2019). Natural history of the aging spine: A cross-sectional analysis of spinopelvic parameters in the asymptomatic population. *Journal of Neurosurgery. Spine*, *32*(1), 63–68. doi:10.3171/2019.7.SPINE181164 PMID:31561232

Bakas, S. (2015, October). GLISTRboost: combining multimodal MRI segmentation, registration, and biophysical tumor growth modeling with gradient boosting machines for glioma segmentation. In *BrainLes 2015* (pp. 144–155). Springer.

Bond, R. R., Novotny, T., Andrsova, I., Koc, L., Sisakova, M., Finlay, D., Guldenring, D., McLaughlin, J., Peace, A., McGilligan, V., Leslie, S. J., Wang, H., & Malik, M. (2018). Automation bias in medicine: The influence of automated diagnoses on interpreter accuracy and uncertainty when reading electrocardiograms. *Journal of Electrocardiology*, *51*(6), S6–S11. doi:10.1016/j.jelectrocard.2018.08.007 PMID:30122457

Chartrand, G., Cheng, P. M., Vorontsov, E., Drozdzal, M., Turcotte, S., Pal, C. J., Kadoury, S., & Tang, A. (2017). Deep learning: A primer for radiologists. *Radiographics*, *37*(7), 2113–2131. doi:10.1148/rg.2017170077 PMID:29131760

Davenport, T., & Kalakota, R. (2019). The potential for artificial intelligence in healthcare. *Future Healthcare Journal*, *6*(2), 94–98. doi:10.7861/futurehosp.6-2-94 PMID:31363513

Esteva, A., Kuprel, B., Novoa, R. A., Ko, J., Swetter, S. M., Blau, H. M., & Thrun, S. (2017). Dermatologist-level classification of skin cancer with deep neural networks. *Nature*, *542*(7639), 115–118. doi:10.1038/nature21056 PMID:28117445

Ford, E., Carroll, J. A., Smith, H. E., Scott, D., & Cassell, J. A. (2016). Extracting information from the text of electronic medical records to improve case detection: A systematic review. *Journal of the American Medical Informatics Association: JAMIA*, *23*(5), 1007–1015. doi:10.1093/jamia/ocv180 PMID:26911811

Gaonkar, B., Beckett, J., Villaroman, M. H. S. D., Ahn, B. S. C., Edwards, B. S. M., Moran, S., Attiah, M., Babayan, D., Ames, C., Villablanca, J. P., Salamon, N., Bui, A., & Macyszyn, L. (2019). Quantitative analysis of neural foramina in the lumbar spine: An imaging informatics and machine learning study. *Radiology. Artificial Intelligence*, *1*(2), 180037. doi:10.1148/ryai.2019180037 PMID:33937788

Gaonkar, B., & Davatzikos, C. (2013). Analytic estimation of statistical significance maps for support vector machine based multivariate image analysis and classification. *NeuroImage*, *78*, 270–283. doi:10.1016/j.neuroimage.2013.03.066 PMID:23583748

Gaonkar, B., Kim, K., & Macyszyn, L. (2020). Ethical issues arising due to bias in Training A.I. algorithms in healthcare and data sharing as a potential solution. *AI Ethics Journal*, *1*(1), 1–9. doi:10.47289/AIEJ20200916

Gaonkar, B., Shinohara, R. T., & Davatzikos, C. (2015). Interpreting support vector machine models for multivariate group wise analysis in neuroimaging. *Medical Image Analysis*, *24*(1), 190–204. doi:10.1016/j.media.2015.06.008 PMID:26210913

Gianfrancesco, M. A., Tamang, S., Yazdany, J., & Schmajuk, G. (2018). Potential biases in machine learning algorithms using electronic health record data. *JAMA Internal Medicine*, *178*(11), 1544–1547. doi:10.1001/jamainternmed.2018.3763 PMID:30128552

Goddard, K., Roudsari, A., & Wyatt, J. C. (2012). Automation bias: A systematic review of frequency, effect mediators, and mitigators. *Journal of the American Medical Informatics Association: JAMIA*, *19*(1), 121–127. doi:10.1136/amiajnl-2011-000089 PMID:21685142

Goodfellow, I., Bengio, Y., & Courville, A. (2016). *Deep learning*. MIT Press.

Halevy, A., Norvig, P., & Pereira, F. (2009). The unreasonable effectiveness of data. *IEEE Intelligent Systems*, *24*(2), 8–12. doi:10.1109/MIS.2009.36

He, K., Zhang, X., & Ren, S. (2017). *Delving deep into rectifiers: surpassing human-level performance on imageNet classification*. https://arxiv.org/pdf/1502.01852.pdf

Jha, S., & Topol, E. J. (2016). Adapting to artificial intelligence: Radiologists and pathologists as information specialists. *Journal of the American Medical Association*, *316*(22), 2353–2354. doi:10.1001/jama.2016.17438 PMID:27898975

Kaggle Data Science Bowl. (2017). https://www.kaggle.com/c/data-science-bowl-2017

Kohli, M., Prevedello, L. M., Filice, R. W., & Geis, J. R. (2017). Implementing machine learning in radiology practice and research. *AJR. American Journal of Roentgenology*, *208*(4), 754–760. doi:10.2214/AJR.16.17224 PMID:28125274

Lakhani, P., Prater, A. B., Hutson, R. K., Andriole, K. P., Dreyer, K. J., Morey, J., Prevedello, L. M., Clark, T. J., Geis, J. R., Itri, J. N., & Hawkins, C. M. (2018). Machine learning in radiology: Applications beyond image interpretation. *Journal of the American College of Radiology*, *15*(2), 350–359. doi:10.1016/j.jacr.2017.09.044 PMID:29158061

Lease, M. (2011). On quality control and machine learning in crowdsourcing. *Human Computation (Fairfax, Va.)*, *11*(11).

Lee, J. G., Jun, S., Cho, Y. W., Lee, H., Kim, G. B., Seo, J. B., & Kim, N. (2017). Deep learning in medical imaging: A general overview. *Korean Journal of Radiology*, *18*(4), 570–584. doi:10.3348/kjr.2017.18.4.570 PMID:28670152

Liu, Y., Gadepalli, K., & Norouzi, M. (2017). *Detecting cancer metastases on gigapixel pathology images*. https://arxiv.org/pdf/1703.02442.pdf

Lori, K. (n.d.). Putting the AI in Radiology. *Radiology Today, 19*(1), 10.

Macyszyn, L., Akbari, H., Pisapia, J. M., Da, X., Attiah, M., Pigrish, V., Bi, Y., Pal, S., Davuluri, R. V., Roccograndi, L., Dahmane, N., Martinez-Lage, M., Biros, G., Wolf, R. L., Bilello, M., O'Rourke, D. M., & Davatzikos, C. (2015). Imaging patterns predict patient survival and molecular subtype in glioblastoma via machine learning techniques. *Neuro-Oncology, 18*(3), 417–425. doi:10.1093/neuonc/nov127 PMID:26188015

Mason, W., Vaughan, J. W., & Wallach, H. (2014). Computational social science and social computing. *Machine Learning, 95*(3), 257–260. doi:10.100710994-013-5426-8

Matheny, M. E., Whicher, D., & Israni, S. T. (2020). Artificial Intelligence in health Care: A report from the National Academy of Medicine. *Journal of the American Medical Association, 323*(6), 509–510. doi:10.1001/jama.2019.21579 PMID:31845963

Office, U. (2020, January 21). *Artificial Intelligence in Health Care: Benefits and Challenges of Machine Learning in Drug Development* [Reissued with revisions on Jan. 31, 2020]. https://www.gao.gov/products/GAO-20-215SP

Oram, A. (2001). *Peer-to-peer. Harnessing the power of disruptive technologies.* O'Reilly & Associates.

Parasuraman, R., Molloy, R., & Singh, I. L. (1993). Performance consequences of automation-induced 'complacency'. *The International Journal of Aviation Psychology, 3*(1), 1–23. doi:10.120715327108ijap0301_1

Prevedello, L. M., Erdal, B. S., Ryu, J. L., Little, K. J., Demirer, M., Qian, S., & White, R. D. (2017, July 3). Automated critical test findings identification and online notification system using artificial intelligence in imaging. *Radiology, 285*(3), 162664. Advance online publication. doi:10.1148/radiol.2017162664 PMID:28678669

Rigby, M. J. (2019). Ethical dimensions of using artificial intelligence in health care. *AMA Journal of Ethics, 21*(2), 121–124. doi:10.1001/amajethics.2019.121

Russell, S., & Bohannon, J. (2015). Artificial intelligence. Fears of an AI pioneer. *Science, 349*(6245), 252. doi:10.1126cience.349.6245.252 PMID:26185241

Samuel, A. L. (1959). Some studies in machine learning using the game of checkers. *IBM Journal of Research and Development, 3*(3), 210–229. doi:10.1147/rd.33.0210

Schwartz, W. B. (1970). Medicine and the computer: the promise and problems of change. In *Use and Impact of Computers in Clinical Medicine* (pp. 321–335). Springer. doi:10.1007/978-1-4613-8674-2_20

Shivade, C., Raghavan, P., Fosler-Lussier, E., Embi, P. J., Elhadad, N., Johnson, S. B., & Lai, A. M. (2014). A review of approaches to identifying patient phenotype cohorts using electronic health records. *Journal of the American Medical Informatics Association: JAMIA*, *21*(2), 221–230. doi:10.1136/amiajnl-2013-001935 PMID:24201027

Sotiras, A. (2016). Machine learning as a means toward precision diagnostics and prognostics. In *Machine learning and medical imaging* (pp. 299–334). Academic Press. doi:10.1016/B978-0-12-804076-8.00010-4

Tripathi, S. (2021). *Artificial Intelligence: A Brief Review.* Analyzing Future Applications of AI, Sensors, and Robotics in Society.

Wei, W. Q., Teixeira, P. L., Mo, H., Cronin, R. M., Warner, J. L., & Denny, J. C. (2016). Combining billing codes, clinical notes, and medications from electronic health records provides superior phenotyping performance. *Journal of the American Medical Informatics Association: JAMIA*, *23*(1), 20–27. doi:10.1093/jamia/ocv130 PMID:26338219

Wong, J., Horwitz, M. M., Zhou, L., & Toh, S. (2018). Using machine learning to identify health outcomes from electronic health record data. *Current Epidemiology Reports*, *5*(4), 331–342. doi:10.100740471-018-0165-9 PMID:30555773

Chapter 5
Reducing Pain Through Affective Computing

Luca Bondin
University of Malta, Malta

Alexiei Dingli
University of Malta, Malta

ABSTRACT

For a long time, the primary approach to control pain in patients involved the use of specially designed drugs. While these drugs have proved to be sufficient to reduce the perception of pain in patients of all ages, they do not come without any potential side effects. The prolonged use of such drugs can have adverse effects on the health of a patient. This research proposes a shift away from such practices and proposes the use of technology as an adjunct tool to help patients cope with pain. Through the adoption of affective computing, this research presents Morpheus results obtained at the time of writing confirm that the approach presented by this research is indeed useful and can achieve results that are in line with the set out as part of this study. The authors firmly believe that the approach presented in this research can lay the foundations for the research and development of similar applications in pain reduction scenarios.

INTRODUCTION

Pain is one of the most urgent concerns for patients undergoing any treatment procedure. Caused by injury, disease or invasive medical procedures, pain offers an experience that is generally exhausting and affects individuals both physically

DOI: 10.4018/978-1-7998-7888-9.ch005

and psychologically. A variety of methods were explored to help treat patients in pain. However, for years, the primary approach to reducing pain in patients involved exclusive medicine and pharmaceuticals. As of 2014, pain medications were the third most written prescriptions, and few pain prescription drugs achieved acceptable pain relief in more than 50% of treated patients (Wiederhold et al., 2014).

The use of medicine and pharmaceuticals for an extended period may also lead to other issues that might have undesired effects on the health of the patient receiving treatment. For example, prolonged use of a particular drug leads to what is known as Tolerance. Tolerance is a person's diminished response to a drug, which occurs when used repeatedly. This causes the body to adapt to the continued presence of the drug, thus reducing its effects. For example, when morphine is used for a long time, larger doses must be taken to produce the same effect. Tolerance develops because the drug's metabolism speeds up, or the strength of the bond between the receptor and the drug decreases. Prolonged use of a drug may also lead to patients' Resistance that refers to the ability of microorganisms or cancer cells to withstand the effects of a drug. The development of Tolerance and Resistance is also compounded by the possibility that drug response is also subject to differences between patients' ages. Creating active drugs across a broad population while ensuring that the risks of developing Tolerance and Resistance are kept to a minimum is challenging. Pain is very much a private emotional experience that varies from one individual to another (Osterweis et al., 1987).

In light of this, we are now witnessing a shift in how professionals are looking at new and novel approaches to help patients cope with pain symptoms. Researchers, amongst others, are exploring psychological methods for reducing pain, such as cognitive-behavioural procedures and hypnosis. Others have turned to technology to provide the answer. Among the technology-based approaches, researchers have started looking at adopting Affective Computing to take healthcare to the next step.

The research presented in this chapter focuses on using Affective Computing and other easily accessible technologies to provide a coping mechanism for patients undergoing painful treatment procedures. We aim to tackle issues that commonly arise when creating such applications, namely the lack of readily available datasets, through the introduction of Federated Learning. More importantly, the research aims to provide a coping mechanism that is enjoyable and safe from any side-effect on the patient's health. This chapter intends to describe the methodology we adopt and discuss the experiments' results as part of this research.

BACKGROUND

Sensing Pain

Processing of pain in humans happens at multiple levels in the human operating process; from the sensation of pain through the pain-sensitive fibres in the skin making up the Peripheral Nervous System, to neuromodulation at the spine level, and finally to the post-spinal modulation that happens inside the brain (Garland, 2012). When noxious stimuli impinge upon the body from external or internal sources, information regarding the damaging impact of these stimuli on bodily tissues is transduced through neural pathways and transmitted through the peripheral nervous system to the central and autonomic nervous systems. This form of information processing is known as nociception, which is how information about actual or potential tissue damage is relayed to the brain. Activation of nociceptors is transduced along the axons of peripheral nerves, which terminate in the dorsal horn of the spine. There, messages are relayed up the spinal cord to the brain, specifically through the spinothalamic tract to output the thalamus. In turn, the thalamus serves as the significant "relay station" for sensory information to the cerebral cortex. These signals are transmitted through "gates" in the spine and are received and processed inside the brain. In this context, we discuss the Gate Control theory of pain.

The Gate Control theory of pain, proposed by Melzak and Wall (1965), proved to be a revolution in pain research. The understanding of the Gate Control theory of pain is relatively intuitive. In simple words, nerves from all over the body run to the spinal cord. The spinal cord is the first main meeting point for the nervous system, and one can imagine that there are a series of gates in it. These gates are the points into which messages about pain arrive from all over the body. Messages from the body pass towards the brain through these gates. If the gates are more open, then more pain messages pass through to the brain, and one is more likely to experience a high level of pain. On the other hand, if the gates are more closed, fewer messages go to the brain, and one is likely to experience less pain.

There are, however, anomalies in this process. For example, literature (Garland, 2012) notes that nociception can occur in the absence of awareness of pain, and pain can occur in the absence of measurably noxious stimuli. This phenomenon is observable in massive trauma cases when victims exhibit a stoic painless state despite severe injuries.

Conversely, individuals with functional pain syndromes report considerable anguish despite having no visible tissue damage. In layman terms, this means that the "gates" might be open on occasions where there is no obvious source of origin for the pain being felt. Even worse, on occasions, these "gates" remain stuck in an open position sending the brain into overdrive and naturally, causing the sensation of immense pain.

Distraction Therapy

Only after understanding how we as human beings perceive pain can we start looking at possible innovative techniques employed as pain coping mechanisms. One of the main contributors to feeling increased pain is the attention focused on it. Focusing on the pain increases the perception of pain by the brain and leads to uncomfortable situations. Researchers proposed the Capacity theory to determine how the opening of gates contributes to the perception of pain. The Capacity theory proposes that each individual has a limited pool of information processing resources inside the brain. Using the capacity for one activity limits their availability for another activity. Therefore, engaging in an attention-occupying activity limits the capacity of public attention and prevents other information from being processed and accessing consciousness. With respect to what was previously discussed in terms of the "gates" in the spinal cord getting stuck in an open position, the ultimate goal of Distraction Therapy is to prevent this from happening avoiding the risk of the brain going into an infinite loop of continuously feeling the sensation of pain.

Most notably, the Capacity theory opens up numerous possibilities regarding the adoption of such coping mechanisms. Pearce (1983) discussed the potential of using cognitive methods to manage pain, because evidence from experimental pain studies showed that cognitive factors such as predictability and control, influence the perceived intensity or distress of pain stimuli. This research is still very much relevant. The way we think and behave play a crucial part in helping close the gates to pain symptoms. Mental factors are key contributors to help to reduce the sensation of pain, and if one can concentrate intensely on something other than the pain, the level of distraction these thoughts afford help to close the gates. In this context, we discuss Distraction Therapy.

Distraction is the process of shifting attention away from something. Distraction Therapy, therefore, can be described as an interventional tool that is used to refocus attention from pain to a pleasant sensory stimulus (Siegele, 1974). Engaging in thoughts or activities that distract attention from pain is one of the most commonly used and highly endorsed strategies for controlling pain (Johnson, 2005). Researchers have used the distraction of attention to modify internal thoughts by introducing extra sensory inputs to divert an individual's attention away from pain symptoms. The use of distraction combines auditory and visual overload, which shields the individual from full awareness of pain. This, in turn, increases pain tolerance. In essence, it does not mean that the pain is no longer present, but rather that this pain is put in the background, and focus can shift to the other activities which make a patient feel more at ease.

The effectiveness of this form of therapy stems from the way we, as humans, are wired. Emotions result in autonomic, endocrine, and immune responses, amplifying the pain through several psychophysiological pathways. For example, it has been scientifically proven that negative emotions bias attention toward pain. Negative emotions are associated with increased activation in brain structures that not only mediate the processing of emotions but are also essential nodes of the pain neuromatrix that tune attention toward pain, intensify pain unpleasantness, and amplify interoception (the sense of the physical condition of the body) (Wiech and Tracey, 2009). This is where distraction comes in. A distraction that evokes positive emotions is overrides the negative emotions, thus reducing the sensation of pain.

The methodology by which distraction is adopted is a topic that researchers have investigated for years. Having established that distraction does indeed work in its intended goal to reduce pain measurements, attention now shifted to determine which approaches and strategies best suited the application of Distraction Therapy. Some of the most common approaches, namely the use of video clips, music and imagery, have been shown to have the ability to alter anxiety, arousal and other human characteristics, which influence the pain experience. In addition, there are suggestions that a distractor that maximises attentional demand will be the most effective, implying that distraction tasks that are more difficult and require more attentional capacity will work best. However, there are more considerations to be made when eventually choosing a distraction method. Since people differ in interests and abilities, the best distractor varies according to the individual. It means that if, for example, an individual has failed in mathematics, a one-size-fits-all approach that would use mathematical problems as a distractor will have adverse effects on an individual, in contrast to using the same distractor with someone who is an A student in the subject. Therefore, the need for an informed choice of method, based on the audience's interests, to perform distraction is crucial to the overall success of Distraction Therapy.

Typical distraction interventions explored to administer the pain symptoms include deep breathing, listening to soothing music, and watching videos that invoke pleasant emotions in an individual. However, while the effectiveness of these approaches has been proven to a certain extent, the rise in popularity of other mediums that afford more interaction and provide higher levels of distraction has led researchers to identify other coping strategies. One of the most popular coping strategies for pain management is the use of Virtual Reality (VR). This chapter discusses an approach whereby we want to take what has already been achieved in terms of Virtual Reality for Distraction Therapy to the next level by introducing concepts associated with Artificial Intelligence (AI), such as Affective Computing.

Affective Computing

The very basic idea behind Artificial Intelligence is to make machines behave the same manner as humans do. Researchers have successfully taught machines how to see things like humans do and make sense of the objects in their field of vision. Others have taught machines how to speak different languages and understand human commands said in different tongues. We have taught machines how to learn to carry out new tasks without human intervention autonomously. While research has made considerable progress in Artificial Intelligence, it is felt that on most occasions, we are still missing the link that would make AI well and truly a tool that could behave with truly human-like capabilities. As humans, we can empathise and experience feelings. While it is true that most of our decisions are based on previous experiences, it is also true that our ability to feel and detect emotions is a crucial element in our decision-making process. Emotions are vital for us to function as rational decision-making human beings. Neurological evidence indicates that emotions are not a luxury, but rather, they are essential for rational human performance (Picard, 2000). However, while this is natural for us humans, it is not natural for most systems we use in our daily life. Very few systems are capable of doing this. Research in this area has started identifying the benefits of adding these capabilities to our machines. However, considerable work is still required to get to a stage where this capability is the norm rather than the exception. This field is generally referred to as Affective Computing.

Affective Computing is the study of assigning computers the human-like capabilities of observation, interpretation and generation of affect features (Tao and Tan, 2005). It is one of the essential topics for harmonious human-computer interaction. It aims to increase the quality of human-computer communication and improve the overall intelligence of the computer. Back in 1997, when the concept was first introduced, Picard remarked that "Computers are beginning to acquire the ability to express and recognise affect". Fast forward to 2020, and over the last two decades, the interest generated by Affective Computing has transformed the field into an influential area for research and industrial development. Nowadays, the software can detect human emotions with remarkable accuracy through sensing manifestations of physiology, speech and body motion, amongst others.

Healthcare is among the application areas where Affective Computing has flourished over the years. Yannakakis (2018) details some of the existing applications where Affective Computing has provided a better experience for patients and caregivers alike. Often through the implementation of affect-enabled serious games, Affective Computing has proven its worth in the creation of tools to help train caregivers who deal with people on the autism spectrum (Akinloye et al., 2020) or in developing tools to help patients who have PTSD (Malgaroli and Schultebraucks, 2021), for example.

Reducing Pain Through Affective Computing

The research presented in this chapter aims to bring together several technologies to provide effective Distraction Therapy to patients undergoing painful treatment procedures. More importantly, the goal is to provide a tool that can be used by people of all ages, which is not "procedure" specific. To achieve this, in addition to Affective Computing, the research also considers the introduction and implementation of a VR game. VR applications in such scenarios is relatively novel but is rapidly gaining popularity. This is evidenced by the ever-growing body of literature detailing the use of VR as a means with which to reduce pain in individuals. The studies undertaken by Chirico et al. (2020) and Lambert et al. (2020) are testament to this. Upon analysis of the characteristics of VR, it is immediately evident why VR can be a potential game-changer in the delivery of Distraction Therapy. In a pain-controlling setting, when one is immersed in a virtual environment, including a patient's visual processing, auditory processing, and physical actions results in an increasing demand for attention. In line with the capacity theory, this results in a reduced sensation of pain symptoms (Hoffman et al., 2006). Since this is perfectly in line with what the research aims to achieve, the introduction of VR as a crucial part of the research is a natural step in achieving the research goals. To further enhance the engagement, the game element is introduced as a form of active participation. Literature suggests that such applications usually consist of passive participation, where the individual is merely a spectator, or active participation, where the player can interact with the virtual world. Loreto-Quijada et al. (2014) investigated the application of active participation in a VR environment in contrast to passive participation. Their experiments show that the active participation environment had a more significant effect on the pain tolerance threshold of patients compared to the results obtained during passive participation. Therefore, this research adopts the former approach through a VR game where the player is placed inside a roller-coaster cart that navigates the world during gameplay. In contrast, the player has to carry out tasks and interact with the world itself.

In summary, this research proposes creating an "affect-enabled" VR-based game, which can immerse a patient in a virtual world and distract the attention resources away from any pain symptoms, effectively administering Distraction Therapy. Literature has established that one can never separate the notion of pain and emotion (Wiech and Tracey, 2009). Therefore, the inclusion of Affective Computing and its capabilities to understand and elicit emotions theoretically make it possible to reduce pain symptoms seamlessly. Furthermore, the Affective Computing component inside the game makes it possible that the VR game understands how the player is feeling at any point in time. Through this, the application can perform real-time alterations to the VR experience to better reflect the affective state of the patients at any given time during the procedure. This real-time adaptation ensures that one remains engaged with what is happening inside the virtual environment instead of focusing on what is causing the sensation of pain. In this manner, distraction levels are kept at a maximum throughout the entire use of the application.

The Affective Loop

There are various approaches to implementing affect-enabled applications. Prevalently, there is a notion of open- v closed-loop implementations. In the context of affect-enabled games, an open-loop implementation implies that players' emotion may be a "side effect" of the game without much conscious thought given to emotion during design. In short, as long as the game is more "fun" than "frustrating", the players remain engaged, and their emotions can be ignored. On the other hand, a closed-loop approach requires that the emotions are sensed and recognised by the system, and some aspect of the game is modified to reflect the player's current state. The approach proposed by this research adopts the closed-loop approach, which implies implementing the "Affective Loop". For a piece of software to be considered "affect-enabled" in this setting, the software must implement a four-phase closed-loop known as the "Affective Loop".

The first stage of the closed-loop is known as the "Affect Elicitation" stage. As the name suggests, the player is faced with specifically designed scenarios to elicit the targeted emotions during this stage. The second stage of the loop is the "Affect Sensing" stage. This stage entails the data gathering about the player's affective state. Having elicited an emotion in an individual during the affect elicitation phase, the software must be equally capable of knowing how to capture that emotion for further processing. Several intertwined issues arise during the implementation of this phase in particular. The first major issue for Affective Computing is that it is impossible to measure cognitive influences since these depend on self-reports that are likely to be highly variable. No one can read what is going on in someone else's mind. While several researchers have proposed an explicit way of data gathering through questionnaires, such approaches tend to be highly subjective and prone to error. Individuals may not express their feelings through questionnaires accurately, and therefore, other approaches had to be explored.

While it is impossible to measure cognitive influences or read people's minds, it is possible to measure physiological responses that often arise during the expression of emotion. Sensing affect by analysing physiological signals has some advantages over explicit data gathering methods because the process eliminates human subjectivity. Emotion is mainly manifested through the bodily or physiological reactions of the individual, and manipulation of these reactions is virtually impossible since they happen without the individual necessarily being aware of their occurrence. However, this approach, in itself, also gives rise to numerous issues and dilemmas.

Perhaps the biggest challenge, in this case, lies in determining what signals should be sensed and later mapped as emotions by the affect-enabled software. Researchers in psychology have devised many different models of emotion that can be roughly subdivided into categorical and dimensional models. In computational studies, categorical models often employ Ekman's (1992) six basic emotions. According to this psychological theory, all human beings share a standard set of cross-culturally basic emotions. Thus, each emotional state of an individual can be unambiguously classified as one of these six categories.

On the other hand, Russell and Mehrabian (1977) propose the Valence-Arousal-Dominance (VAD) model. Contrary to Ekman's theory which models emotion into either anger, disgust, fear, joy, sadness or surprise, according to this model, emotional states can be described relative to three fundamental emotional dimensions. The three emotional dimensions include valence, the degree of pleasure or displeasure of emotion, arousal, i.e., the level of mental activity, ranging from low engagement to ecstasy, and dominance, which is the extent of control felt in a given situation. This research takes a leaf out of Russel and Mehrabian's theory and maps emotion according to arousal levels. Russel and Mehrabian's methods complement the theory of "Flow", proposed by Mihalyi Csikszentmihalyi (2014). In general, Csikszentmihalyi's theory explains that while carrying out some activity, a person can either be "engaged", "aroused", or "bored". When a person is engaged, it is said that the person is in a state of "flow" where maximum distraction occurs. Therefore, the task, in this case, measures the engagement levels of an individual. In turn, this task is made attainable by measuring the physiological signals emitted by the individual, which are the results of sympathetic arousal happening in the individual's physiological system.

This research proposes the use of non-invasive wearable sensors to measure physiological reactions provided by the individual. For this research, physiological signals are measured using sensors worn on the player's wrist. Wearable sensors enable long-term continuous physiological monitoring, which provides our platform with enormous capabilities and increased accessibility. Also, the use of a wearable device worn as a smartwatch reduces the feeling that the player is being "watched", which, in turn, could result in a skewed representation of the player's emotional state during gameplay. For reading the physiological signals, the wearable device records the player's heart rate data during gameplay. More specifically, the device reads Heart Rate Variability (HRV) signals and BPM signals to determine the player's current affective state. HRV, in particular, is an excellent indicator of sympathetic arousal, where low HRV reading is an indication of high arousal and vice-versa.

Therefore, a successful closed-affective loop can be made through three elements; the VR game, the wearable device that reads physiological signals from the player, and, finally, the player (See Figure 1).

Figure 1. Main actors in the framework proposed by this research (Source: Self)

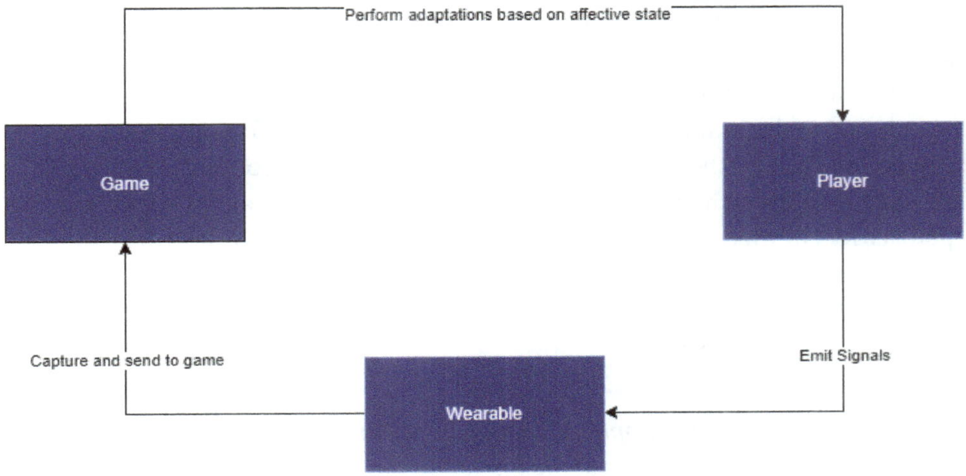

The third phase in the affective loop consists of the "Affect Modeling" phase. In line with what Calvo and Mello (2010) propose, this phase is implemented in three stages; signal processing, feature extraction, and machine learning. In this phase, this research proposes a novel approach that steers away from what is usually the norm in such applications. For example, in traditional applications where machine learning is implemented as part of the system, signal processing, feature extraction and model training is usually carried out on one curated body of data. On the other hand, the researchers in this work take a different route.

To begin with, gathering a large body of data upon which a model can be trained is a challenging task to carry out in a lab scenario. The nature of the data being read by the application makes it necessary to play the game for a long time to record a substantial amount of data from one player. In order to make the data more representative, the process would have to be repeated many times with many different players. Such a process would have been unfeasible to carry out. Secondly, this research is based on the belief that each person reacts differently to various situations. Therefore, introducing a "one-size-fits-all" approach with a static model used across all users of the application most likely decreases the efficiency and effectiveness of the whole approach. Physiology across different individuals varies extensively, and whatever excites one individual might not entice someone else.

As a result, creating a player-specific model is imperative if maximum analgesia through the game is achieved. This research takes this proposition a step further by focusing on Charles et al.'s (2005) statements on creating a player model and proposes a tweaked approach to the "Affect Modeling" stage.

The first few minutes of playtime is crucial for the successful execution of this phase. Then, behind the scenes and completely hidden from the player, the game starts gathering and tagging training data accordingly. The application starts by reading new RR and BPM data every second. Upon the completion of each 30-second window, the algorithm calculates an RMSSD value from the RR readings. While the conventional minimum recording is often reported to be 5 minutes, researchers have proposed ultra-short-term periods of 10 seconds, 30 seconds, and 60 seconds. For what this research aims to achieve, this research adopts a 30-second window approach for HRV measurements. A 60-second window is used for BPM displacement measurements. Then, upon completion of 60-second time windows, the algorithm calculates the average displacement of BPM readings from the starting heart rate reading during the 60-second window.

Figure 2. Data gathered by application to build the affect model. Note the formation of a cluster to the lower right and the top left of the graph. (Source: Self)

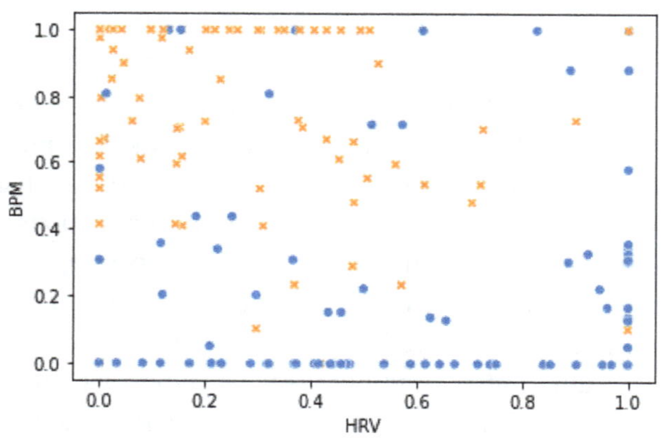

Perhaps the most significant novelty presented in this research lies herein. In line with Charles et al.'s statements on the importance of an evolving model, since the use of a generic model had been excluded from the start, some intelligent thinking was required. In order to build an accurate affect model, a large amount of data needs to be gathered. Otherwise, there is a severe risk that the algorithm might overfit, resulting in abysmal performance when working on unseen data. Furthermore, gathering enough data possibly meant that the player would need to play for a very long time before the model could start making its predictions. Given that the research wants to target patients receiving a wide variety of treatment procedures which could take from a couple of minutes to a couple of hours, the task facing the researchers demanded that a solution be found where somehow the model could be trained on a large body of data in a short period of time. The solution to this challenge comes in the form of Federated Learning.

Federated Learning (Konečný et al., 2016) is a relatively new concept presented by Google. The main idea behind Federated Learning, as initially presented, is that whereas in traditional settings, data is housed on one machine where the training occurs, a Federated learning scenario builds a machine-learning model based on datasets that are distributed across multiple devices. Federated Learning models make it possible to train a shared model by aggregating locally computed updates via a central coordinating server. In the context of this research, the implementation of Federated Learning makes it possible that the affect model inside the affective game learns to make decisions backed by a large body of training data in a short period. In addition, the adoption of Federated Learning comes with added benefits that are pivotal in the creation of intelligent systems, especially when such systems are to be deployed in sensitive areas such as healthcare. Federated Learning makes it possible to train models on large bodies of data without sharing the data itself. Human-related data is very sensitive, and privacy is often the primary concern when using such data. In light of data privacy-preserving laws, such as the General Data Protection Regulation (GDPR) enforced by the European Union, the importance of implementing privacy-preserving machine learning implementations has never been more significant. The implementation of Federated Learning as part of this research is as follows;

1. A global model is initialised with weights after training on a body of data and stored on the Federated Server.
2. Each agent connected to the server downloads a global model from the server and initialises the local model with downloaded weights.
3. Each agent receives new local data and retrains a model to reflect the newly seen data.
4. Repeat Step 3 for *N* times until the local model has been trained on a substantial amount of data.
5. After repeating for *N* times, calculate the weight differences between the new local model and the model downloaded from the Federated Learning server.
6. Upload the weight changes to the server where weighted aggregation occurs between weight change updates from individual agents connected to the Federated Learning loop and update the global model.

7. Repeat steps 2-6 until the process is explicitly terminated and the Federated Learning loop is disrupted.

Figure 3. Federated Learning as implemented by the proposed affect-enabled application (Source: Self)

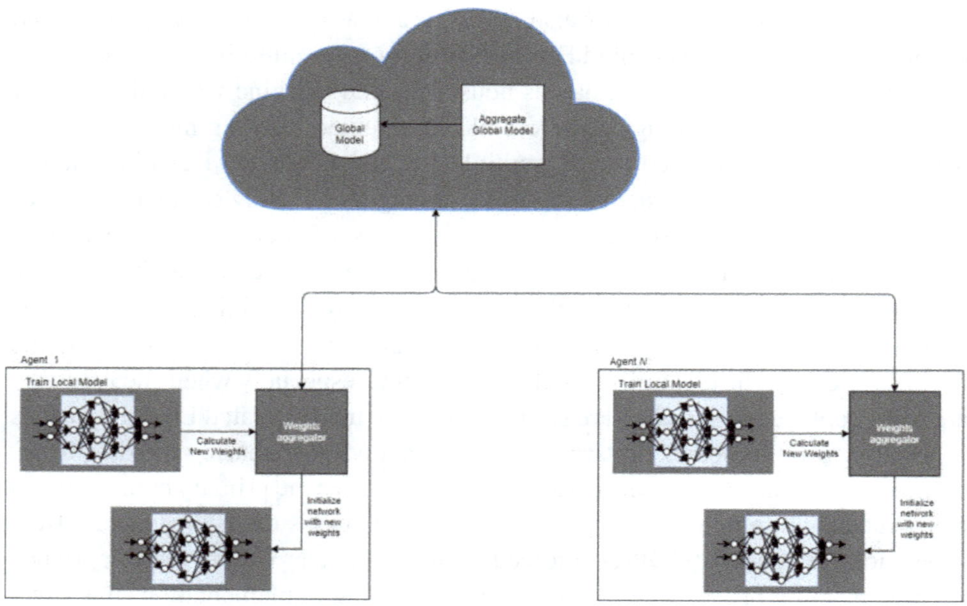

Finally, the "Affect-driven Adaptation" phase closes off the Affective Loop. In this phase, the application is constantly reading bio-signals off the player and reacting accordingly. In line with the previously discussed "Flow" theory, the main objective at this point is to keep the player engaged by adapting the game in real-time to avoid the player slipping into boredom or becoming too anxious, thus achieving maximum distraction.

Results

In evaluating the approach adopted by Morpheus, various components need to be taken into consideration to build a clear picture of the strengths and weaknesses of the chosen approach. Therefore, the system's components first need to be evaluated in isolation to pinpoint any shortcomings of the overall approach.

The main objective of application is to deliver Distraction Therapy through the use of Affective Computing and affect-enabled applications. In order to gauge the level of distraction analgesia administered by the application, people were invited to take part in a pain tolerance experiment. The experiment aims to determine whether Affective Computing performs better in this scenario than standard distraction techniques in pain controlling scenarios. It also aims to determine how pain tolerance increases when using such technologies instead of not using any distraction method at all. Twenty individuals were invited to participate in this experiment again, aged between 13 and 30. Participants were required to sit with their feet in cold water three times. The first-time participants were asked not to make use of any distraction tool. The second time participants were given a VR game with no affect-driven adaptations, which we note as "Passive Distraction". Finally, participants were allowed to use the application designed by this research, which we note as "Active Distraction". Participants were not informed of the experiment's main goal to mitigate order effects, and different orders were tried. We recorded the time each participant spent with feet in cold water for evaluation purposes. To induce pain sensation, water was kept at a temperature of 15°C and participants were asked to terminate the experience when the sensation of pain became unbearable. At 15°C, receptors in the body start to send pain messages to the brain (Woods et al., 1967). Because of this procedure, it was decided that individuals aged less than 13 years would not be involved in this first iteration of the experiment.

The results achieved from this experiment were quite interesting. In particular, this part of the evaluation was interested in determining whether the affect driven application adopted by this research improves the pain reduction capabilities offered by non-adaptive VR applications. From their experiments, Sato (2010) report that individuals using VR as a distraction tool reported a drop of 50% in pain scores. Therefore, we use this study as a baseline to determine the effectiveness of our approach. Upon analysis of the results, we note that the time individuals spent with feet in cold water while using the adaptive VR approach are, on occasions, 23% higher compared to the time individuals spent with feet in cold water when using non-adaptive VR. To further analyse this approach's statistical significance, we analyse the statistical significance of this result by carrying out a one-way within-subjects ANOVA test. Furthermore, upon conducting Post hoc tests using the Bonferroni correction, there was a statistical significance in the result with $p < 0.05$, thus indicating that the increase was not down to chance.

CONCLUSION

The work done in by this research contributes significantly to the application of Affective Computing and Distraction Therapy for pain reduction. While the study is still ongoing, the results are highly encouraging and point to a bright future in developing such applications. Furthermore, the statistically significant increase in pain tolerance registered by the experiment participants when using the designed application, instead of using non-adaptive VR, already provides significant encouragement that the adopted approach is effective.

The work done is also revolutionary as it contributes to literature by introducing Federated Learning in this setting. Through its introduction, Federated Learning has helped overcome problems that would otherwise have been considered show-stoppers, and therefore its impact cannot be understated. In light of the existing achievements, there is great confidence in the research that the approach undertaken is yielding results that align with the objectives of this study. We believe that the work being done by this research can prove to be a game-changer in developing affect-enabled software that will help significantly improve patients' lives during some of the most challenging periods of their lives.

ACKNOWLEDGMENT

This research is supported by the Epic for Good Foundation.

REFERENCES

Akinloye, F. O., Obe, O., & Boyinbode, O. (2020). Development of an affective-based e-healthcare system for autistic children. *Scientific American*, *9*, e00514.

Calvo, R. A., & D'Mello, S. (2010). Affect detection: An interdisciplinary review of models, methods, and their applications. *IEEE Transactions on Affective Computing*, *1*(1), 18–37. doi:10.1109/T-AFFC.2010.1

Charles, D., Mcneill, M., McAlister, M., Black, M., Moore, A., Stringer, K., ... Kerr, A. (2005). *Player-centred game design: Player modelling and adaptive digital games*. Academic Press.

Chirico, A., Maiorano, P., Indovina, P., Milanese, C., Giordano, G. G., Alivernini, F., Iodice, G., Gallo, L., De Pietro, G., Lucidi, F., Botti, G., De Laurentiis, M., & Giordano, A. (2020). Virtual reality and music therapy as distraction interventions to alleviate anxiety and improve mood states in breast cancer patients during chemotherapy. *Journal of Cellular Physiology*, *235*(6), 5353–5362. doi:10.1002/jcp.29422 PMID:31957873

Csikszentmihalyi, M. (2014). Play and intrinsic rewards. In *Flow and the foundations of positive psychology* (pp. 135–153). Springer.

Dubner, R. (Ed.). (2013). *The neural basis of oral and facial function*. Springer Science & Business Media.

Ekman, P. (1992). An argument for basic emotions. *Cognition and Emotion*, *6*(3-4), 169–200. doi:10.1080/02699939208411068

Garland, E. L. (2012). Pain processing in the human nervous system: A selective review of nociceptive and biobehavioral pathways. *Primary Care: Clinics in Office Practice*, *39*(3), 561–571. doi:10.1016/j.pop.2012.06.013 PMID:22958566

Goldscheider, A. (1894). *Ueber den schmerz in physiologischer und klinischer hinsicht: nach einem vortrage in der Berliner militärärztlichen gesellschaft am 22. januar 1894*. Hirschwald.

Hoffman, H. G., Seibel, E. J., Richards, T. L., Furness, T. A., Patterson, D. R., & Sharar, S. R. (2006). Virtual reality helmet display quality influences the magnitude of virtual reality analgesia. *The Journal of Pain*, *7*(11), 843–850. doi:10.1016/j.jpain.2006.04.006 PMID:17074626

Johnson, M. H. (2005). How does distraction work in the management of pain? *Current Pain and Headache Reports*, *9*(2), 90–95. doi:10.100711916-005-0044-1 PMID:15745617

Kahneman, D. (1973). *Attention and effort* (Vol. 1063). Prentice-Hall.

Konečný, J., McMahan, H. B., Ramage, D., & Richtárik, P. (2016). *Federated optimisation: Distributed machine learning for on-device intelligence*. arXiv preprint arXiv:1610.02527.

Lambert, V., Boylan, P., Boran, L., Hicks, P., Kirubakaran, R., Devane, D., & Matthews, A. (2020). Virtual reality distraction for acute pain in children. *Cochrane Database of Systematic Reviews*, 10. PMID:33089901

Liutsko, L. (2014). Differential effects of two virtual reality interventions: Distraction versus pain control. *Cyberpsychology, Behavior, and Social Networking*, *17*(6), 353–358. doi:10.1089/cyber.2014.0057 PMID:24892197

Loreto-Quijada, D., Gutiérrez-Maldonado, J., Nieto, R., Gutiérrez-Martínez, O., Ferrer-García, M., Saldana, C., Fusté-Escolano, A., & Liutsko, L. (2014). Differential effects of two virtual reality interventions: Distraction versus pain control. *Cyberpsychology, Behavior, and Social Networking*, *17*(6), 353–358. doi:10.1089/cyber.2014.0057 PMID:24892197

Malgaroli, M., & Schultebraucks, K. (2021). Artificial Intelligence and Posttraumatic Stress Disorder (PTSD). *European Psychologist*.

Melzack, R., & Wall, P. D. (1965). Pain mechanisms: A new theory. *Science*, *150*(3699), 971–979. doi:10.1126cience.150.3699.971 PMID:5320816

Moayedi, M., & Davis, K. D. (2013). Theories of pain: From specificity to gate control. *Journal of Neurophysiology*, *109*(1), 5–12. doi:10.1152/jn.00457.2012 PMID:23034364

Osterweis, M., Kleinman, A., & Mechanic, D. (1987). Measuring pain and dysfunction. In *Pain and Disability: Clinical, Behavioral, and Public Policy Perspectives*. National Academies Press.

Pearce, S. (1983). A review of cognitive-behavioural methods for the treatment of chronic pain. *Journal of Psychosomatic Research*, *27*(5), 431–440. doi:10.1016/0022-3999(83)90082-X PMID:6366219

Picard, R. W. (2000). *Affective Computing*. MIT Press. doi:10.7551/mitpress/1140.001.0001

Russell, J. A., & Mehrabian, A. (1977). Evidence for a three-factor theory of emotions. *Journal of Research in Personality*, *11*(3), 273–294. doi:10.1016/0092-6566(77)90037-X

Sato, K., Fukumori, S., Matsusaki, T., Maruo, T., Ishikawa, S., Nishie, H., Takata, K., Mizuhara, H., Mizobuchi, S., Nakatsuka, H., Matsumi, M., Gofuku, A., Yokoyama, M., & Morita, K. (2010). Nonimmersive virtual reality mirror visual feedback therapy and its application for the treatment of complex regional pain syndrome: An open-label pilot study. *Pain Medicine*, *11*(4), 622–629. doi:10.1111/j.1526-4637.2010.00819.x PMID:20202141

Shaffer, F., & Ginsberg, J. P. (2017). An overview of heart rate variability metrics and norms. *Frontiers in Public Health*, *5*, 258. doi:10.3389/fpubh.2017.00258 PMID:29034226

Sharma, N., & Gedeon, T. (2012). Objective measures, sensors and computational techniques for stress recognition and classification: A survey. *Computer Methods and Programs in Biomedicine*, *108*(3), 1287–1301. doi:10.1016/j.cmpb.2012.07.003 PMID:22921417

Siegele, D. S. (1974). The gate control theory. *AJN The American Journal of Nursing*, *74*(3), 498. PMID:4361027

Tao, J., & Tan, T. (2005, October). Affective Computing: A review. In *International Conference on Affective Computing and intelligent interaction* (pp. 981-995). Springer. 10.1007/11573548_125

Wiech, K., & Tracey, I. (2009). The influence of negative emotions on pain: Behavioral effects and neural mechanisms. *NeuroImage*, *47*(3), 987–994. doi:10.1016/j.neuroimage.2009.05.059 PMID:19481610

Wiederhold, B. K., Gao, K., Sulea, C., & Wiederhold, M. D. (2014). Virtual reality as a distraction technique in chronic pain patients. *Cyberpsychology, Behavior, and Social Networking*, *17*(6), 346–352. doi:10.1089/cyber.2014.0207 PMID:24892196

Woods, P. J., Griffith, B. A., Page, R. P., & Rodier, P. M. (1967). Human responses to various conditions of water temperature. *Perception & Psychophysics*, *2*(4), 157–160. doi:10.3758/BF03210311

Yannakakis, G. N. (2018). Enhancing health care via affective. *Computing*.

Chapter 6
Ethical Considerations of Using VR in Mental Health Training

Andrew Cachia
University of Malta, Malta

Vanessa Camilleri
University of Malta, Malta

Alexiei Dingli
University of Malta, Malta

Michael Galea
University of Malta, Malta

Paulann Grech
University of Malta, Malta

Alexei Sammut
University of Malta, Malta

Josianne Scerri
University of Malta, Malta

ABSTRACT

Mental health students, who are still undergoing training, might find it challenging to visualise and fully understand what their patients experience. For this reason, the authors created a virtual reality simulator which mimics the symptoms of a person suffering from schizophrenia at a virtual workplace. The simulation is managed by an artificial intelligence system which asks the user to attempt simple tasks, while simultaneously facing both visual and auditory hallucinations. The AI also adapts the storyline and character behaviour dynamically to increase the immersiveness of the experience. A pilot study was carried out, and the initial results were very encouraging. In fact, the absolute majority of the users stated that the simulation has helped increase their understanding of schizophrenia. In this chapter, the authors evaluate this experiment but from a different perspective. They focus mainly on the use of emerging technologies such as AI and VR and discuss the ethical considerations of their use within the field of mental health.

DOI: 10.4018/978-1-7998-7888-9.ch006

INTRODUCTION

The amount of people that suffer from mental health illnesses is around 13% of the global population according to the Global Health Metrics published by the Institute for Health Metrics and Evaluation (IHME) at the University of Washington. Of course, this was before the 2020 global pandemic hit us. Today, the world is currently experiencing a surge in mental health issues (Torales et al., 2020, Gruber et al., 2020, Cullen et al., 2020) and because of this, it is extremely important that governments invest in Mental Health professionals capable of supporting all those people in need. To do so, we need to train students in a professional yet timely manner. Educational institutions are doing their best to satisfy these needs, yet they have their own limitations. Students cannot simply gain access to patients as they please but have to go through rigorous processes in order to safeguard their own well-being and that of their patients.

A work around this issue would be to use emerging technologies such as Artifcial Intelligence (AI) and Virtual Reality (VR) to simulate virtual patients, environments and situations. AI can give virtual characters a personality and make them act and interact in specific ways using natural languages such as English or French. It can adjust the environment based upon the needs of the simulation and ensure that the reactions experienced by the users are realistic enough. So if the user needs to collect an object, the virtual object is placed in the room and it is ensured that the user can interact with it. Finally, the AI can orchestrate particular situations and trigger them based upon specific needs. This might include a phone ringing when the user approaches it or even the triggering of the hallucinations based upon the progression within the story line. VR is a very powerful technology and several studies (V. Camilleri et al., 2017,J. Camilleri et al., 2016,V. Camilleri et al., 2019) have shown that not only are users much more immersed in the experience if they use VR simulations, but they also tend to alter their perspective. When one walks in another person's shoes, the person's empathy increases and they better understand what another person is experiencing because they can relate to the issues directly.

In this project, that is what we tried to achieve. We aimed to assist the students to better understand what their patients are experiencing, whilst enabling them to become more empathic. To do so, we decided to simulate a mental health condition commonly referred to as Schizophrenia, which is characterized by a distorted perception of reality. This may include hallucinations, confused thinking, hearing voices, and distorted emotions. We chose this specifically because the visual and auditory simulations can be easily simulated using VR technologies.

Even though there have been various attempts in the past to use AI and VR in such a domain, the results were rather limiting. The major reason for this was that both technologies were not mature enough to handle such a task. AI has been around for almost 70 years, however in the past decade, this eld of study experienced giant leaps with the development of powerful hardware and software algorithms capable of going beyond human capabilities in several domains. On the other hand, past VR headsets were bulky and they were responsible for health-related issues such as eye strain, headaches, dizziness and nausea. This made them uncomfortable to use and in reality, very few people adopted them. Today, most of the health-related issues concerning VR headsets have been severely reduced and the headsets are becoming more comfortable.

Notwithstanding this, the application of these two technologies with regards to schizophrenia is rather limited. Creating an immersive experience using a combination of these two technologies will provide the students with a powerful experience which can help them understand and feel what a person suffering from schizophrenia experiences throughout his daily life. It will also give the user more insight on how to best assist the person suffering from those symptoms.

This project is part of an ongoing collaboration between the Department of AI and the Department of Mental Health at the University of Malta. It aims to provide support and foster empathy for patient care. The intended audience for the project were mainly mental health nurses, who are trained in dealing with patients having mental health illnesses. In the following sections, we will first have a look at the emerging technologies used in the project. Then we will venture in the use of VR for mental health, education, and treatment. Finally, we will discuss the ethical considerations with regards to this project while discussing the case study at hand. We will then conclude by providing some recommendations for consideration to those who would like to use such technologies in mental health applications.

EMERGING TECHNOLOGIES

Artificial Intelligence

Artificial Intelligence has been used in a wide range of medical applications such as health management systems, managing health records and assisting physicians Hamet and Tremblay, 2017. According to Intel Corporation, 2018, 37% of US Healthcare leaders are already using some elements of AI, and 54% of them are expecting widespread adoption in the coming years. Notwithstanding the lack of trust, that still exists, AI is already extensively used in mental health applications.

Maybe the most famous example is, without doubt, the 1966 ELIZA, described in Weizenbaum, 1966. ELIZA is most probably one of the first chatbots in existence. It made use of a language analyser to process text and generate a plausible reply using predefined patterns. Essentially, it tried to simulate a Rogerian psychotherapist.

Even though ELIZA did not form part of any actual therapy, the people who used it were quite amazed. Professor Weizenbaum, its creator, found these human reactions disturbing and eventually wrote Weizenbaum, 1976 to try to explain the limits of such systems. However, the use of natural language processing in this domain did not end there, and there were various applications throughout the years.

Countries like the UK are introducing chat-bots such as O'Hear, 2017 within their National Health System to diagnose patients. They hope to reduce the amount of primary-care appointments required to diagnose a patient with a mental health condition to just one appointment. Studies like Bedi et al., 2015, Corcoran et al., 2018 and Rezaii et al., 2019 identified that by using linguistic markers and machine learning, they can predict which people will develop psychosis with very high accuracies spanning beyond 90%. Other studies such as Lup et al., 2015, Katchapakirin et al., 2018 and Wongkoblap et al., 2017 made use of pictures posted on social media to detect signs of mental health conditions. These studies used features such as colours or facial expressions and were able to achieve more than 70% accuracy. Just et al., 2017 used machine learning techniques to analyse MRI images to distinguish between people with suicidal thoughts versus the rest. The system identified these people with 91% accuracy and also managed to spot others who had attempted suicide with 94% accuracy.

However, even though the use of AI in diagnostics has made considerable strides in the past decades, AI for psychological treatment is still rather controversial since the patient's health is at stake. The approach which AI researchers are taking is to create tools which augment the work of the healthcare professionals rather than replace them. One such example is Ewbank et al., 2020, where they trained an AI system on therapy scripts of around 17,500 patients. The experiments found that there was a direct association between clinical out-comes and the therapist's utterances. Therapists who followed certain protocols helped the patient to improve more than those that did not. However, the de-tailed monitoring of therapists is costly and rather time-consuming. Evaluation is an area where the AI can help since it can monitor the therapists in real-time, provide them with adequate feedback and guide them towards achieving effective interactions with the patient. The use of a data-driven understanding of mental health treatment is still in its infancy, but it is showing some promising results.

Large companies too are investing heavily in the use of AI in psychiatry. IBM research[1] is building tools to detect early indicators of mental health. Speech is being analysed for patterns which provide early signs of developmental disorders, mental illnesses and other diseases. Early detection of mental health issues is essential when one considers that around 1 in 5 adults is experiencing a mental health condition, and the cost of these conditions will rise to US$ 6.0 trillion by 2030. Textual analysis is at the forefront of this research, and machine learning techniques help to provide an overview of the patient's mental health. This technology together with the harvesting of social media posts Chrunch, 2018 is compelling since the state of the person, is identified in quasi-real-time, and negative thoughts can be tagged almost immediately. Chat-bots too will become more popular in the coming years, but they will focus on providing ancillary services which can still help the patients. Systems such as Woebot Fitzpatrick et al., 2017 offers cognitive-behavioural therapy online via Facebook Messenger. According to one of the experiments reported in the study, when compared to a control group, patients who used Woebot experienced a significant reduction in symptoms after just two weeks of using the Chat-bot. Computer vision is also extensively used in experiments such as Gattupalli et al., 2017 and Sayed et al., 2019 where the data from people (in this case children) performing tasks is being analysed using AI to assess aspects such as decision making, attention spans and emotional management. Fabiano et al., 2020 on the other hand, analyses micro-movements associated with the gaze of a child. It then trains a machine learning system specialised in detecting abnormalities which eventually tags children with autism.

It is very evident from these different use-cases that the future of AI in mental health offers a lot of potential. The reason why it is garnering so much success in this eld is rather simple. AI is exceptionally good at detecting patterns in data. Cues identified by the naked eye of a professional are verified by an AI, thus helping them in their work. However, an AI can quickly spot micro-patterns (syntactical cues, gaze abnormalities, etc.) which an expert can easily miss. The future of AI in mental health is obvious. It is all about augmenting the work of the professional, helping them reduce their errors to an absolute minimum and assisting them in the monitoring of patients even after the therapy session, when the patient goes about their daily life.

Virtual Reality

The term Virtual Reality (VR) as coined by Jaron Lanier in 1987 Lanier, 1992, referred to a reality that goes beyond a 360-degree environment and explores ways of communication that exceed fantasy. The notions held by the man (who has been hailed as the visionary father figure of VR), regarding the level of immersion humans experience whilst in this environment, do not support as much dependence on technology as communication on the visceral level, which the human can establish with the technology Lanier, 2017. One of the concepts proposed by Lanier, and which other VR visionaries such as Chris Milk propagate through their projects, is that the main focus of VR should go beyond the use of the medium and the technology developed, to extend to the impact on the human Milk, 2015. More often than not, this implies the extent of identification of the human user with the context of the virtual environment and with other virtual characters that may form part of it. VR is often represented by a set of artificially produced sensory stimuli (such as those produced for vision, sound, and touch) that are projected as part of a 360-degree virtual environment. How-ever, this experience needs to be complemented by some form of interaction by the human, and this interaction might partially or fully determine what happens in that environment.

In an optimally set VR experience, human users might be able to walk around, explore the virtual area, and be able to control and manipulate objects within that artificially reproduced environment as though it was real. Jaron Lanier Lanier, 2017 describes the sense of embodiment that he experienced the first time that he explored the VR environment and the sensations that he went through as he identified with the virtual hand that was visible in the VR environment. Even though he described that hand as being gargantuan in proportion to the rest of the environment, he could still somehow experience a personal association with that hand.

In a similar manner, when in 2010, Nonny de la Pena, came up with the immersive journalism project, people were identifying and associating with the objects of the re-created virtual environment, despite the fact that some of that environment was clearly digitally reconstructed De la Pena et al., 2010. For her project, the award-winning journalist, transformed a story about homeless people queueing in for food at a shelter, into a VR environment constructed from digitally recreated avatars in a virtual location, coupled with real audio from everyday captures. The result was a surprisingly immersive experience for the human users, who could associate with the setting in a way that triggered empathy. Feedback from people who went through the virtual reconstruction, indicated that they clearly showed signs of visible emotion as they tried to help the avatar who was in critical difficulty.

Tracing back to the 1960's, the immersive nature of a sensory machine was already being explored by Ian Sutherland, who proposed the 'Ultimate Display'. This was a sensory-machine connected to a computer and for which a computer would have control over matter. In this room, a virtual chair would look as good as a real chair to the user. This laid the conceptual foundation of both Augmented and Virtual Reality.

Chris Milk, co-founder and CEO of Within (Virtual Environment), focuses on the key element of communication for an effective VR design Milk, 2015. This means that the way the experience is brought across to the users, paves the way for a communication which on the one hand mirrors the physics of the world, and on the other stimulates a visceral form of emotion. As an example, when in VR, whilst on the one hand the brain needs to understand that a ball bouncing in the VW follows the same physical rules as in the physical world, the whole sequence of events needs to bring forward the same adrenaline rush as that which one gets when one is playing a game of basketball. VR is about bringing forward those same set of emotions naturally, without one having to think about the medium or the way in which the experience is unfolding.

There is another form of communication which VR can exploit and use to increase its impact on human behaviour. This is the indirect form of communication where the brain interprets the signals it gets, according to the way in which these are associated either to past or new memories. In this way, VR designers may target an audience, and apply mental models to the environment design to communicate a message Giroux et al., 2019. Mental models are conceptualisations built by users according to their perceptions of how a specific system might work. Therefore, a target audience sharing similar experiences can also share their perceptions of how a problem can be solved Zhang et al., 2010.

Following VR's potential for increased immersion and presence, the medium can be used to construct authentic experiences. There are four illusions of presence that the brain can construct to contribute to creating authentic experiences for the user. These are the illusions of a stable space, of self-embodiment, of physical interaction and of social communication Gonzalez-Franco and Lanier, 2017. The illusions of presence support the perception that a user is indeed part of the overall experience Slater, 2018. It is through the perception system that the body responds and reacts, whilst the cognitive system raises the awareness that what the user is experiencing is not 'real'. Although fidelity in graphics may carry their importance, this does not necessarily mean that for VR to be immersive there needs to be realism in graphics. One of the most important aspects sustaining perception is the predictive ability resulting from users' association to previous experiences. Therefore, one of the strong points of a highly immersive VR environment is the multisensory integration coupled with complex brain processes and cognitive functions dealing with predictions. This implies that the content and the context of the VR, together with the multisensory function integration, in particular vision, may contribute to a more immersive experience for the user.

The immersive nature of VR and its potential to support empathy extends the functionalities of the medium to a more diverse range of applications. Its potential to move beyond low fidelity simulations to integrate a more complex approach to display different realities make it ideal as an emerging technology to be used in education and training, especially in areas that involve patient care as demonstrated in the following section.

APPLICATIONS OF VIRTUAL REALITY FOR MENTAL HEALTH TREATMENT AND EDUCATION

Treatment

The exponential increase in articles on VR in mental health with recent studies on VR with autism and other illness indicates that it could be beneficial to use the VR technique for recreating scenarios in a laboratory environment Valmaggia, 2017. This section focuses on the specifuc application of VR to the management of psychosis.

The use of VR in psychosis shows promise. The term psychosis refers to conditions that affect the mind, where there has been some loss of contact with reality. During a period of psychosis, a person's thoughts and perceptions are disturbed and the individual may have difficulty understanding what is real and what is not. Symptoms of psychosis include delusions (false beliefs) and hallucinations (seeing or hearing things that others do not see or hear) of Mental Health, 2020.

VR, which can allow patients to talk to an avatar of their hallucinations, explore locations that give them anxiety, and practice talking to others in a variety of threatening or non-threatening situations, gives patients the chance to work through their own fears in a no-risk environment. The added element of AI takes the software a step further by enabling the system to learn, reason, perceive and execute tasks that have the best chance of achieving a specific goal.

So far, research related to VR, AI and psychosis has been targeted at im-proving function, and studies have been conducted to examine methods for improving cognition, social skills, job interview skills, and to augment cognitive behavioural therapy (CBT) in schizophrenia or other mental disorders with psychosis.

Currently there are four pioneering research centers in VR research in relation to mental health with specific focus on psychosis. Oxford VR[2], which is a spinout company from Oxford University is led by Freeman who has established the use of VR in mental health and is a pioneer in developing automated immersive technologies to increase access to evidence-based psychological therapies. Oxford VR builds on Freeman's research into the use of VR to understand and treat psychological disorders. In 2019, Freeman launched an ongoing trial called 'THRIVE'. In this trial, multiple centers are exploring the use of therapy through VR to people with persecutory delusions. This involves the use of virtual social situations, which are graded in difficulty and which patients need to navigate through Freeman et al., 2019. Whilst doing this, an automated avatar coach provides cognitive therapy. In this manner, the need for a therapist to be physically present may not be required and the treatment is scalable to include different contexts, and scenarios. Furthermore, Freeman and colleagues have just initiated a new trial called 'Game Change'. The objective is to place patients with schizophrenia into VR recreations of real-world situations they might find difficult, like getting on a bus or walking down the street. Many patients with psychosis experience everyday social situations as anxiety-provoking. Fear can lead patients to withdraw from activities, and this isolation leads to a cycle of worsening physical and mental health. Breaking this cycle requires highly active treatment directly in the troubling situations so that patients learn that they can safely and confidently enter them. However, patients with psychosis seldom receive such life-changing interventions. To solve this problem, Freeman developed an automated psychological treatment delivered in virtual reality. The idea is that spending time in virtual versions of stressful situations may help people better cope with the real thing.

King's College is another center which has been involved in VR and mental health research. The team led by Valmaggia had conducted earlier studies in the early 2000s, with the aim of assessing the safety aspect and the use of VR with the symptoms of psychosis (and other mental illnesses). In those early studies, it was established that people were able to distinguish between physical reality and VR. This gave positive indications that participation in virtual experiences does not make the symptoms worse.

Intricate detailing and planning go into designing a VR environmental situation Valmaggia, 2017. The VR lab at King's College London has an in-house programmer to assist in the creation of VR experiences which are developed alongside people that have the real-life experience, specifically psychosis.

The research team led by Craig at the University of Manchester has also been influential in this eld. Together with researchers from University College London, and King's College London, a VR treatment called AVATAR therapy for distressing auditory hallucinations was compared to traditional supportive counselling Rus-Calafell, Garety, Sason, Craig, et al., 2018a. AVATAR therapy is an experimental therapy which involves a face-to-face discussion between a person with schizophrenia and an avatar representing their auditory hallucination. The primary outcome of this therapy was a reduction in auditory verbal hallucinations at 12 weeks.

On similar lines, Peter Yellowlees, a psychiatrist at the University of Queensland in Brisbane, built a prototype 3D VR simulation that shows a typical living room projected onto a wrap-around screen Banks et al., 2004. The virtual setting can be modified to mimic common hallucinations. At the same time, a soundtrack gives an abusive running commentary, which is typical of many schizophrenic hallucinations. Yellowlees and his fellow researchers have also created a virtual psychotic environment based on photographs of an inpatient ward and hospital furnishings at UC Davis Medical Center. The team constructed simulations of auditory and visual hallucinations based on recorded audio samples and digital images described in interviews with schizophrenia patients. The researchers then inserted the hallucinations as individual objects that would appear automatically throughout the ward. Whilst Yellowlee's work holds promise, all his e orts in this eld seem to be dated between 2002 and 2006 with no recent updates.

In one of the most recent comprehensive systematic reviews on the topic of VR and mental health, Freeman et al., 2017 explored the application of virtual reality to the prominent mental illnesses. The findings highlighted the overwhelming application of this technology to anxiety disorders with 129 intervention studies being dedicated to this cause. The majority of the studies focus on phobia, with a minority of others being dedicated to Obsessive Compulsive Disorder. Most of the interventions were based on exposure and overall, the virtual reality treatment was comparable to face-to-face interventions in terms of efficacy. The review identified 44 virtual reality research studies that have explored the application of VR to schizophrenia and related issues, including 23 focusing on theory building, 15 on evaluation, and six on therapy testing. The research has mostly employed virtual reality to analyse psychotic episodes in attempt to figure out what causes them. Treatment trials are typically modest and limited in number, but the findings are highly promising. In another recent systematic review, Rus-Calafell, Garety, Sason, Craig, et al., 2018 described how the most significant additional advantages of VR as applied to psychosis, may turn out to be for therapy. In this view, VR allows professionals to assist patients in observing and changing their emotions, cognitions, and behaviours in real-time, in carefully controlled situations. Three of the eight treatment studies found that participants enjoyed using new technologies in the clinical setting, that it increased their motivation for treatment (Park et al., 2011) and that it was more interesting and useful than traditional training (Tsang and Mann, 2013). Clearly, this research is still in its infancy and the limited studies available cannot yet indicate whether VR is more efficacious than alternative therapies with similar goals that require less technological resources. Notably, the effect sizes for target symptom improvement are promising in several of the existing studies (Rus-Calafell, Garety, Sason, Craig, et al., 2018b)

Surprisingly, in their systematic review, Freeman et al., 2017 reported that they could only locate two studies on the application of virtual reality to de-pression. Virtual reality has also been applied successfully to substance misuse. The authors discussed how virtual reality has the ability to o er individuals with simulations of the signals that lead to cravings, which drive subsequent harmful behaviours like drug abuse or alcohol abuse. To this extent, there have been 22 virtual reality research studies on substance abuse, with 15 focusing on evaluation, five on therapy, and two on theory building. The final mental illness explored during the systematic review by Freeman et al., 2017 concerned the area of eating disorders. In this area, reduced food cravings, improved body im-age, and improved emotional control abilities are all apparent objectives for VR. Ten of the studies on VR as applied to eating disorders dealt with therapy, seven with assessment, and one with theory building. The authors of the systematic review noted that one of the most interesting studies in this area was carried out by Keizer et al., 2016 who facilitated the experience of a healthy Body Mass Index by individuals with anorexia nervosa. The results showed that for at least two hours after the VR exposure, the participants had a reduction in body size overestimation. Other recent research on the application of VR to mental health includes that by Browning (2020) who demonstrated how nature exposure in VR can enhance emotional well-being in those who do not have access to the outdoors. In another study by Tsung-Yi et al., 2020, the researchers explored the physical and mental health effects of a combination of virtual reality and horticultural therapy on older adults in an institution. The results suggested that a 9-week program schedule is enough to lead to an improved health status, life meaning, loneliness, perceived mattering and depression amongst this population group.

Despite the obvious advantages of VR, it is important to remember that the current data has limitations. The main limitations noted are:

VR has been defined differently within existing studies, ranging from a computer screen that is used to create a 2D virtual world to 3D immersive head-mounted displays
Varying levels of immersion
Small sample sizes
The process involved in VR-assisted therapy is not adequately explored
Limited follow-up periods
Reliability and validity tests lack robustness
The combined use of Artificial Intelligence and Virtual Reality

In identifying the existing research gaps in this area, Freeman et al., 2017, identified three questions that need to be answered:

1. "What is the best way to immerse individuals in VR so that learning most readily transfers to the real world, balancing the need to use affordable equipment?"
2. "Can key theory-driven psychological treatment techniques (beyond simple exposure) be successfully delivered in VR?"
3. "Do engaging, personalized, theory-driven treatments implemented in affordable VR, with limited use of clinicians, produce large real-world benefits for patients?"

Education

The technological advancements and accessibility of sophisticated handheld Virtual reality devices is now more than ever providing an opportunity to expand the reach and depth of technology in healthcare education. Despite the advantages of virtual reality technologies for education, the development in this area is rather poor. Warburton, (2009) reports that such development may be hindered by the barriers of use including technical complexity, difficulty in establishing a sense of identity in collaborative virtual environments, the development of cliques amongst users of virtual technologies, time and money issues and the proliferation of platforms and standards that make inter-operability be-tween simulations di cult which, in turn, reduces opportunities for sharing these resources. Loughlin (2017) further reports more obstacles that limit the development of VR technologies in healthcare education, namely the self-perceived lack of technological support and skills amongst educators and students. This highlights the need of supportive guidance and clear instructions (Warburton, 2009).

It must be acknowledged that although the cost to development a simple VR simulation is not prohibitive, the cost for development VR simulations for an educational institution, including the devices necessary to enable usage is relatively higher. Fortunately, the accessibility and ownership of mobile handheld devices amongst students may contribute to a more accessibility and personalised used of this technology. A need arises for the development and deployment of providing online access to practice simulation in high quality healthcare education using Virtual Reality as this has the potential to further widen the access to healthcare education. Falconer, (2013) describes that the use of virtual reality in education justify the financial costs as such technology enables the students to experience a sense of place in the virtual environment which would influence their studies in a wider context than the specific simulation. The potential benefits of place and identity experience for healthcare students is significant. Virtual reality can provide a range of place educational opportunities, including familiarisation experiences of their clinical work placements prior to the even before they commencement of their clinical placements, as well as the experience of potential clinical scenarios which may be discussed during the theoretical component. This allows for the practice of aspects such as skills in a safe setting, which students might find challenging or rarely encounter in practice. Also the repeated practice using VR strengthens the knowledge and skills previously learned. Multi-user Virtual Reality Learning Environments (VRLE) further allow the bridging of the theory practice gap by engaging students in co-learning through professional and/or a multi-disciplinary group. Such examples include case conferences, or experiencing of procedures with other real life healthcare workers such as clinical assessments or triage. Results emerging form a pilot study conducted by King et al. (2018) investigating the use of virtual reality learning environments in healthcare education to bridge the theory practice gap and improve patient safety identifies that students found the option of learning using VRLEs as a valuable addition to their learning and that VRLE increased their knowledge, confidence and reasoning as well as had a positive impact on the quality of care provided to their patients in clinical practice. The technical complexity of creating and running VR simulations means that partnerships with developer companies are often a feature of these approaches to educational uses of VR. Such partnerships provide significant creative opportunities for the development of educational experiences, and also o er operational opportunities for knowledge exchange between educators and developers. This co-operation in design between healthcare academics, clinical practitioners, technical researchers and developers must ensure that the VRLEs created are sustainable, trusted and valued by all parties involved. Moreover, whilst such technology presents with a host of benefits, it also raises ethical considerations that need to be considered before applying VR as a tool in mental health education and training.

Ethical Issues in Mental Health Education and Training

The incorporation and presence of technology in our environment, has an influence on the way we think, perceive the world around us and how we behave. The Stanford Prison Experiment Haney et al., 1973 and Milgram's obedience experiments Milgram, 1974 are two eminent examples in the long list of related studies that demonstrate how human behaviour relates to our environment, and consequently, how flexible in its adjustment and response is the human mind. VR has considerable potential in instigating both positive and negative experiences, such as stimulating pro-social emotions or biased and inaccurate representations that can alter perceptions of persons or groups Ford, 2001. In settings where it is virtually impossible to undergo the full clinical experience, VR can also o er learners a controlled simulation environment which is interactive and which can extend their imagination, thus increasing their cognitive skills via situational awareness. However, besides instigating emotional responses, there is evidence that the use of VR can also have an impact on the users' behaviour that might have permanent or semi-permanent effects. A study by Yee and Bailenson Yee and Bailenson, 2007 investigated users' change in behaviour following the illusion of embodiment in VR. Participants who were assigned an avatar in the VR and who saw themselves as this avatar during the virtual session, exhibited changes in their behaviour that were in accordance with their perceived stereotypes of the character. Hence, when participants were assigned avatars belonging to a minority group, such as a short, dark skinned female avatar, their reactions reflected their preconceived concepts of how such a person would respond in a given circumstance. This became known as the 'Proteus Effect' and is an ethical concern that has to be considered when designing VR experiences, especially when applied to education, and more so when the eld is that of mental health education.

There is a substantial body of research exploring the application of VR in the eld of mental health, targeting treatment and/or cure of a number of disorders Spiegel, 2018. Such benefits relate to the therapeutic applications of VR for a wide range of conditions including social phobias, panic attacks, body-image disturbances and post-traumatic stress disorder. However, studies relating to this eld pay particular attention to participant recruitment, for which screening is required both in the recruitment of study participants and in excluding others who may be at risk of aggravating an extant psychological condition or who may have an undetected psychiatric vulnerability Madary and Metzinger, 2016. Although VR treatments have demonstrated some promising results, it is not clear whether such therapies will ultimately be more effective than traditional therapeutic regimens Gregg and Tarrier, 2007; Parsons and Rizzo, 2008. Moreover, the perception of VR as a 'novel' form of treatment in comparison to what is traditionally practiced, may actually lead patients to interpret its success more favourably and also further strengthen any false hopes or 'therapeutic misconceptions' that patients may entertain. Hence, when exploring the therapeutic application of VR with persons having mental health illnesses, the services of a certified professional specialized in the area is required.

However, some contemporary research is also exploring the application of VR in the eld of mental health education. Professionals are exploiting the affordances of VR including complex simulations that lead to increased presence and immersion. In fact, an association has been demonstrated between VR simulation and improvements in attitudes, knowledge and empathy in users Wan and Lam, 2019. This highlights the need for discussions about ethical issues and considerations that need to be taken into account before experimenting with VR in Mental Health Education. The creation of a framework for supporting the correct ethical use of VR in Mental Health Education is therefore an important task for research in this novel domain.

The Belmont Report is one such framework that can be adopted and adapted for the context of VR. This consists mainly of three meta-categories: (1) non-maleficence and beneficence, (2) autonomy, and (3) justice.

The first principle of non-maleficence can be exemplified when the user experiences harm that goes against the innate principle of beneficence. A simplified rule for non-maleficence can be summarised in terms of experimentation. VR experiments involving any possible serious or long-lasting harm to the user should not be conducted. The blurring of the distinction between the real and illusory may pose mental health risks such as depersonalization and derealization dissociative disorders Madary and Metzinger, 2016. Depersonalization incorporates an experience of detachment from the bodily self i.e., from one's own feelings, thoughts or actions, whilst derealization is marked by a sense of detachment or feeling of unreality with respect to one's environment. Such a detachment from one's environment has also been further associated with a loss of certain social skills such as face-to-face communication that is basic for interpersonal relationships. Some VR users also struggle with lasting cognitive, emotional and behavioural consequences relating to a prolonged difficulty in readjusting and 'returning' to the physical world Hersh eld et al., 2011, where in some instances, doubts also arise regarding whether the real world is at all real. Therefore, each environment needs to be designed for the bene t of the users. When this is framed in terms of a mental health educational environment, there needs to be a balance between immersing learners in the world of the patients and mitigating the risks for the VR users.

The second principle of autonomy signifies that participants should have autonomy and control over their participation in the VR environment. In support of this, all potential participants should be presented with coherent and accurate information detailing the bene ts and possible risks of participating in a VR experience. This incorporates coherent statements to the effect that the VR experience can have lasting behavioural consequences on them, and that there may even be some presently unknown risks tied to such experiences. The per-son's right to decline participation or to withdraw from the study at any point throughout the study should be respected. Researcher/s should also ensure that no person feels coerced to participate due to the investigator being in a position of authority and power over the participant Meltzo, 2005. Furthermore, all procedures must conform to the standards laid down in applicable law and as required by any relevant authority (such as a professional body). The informed consent process includes a formal acknowledgement from the participant/client to the researcher or practitioner. Participants should also be provided with de-brie ng following the procedure that can serve as a guided re-entry procedure to avoid possible cognitive, emotional and/or behavioural trauma and ill effects Behr et al., 2005.

The third ethical principle of justice in the context of this analysis, implies that researchers using VR to explore mental health issues need to be free from biases, to enable proper investigations into a phenomenon. This is of particular relevance in a scenario, where persons with severe mental illnesses often encounter stigmatising attitudes as a consequence of misperceptions, stereotypical beliefs and prejudice associated with mental illness Morgan et al., 2018. Moreover, justice also incorporates the aspect of fairness in subject selection, indicating that persons with a mental illness should not be included in any research simply on the basis of easy accessibility, vulnerability or increased manipulability.

The VR environment also lends itself to a number of other risk factors for which correct ethical procedures and guidelines need to be in place. When experiencing VR, one major risk is that users might be subject to motion sickness, also known as 'Cybersickness'. In such cases, users may experience nausea, vomiting, fatigue, dizziness, headaches and body distortions LaViola, 2000. Various factors have been identified that may predispose persons to motion sickness, such as the ingesting of particular pharmacological agents and hence, the importance of screening persons prior to their VR experience. Aside from screening, studies by Kim et al., 2018 have emerged with a Virtual Reality Sickness Questionnaire (VRSQ) which participants can take as a test in the VR environment prior to the actual VR experience. Target selection is one of the primary components of the VRSQ, in a bid to support hand-to-eye coordination tasks in VR that possibly may mitigate Cybersickness symptoms. Cybersickness may also occur when there is a mismatch between the sensory information received and the participants' perceptual system. Design factors ensuring that the virtual environment reflects the physics of the real world allowing for user interaction and control and in general increasing the sense of presence in the world, may help lessen such Cybersickness Weech et al., 2019. However, research in this area is still quite novel and ongoing.

Another risk factor is that of having a sensory information overload, that may arise due to the volume and nature of the information received through a VR experience. Such information may present as complex and/or confusing and may overtax the users' cognitive ability to process and store any relevant information. This may occur for instance, when users are exposed to a vivid VR experience such as exposure to the auditory and visual hallucinations experienced by persons having schizophrenia. The user may consequently be exposed to a higher degree of immersion and intensity, that may strain and endanger their well-being. Any discussion relating to ethical issues in the use of VR in mental health should also bear in mind the part that cultural diversity may play. For example, the present albeit very limited research that is occurring on this topic, is cross-cultural or mostly limited to the Western hemisphere. We need to be aware of the risk of generalizing our perspective to other people who may perceive and interpret matters in a different manner. Nonetheless, despite the concerns flagged around the use of VR and ethical considerations, one must still assert the positive results from such usage, and that the future still holds much promise for alleviating mental health symptoms and challenges. It is in being open and receptive, but also reasonably cautious, that we can ensure that VR use adheres to ethical regulations without impinging on its potential relating to empowerment of the human being and the containment and eventual cure of various mental illnesses that still puzzle us today. As with many things related to health, where balance in usage is attained, there is room for improvement and for a healthy outcome.

The following section presents a case study applying VR in the elds of education and health care and also discusses the ethical issues relevant to the case study.

Case Study: Training in VR for Dealing with Hallucinations in Psychosis

A research team from the University of Malta have collaborated on a project to create a virtual simulation that will allow the user to experience specific symptoms of a patient suffering from psychosis, including visual and auditory hallucinations. This project is part of an ongoing collaboration between the Department of AI and the Department of Mental Health at the University of Malta, to provide support and foster empathy for patient care. This involves exploring new and innovative technologies as part of the approach to enhance the student's learning experience and to allow the user to walk in the shoes of a person suffering from these illnesses or disorders. Only by appreciating the challenges faced by the patients, can the students fully understand more about the disorder, and be in a position to give better assistance.

Artificial Intelligence, AI, was adopted in the present case study to support the interactive narrative which is used to make the simulation more realistic. The outcome of the story is influenced by the user's actions and decisions, as the Autonomous Agents (AA), take the appropriate actions based on these decisions. The visual and auditory hallucinations are part of the AA, and these will also react to the user's actions and responses. From a more technical point of view, the innovative combination of VR and AI, required extensive thought and planning. Combining these two technologies in an effective manner to enhance the experience in a way that is relevant to the subject matter and to enrich the narrative of the simulation, was quite challenging. VR is all about the user experience, so the role of AI would be to improve that experience for the user. The value of an experience is quite subjective and therefore this is hard to quantify and measure. The content captured within the VR is important for the user experience. In this case study, the participants needed to be engaged with the patient suffering from psychosis including hallucinations. This is not trivial since emotions vary between different users and this affects their level of engagement. We used AI to personalise experiences for different users, so as to support a greater engagement with the experience.

By using a virtual reality headset, the user is immersed in a virtual environment, and is able to experience the surroundings from the perspective of a patient suffering from psychosis. The project team took into account that the VR simulation had to be developed for a group of mental health trainee nurses, studying at the University. Therefore, the design emphasised roles, and contexts which the trainee nurses could identify and associate with. The context of the virtual simulation was taken to be in an office location to better illustrate how persons affected by psychosis would interact in a work environment. The objective of the VR is to enable the user to navigate the virtual world, attempt to perform simple tasks and attempt to interact with the virtual characters in-habiting the world, whilst being subject to visual and auditory hallucinations.

Participants were briefed before taking the VR experience, and they were also informed of how data would be collected. The Oculus Rift was used as the headset device for the VR experience. This was set up in a dedicated lab, and participant sitting was limited to one person per time taking the experience. A survey was given to the participants following their VR experience to collect their feedback following their VR experience. A standardized tool for VR to measure user experience in immersive virtual environments developed by Tcha-Tokey et. al. (2016) was used. Additional items were added to the questionnaire to gain more insights into the effect of AI (visible through the adaptive storyline, hallucinations and dialogue) on the level of engagement of the participants with the experience. From the results obtained there was a positive indication that the participants felt engaged with the VR experience. Positive feedback was also received for the natural ow of the storyline and interactive narrative, as well as for the hallucinations. This gave an indication that the AI used for adaptation and personalisation, affected the experience in a positive manner.

Figure 1. Screenshot of the reception scene. If the user avoids speaking to the receptionist on the left, the colleague on the right will prompt the user to go back and speak to the receptionist. However if the user has already spoken to the receptionist, the agent will be aware and thus the character will say something else (Source: Self).

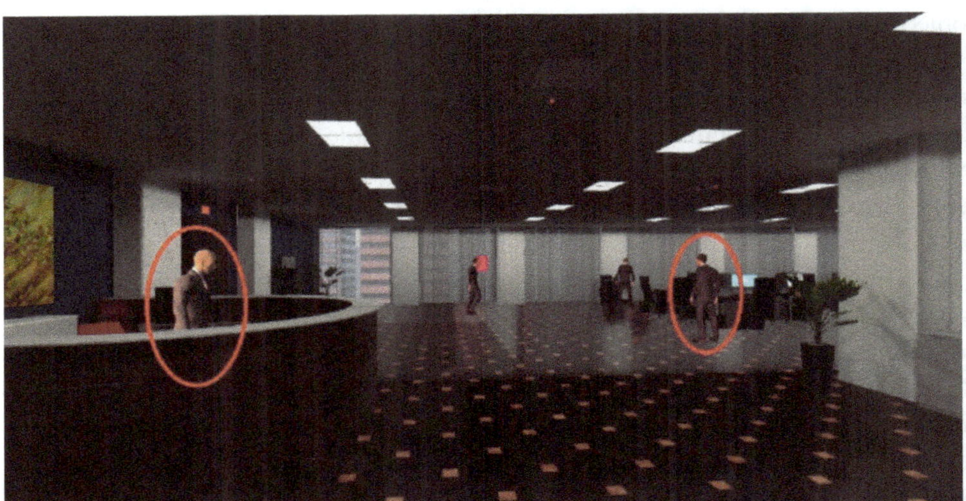

The use of autonomous agents driving the storyline, operating through the use of a Heuristic Search Planner (HSP), was effective in creating a dynamic narrative.

Throughout multiple different trials of the simulation, different actions would be taken by the various characters within the virtual environment depending on the actions and decisions taken by the users trialling the system. This approach and architecture also proved to be very scalable. An infinite amount of new possible storylines can be created by simply adding new actions to the NPCs and specifying their pre-conditions and effects, without needing to specify when or where or with whom they should occur.

In the present case study, the user becomes the patient, going through the motions of a day at the office. There is the morning greeting, simple tasks, such as answering the phone and going to the office of the boss. The user interacts using voice, as well as hand gestures for manipulation of objects.

A challenge posed by the study however, involved user experience with VR. Since for many, VR is still a relatively new technology, a substantial number of participants, had never experienced it before. Experiencing certain negative consequences such as motion sickness, dizziness or nausea are very common when using VR applications, and even more so for users new to the technology and who are not familiar with it. Feeling dizzy and nauseous whilst using Virtual Reality applications has been reported in a number of previous studies Clarke et al., 2016; Egan et al., 2016; Mosadeghi et al., 2016. Therefore, care was taken to ensure as smooth an experience as possible, to prevent users from experiencing motion sickness. Otherwise, not only is the motion sickness a problem in and of itself, but it might cause users to stop early and prevent them from paying attention to the intended objectives of the simulation.

As outlined in the previous sections however, when designing this immersive experience various ethical issues come into play due to the sensitive nature of the study. Thus, the principle of autonomy was safeguarded by providing participants with an information sheet that provided full details of the study including the bene t and risks of participation and their right to withdraw from the study at any point in time, without the need for justification. This enabled the participants to give informed written consent if they were willing to participate. In addition, potential participants were initially approached by a group of intermediaries and not by the researchers to avoid any experience of coercion. To overcome the challenge posed by the principles of non-maleficence and beneficence, staff from the Department of Mental Health were available at all times throughout the evaluations, and in the case that a student experiences any form of distress, student participation would stop immediately. Following the evaluations debriefing was provided and the services of a clinical psychologist could still be availed of should the participant express the need for further assistance.

Although the results of this project cannot be generalised to different categories of users, this case study provides an interesting insight into how VR and AI can merge

Figure 2. Screenshot of the office scene. The agents need to direct the user towards the manager's office at the back of the room. If the user takes the left path he will be prompted by the phone. If the user takes the right path, he will be prompted by another colleague. The agents are aware of the storyline and will only act at the appropriate times and if required (Source: Self).

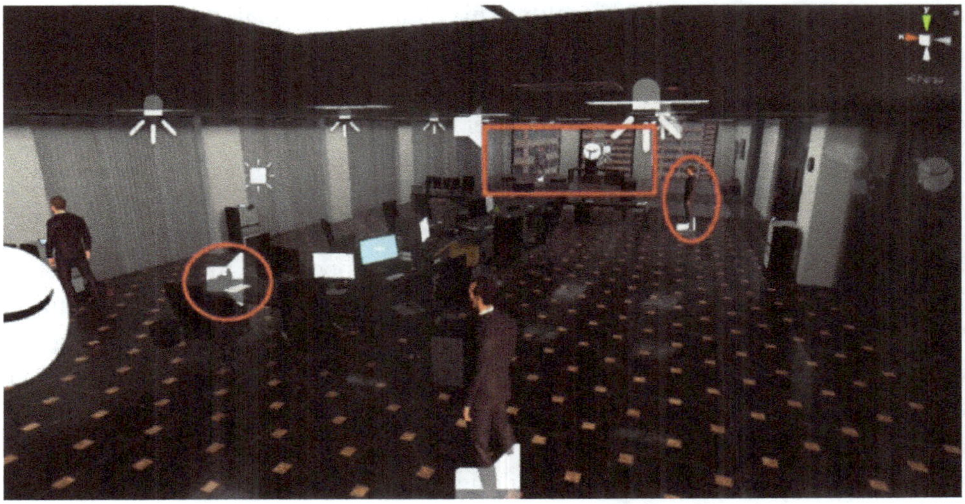

for an interactive immersive narrative in mental health education and training. Our evaluation has also shown that people with previous experience in VR found it easier to use the system and navigate through the Virtual Environment. We can predict that as VR becomes more mainstream, users will begin to feel more comfortable and thus be more receptive to using these technologies as part of their training.

RECOMMENDATIONS

This case study has shown that VR systems enhanced by AI can be a useful adjunct to traditional mental health teaching methods. However, a number of recommendations are being postulated in order to enhance the combination of such methods. As a starting point, it has to be acknowledged that VR environments have the potential to traumatise students due to the inclusion of elements that can be frighteningly realistic. Whilst closeness to reality is a desired element of a VR system, the undertaking of immersive fictional recreations by students needs to be supported with mental health monitoring and support.

Another aspect that needs to be considered is that the patients who feature in VR teaching methods are not equivalent to real patients and so clinic-based teaching has to remain at the lead in facilitating students' appreciation and understanding of mental health symptoms. Whilst AI offers the benefit of an interactive and reactive interface, it does not cater for all the possible scenarios that may present during the face-to-face interaction between a care provider and a care receiver. The 'serendipity' element that often characterises therapeutic interchanges is di cult to replicate in a lab environment using virtual reality. This element is crucial in the education of mental health care professionals since it prompts them to 'think on the spot', be creative and become competent in 'therapeutic flexibility', which is an important element in person-centred care. This refers to the ability to adapt to person and circumstance in a manner that remains therapeutic and that caters to a particular person's needs Santana et al., 2018.

Another aspect to consider is the need to provide feedback to students. Since VR-AI-based settings can be accessed remotely (as opposed to traditional teaching in a classroom setting), self-discipline and enthusiasm for learning must be retained. This can be challenging if there is no interaction with teachers or students during the experience. Thus setting up a feedback system is important. This can be achieved through online platforms or by following up the virtual reality experience with a classroom-based discussion Combs and Combs, 2019.

Another consideration applies to the design of the VR experience. If consideration is not made to represent population and cultural diversity, bias can ensue Combs and Combs, 2019. Thus, if all the virtual patients in a given virtual environment characterise a particular ethnic group, this can result in teaching and learning flaws. This is brought about by the fact that the student may be failing to understand that mental health symptoms may present differently across cultures and that this must be catered for during the assessment and management processes. Thus, during the construction of a VR system, the opinions of the computer scientists combined with the mental health professionals must be sought since these can aggect the outcome.

CONCLUSION

This chapter presented an overview of literature related to the use of VR in the simulation of the symptoms of psychosis, as a treatment medium and as an educational tool in the eld of psychosis. A discussion on the ethical issues related to the use of this technology ensued, which highlighted the crucial considerations and safeguards that have to be in place during the application of VR and AI to the mental health sector. In particular, awareness of the Proteus effect, the need for psychological assistance during exposure and potential de-personalisation/derealisation effects are amongst the issues that were addressed. Subsequently, the creation of a framework for supporting the correct ethical use of VR in mental health education was strongly suggested. Following this discussion, a case study on the use of a VR and artificial intelligence (AI) based application for the symptoms of psychosis was presented. This was based on a project that was carried out at the University of Malta through the joint collaboration of the Department of Mental Health and the Department of Artificial Intelligence. The aim of this project was to develop a VR and AI-based experience that simulates the visual and auditory hallucinations of psychosis for use as an educational tool for mental health students. The experience was developed by the University of Malta team placing the viewer in first person as one suffering from auditory and visual hallucinations. The application was piloted on a small group of mental health nursing students and data was collected in relation to the students' experience and perception of the application. The findings showed that the students appreciated the immersive experience as it added a realistic angle to the understanding of psychotic symptoms. However, motion sickness, dizziness and nausea were reported by some as being factors that somewhat limited the experience. Whilst this was probably related to the fact that many of the users had never made use of such technology, it is a consideration that has to be kept in mind when applying such technology to mental health. Conclusively, a number of recommendations were provided for improvement of the application and for applying VR and AI based technologies in an effective and ethically sound manner in the mental health area. Whilst the effectiveness of such technologies when compared to traditional treatment and educational means has to be established, this area certainly holds promise both for treatment and education. As discussed, it is not without its risks and so thorough consideration by professionals has to be made in order to protect the user's well-being.

REFERENCES

Banks, J., Ericksson, G., Burrage, K., Yellowlees, P., Ivermee, S., & Tichon, J. (2004). Constructing the hallucinations of psychosis in virtual reality. *Journal of Network and Computer Applications, 27*(1), 1-11. doi:10.1016/S1084-8045(03)00031-6

Bedi, G., Carrillo, F., Cecchi, G. A., Slezak, D. F., Sigman, M., Mota, N. B., Ribeiro, S., Javitt, D. C., Copelli, M., & Corcoran, C. M. (2015). Au-tomated analysis of free speech predicts psychosis onset in high-risk youths. *NPJ Schizophrenia, 1*, 15030.

Behr, K., Nosper, A., Klimmt, C., & Hartmann, T. (2005). Some practical considerations of ethical issues in vr research. *Presence, 14*(6), 668- 676.

Camilleri, J., Scicluna, D., Bria, V., Camiller, V., Dingli, A., & Montebello, M. (2016). *If you aren't experiencing it, you're not understanding it! using virtual reality to understand migrants*. Academic Press.

Camilleri, V., Haddod, F., Montebello, M., Camilleri, J. C., Dingli, A., & Bria, V. (2019). Virtual reality (vr) applications in learning: living autism. In *Cases on immersive virtual reality techniques*. IGI Global.

Camilleri, V., Montebello, M., Dingli, A., & Bria, V. (2017). Walking in small shoes: Investigating the power of vr on empathising with children's dificulties, In *2017 23rd international conference on virtual system & multimedia (vsmm)*. IEEE.

Chrunch, T. (2018). *Facebook rolls out ai to detect suicidal posts before they're reported*. https://newsroom.intel.com/news- releases/u- s- healthcare- leaders-expect-widespread-adoption-arti cial-intelligence-2023/

Clarke, D., McGregor, G., Rubin, B., Stanford, J., & Graham, T. (2016). Arcaid:addressing situation awareness and simulator sickness in a virtual reality pac-man game. *Proceedings of the 2016 Annual Symposium on Computer-Human Interaction in Play Companion Extended Abstracts*, 39-45.

Combs, C., & Combs, F. (2019). Emerging roles of virtual patients in the age of ai. *AMA Journal of Ethics, 21*(2), 153. amajethics.2019.153 doi:10.1001/

Corcoran, C. M., Carrillo, F., Fernandez-Slezak, D., Bedi, G., Klim, C., Javitt, D. C., Bearden, C. E., & Cecchi, G. A. (2018). Prediction of psychosis across protocols and risk cohorts using automated language analysis. *World Psychiatry, 17*(1), 67-75.

Corporation, I. (2018). *Us healthcare leaders expect widespread adoption of ai by 2023*. Accessed on 22nd May 2020. https://newsroom.intel.com/news- releases/u-s- healthcare- leaders-expect-widespread-adoption-arti cial-intelligence-2023/

Cullen, W., Gulati, G., & Kelly, B. (2020). Mental health in the covid-19 pandemic. *QJM: An International Journal of Medicine, 113*(5), 311-312.

De la Pena, N., Weil, P., Llobera, J., Giannopoulos, E., Pomes, A., Spanlang, B., Friedman, D., Sanchez-Vives, M., & Slater, M. (2010). Immersive journalism: Immersive virtual reality for the rst-person experience of news. *Presence: Teleoperators and Virtual Environments, 19*(4), 291-301.

Egan, D., Brennan, S., Barrett, J., Qiao, Y., Timmerer, C., & Murray, N. (2016). An evaluation of heart rate and electrodermal activity as an objec- tive qoe evaluation method for immersive virtual reality environments. *Eighth International Conference on Quality of Multimedia Experience (QoMEX)*, 1-6.

Ewbank, M. P., Cummins, R., Tablan, V., Bateup, S., Catarino, A., Mar-tin, A. J., & Blackwell, A. D. (2020). Quantifying the association be-tween psychotherapy content and clinical outcomes using deep learning. *JAMA Psychiatry, 77*(1), 35-43.

Fabiano, D., Canavan, S., Agazzi, H., Hinduja, S., & Goldgof, D. (2020). Gaze-based classi cation of autism spectrum disorder. *Pattern Recognition Letters*.

Fitzpatrick, K. K., Darcy, A., & Vierhile, M. (2017). Delivering cognitive behavior therapy to young adults with symptoms of depression and anxiety using a fully automated conversational agent (woebot): A randomized controlled trial. *JMIR Mental Health*, *4*(2), e19.

Ford, P. (2001). A further analysis of the ethics of representation in virtual reality: Multi-user environments. *Ethics and Information Technology, 3*, 113-121.

Freeman, D., Lister, R., Waite, F., Yu, L.-M., Slater, M., Dunn, G., & Clark, D. (2019). Automated psychological therapy using virtual reality (vr) for patients with persecutory delusions: Study protocol for a single-blind parallel-group randomised controlled trial (thrive). *Trials*, *20*(1). https://doi.org/10.1186/s13063-019-3198-6

Freeman, D., Reeve, S., Robinson, A., Ehlers, A., Clark, D., Spanlang, B., & Slater, M. (2017). Virtual reality in the assessment, understanding, and treatment of mental health disorders. *Psychological Medicine, 47*, 2393-2400. doi:10.1017/S003329171700040X

Gattupalli, S., Ebert, D., Papakostas, M., Makedon, F., & Athitsos, V. (2017). Cognilearn: A deep learning-based interface for cognitive behavior as-sessment. *Proceedings of the 22nd international conference on intelligent user interfaces*.

Giroux, M., Barra, J., Gra, C., & Guerraz, M. (2019). Illusory perception of one's own movements in virtual reality. *Neurophysiologie Clinique*, *49*(6), 437.

Gonzalez-Franco, M., & Lanier, J. (2017). *Model of illusions and virtual reality*. Academic Press.

Gregg, L., & Tarrier, N. (2007). Virtual reality in mental health: A review of the literature. *Social Psychiatry and Psychiatric Epidemiology, 42*, 343-354.

Gruber, J., Prinstein, M. J., Clark, L. A., Rottenberg, J., Abramowitz, J. S., Albano, A. M., Aldao, A., Borelli, J. L., Chung, T., & Davila, J. (2020). Mental health and clinical psychological science in the time of covid-19: Challenges, opportunities, and a call to action. *American Psychologist*.

Hamet, P., & Tremblay, J. (2017). Artificial intelligence in medicine. *Metabolism, 69*, S36-S40.

Haney, C., Banks, W., & Zimbardo, P. (1973). Study of prisoners and guards in a simulated prison. *Naval Research Reviews, 9*, 1-17.

Hershfield, H., Goldstein, D., Sharpe, W., Fox, J., Yeykelis, L., & Carstensen, L. (2011). Increasing saving behavior through age-progressed renderings of the future self. *Journal of Marketing Research, 48*, S23-S37.

Just, M. A., Pan, L., Cherkassky, V. L., McMakin, D. L., Cha, C., Nock, M. K., & Brent, D. (2017). Machine learning of neural representations of sui-cide and emotion concepts identi es suicidal youth. *Nature human Behaviour, 1*(12), 911-919.

Katchapakirin, K., Wongpatikaseree, K., Yomaboot, P., & Kaewpitakkun, Y. (2018). Facebook social media for depression detection in the Thai community. In *2018 15th international joint conference on computer science and software engineering (JCSSE)*. IEEE.

Keizer, A., Van Elburg, A., Helms, R., & Dijkerman, H. (2016). a virtual reality full body illusion improves body image disturbance in anorexia nervosa. *PLoS One, 11*, e0163921.

Kim, H. K., Park, J., Choi, Y., & Choe, M. (2018). Virtual reality sickness questionnaire (vrsq): Motion sickness measurement index in a virtual reality environment. *Applied Ergonomics, 69*, 66-73.

Lanier, J. (1992). An insider's view of the future of virtual reality. *Journal of Communication, 42*, 150-172.

Lanier, J. (2017). *Dawn of the new everything: Encounters with reality and virtual reality*. Henry Holt, Co., Inc.

LaViola, J. (2000). A discussion of cybersickness in virtual environments. *SIGCHI Bulletin, 32*, 47-56.

Lup, K., Trub, L., & Rosenthal, L. (2015). Instagram# instasad? Exploring associations among instagram use, depressive symptoms, negative social comparison, and strangers followed. *Cyberpsychology, Behavior, and Social Networking, 18*(5), 247-252.

Madary, M., & Metzinger, T. (2016). Real virtuality: A code of ethical conduct. recommendations or good scientific practice and the consumers of vr-technology. *Frontiers in Robotics and AI, 3*. frobt.2016.00003 doi:10.3389/

Meltzo, J. (2005). *Ethics in research*. Academic Press.

Milgram, S. (1974). *Obedience to authority. an experimental view*. Tavi-stock.

Milk, C. (2015). *How virtual reality can create the ultimate empathy machine* [TED Talk]. https://www.ted.com/talks/chris milk how virtual reality can create the ultimate empathy machine

Morgan, A., Reavley, N., Ross, A., Too, L., & Jorm, A. (2018). Interventions to reduce stigma towards people with severe mental illness: Systematic review and meta-analysis. *Journal of Psychiatric Research, 130*, 120-133.

Mosadeghi, S., Reid, M., Martinez, B., Rosen, B., & Spiegel, B. (2016). Feasibility of an immersive virtual reality intervention for hospitalized patients: An observational cohort study. *JMIR Mental Health, 3*, 1-10.

O'Hear, S. (2017, Jan. 4). Babylon health partners with uk's nhs to replace telephone helpline with ai-powered chatbot. *TechCrunch*.

Park, K., Ku, J., Choi, S., Jang, H., Park, J., Kim, S., & Kim, J. (2011). A virtual reality application in role-plays of social skills training for schizophrenia: A randomized, controlled trial. *Psychiatry Research, 189*, 166-172.

Parsons, T., & Rizzo, A. (2008). Affective outcomes of virtual reality exposure therapy for anxiety and specific phobias: A meta-analysis. *Journal of Behavior Therapy and Experimental Psychiatry, 39*, 250-261.

Rezaii, N., Walker, E., & Wol, P. (2019). A machine learning approach to predicting psychosis using semantic density and latent content analysis. *NPJ Schizophrenia, 5*(1), 1-12.

Rus-Calafell, M., Garety, P., Sason, E., Craig, T. J. K., & Valmaggia, L. R. (2018). Virtual reality in the assessment and treatment of psychosis: A systematic review of its utility, acceptability and effectiveness. *Psychological Medicine, 48*(3), 362-391.

Santana, M., Manalili, K., Lu, M., Jolley, R., & Zelinsky, S. (2018). How to practice person-centred care: A conceptual framework. *Health Expectations: An International Journal of Public Participation in Health Care and Health Policy, 21*(2), 429. .1111/ hex.12640 doi:https://doi.org/https://doi.org/10

Sayed, S. I., Tsiakas, K., Bell, M., Athitsos, V., & Makedon, F. (2019). Cognitive assessment in children through motion capture and computer vision: The cross-your-body task. *Proceedings of the 6th international workshop on sensor-based activity recognition and interaction*.

Slater, M. (2018). Immersion and the illusion of presence in virtual reality. *British Journal of Psychology, 109*(3), 431-433.

Spiegel, J. (2018). The ethics of virtual reality technology: Social hazards and public policy recommendations. *Science and Engineering Ethics, 24*, 1537-1550.

Torales, J., O'Higgins, M., Castaldelli-Maia, J. M., & Ventriglio, A. (2020). The outbreak of covid-19 coronavirus and its impact on global mental health. *The International Journal of Social Psychiatry*.

Tsang, M., & Mann, D. (2013). A virtual reality-based vocational training system (vrvts) for people with schizophrenia in vocational rehabilitation. *Schizophrenia Research, 144*, 51-62.

Tsung-Yi, L., Huang, C., Hsu, H., Liao, J., Cheng, V., Wang, S., & Guo, J. (2020). Effects of a combination of three-dimensional virtual reality and hands-on horticultural therapy on institutionalized older adults' physical and mental health: Quasi-experimental design. *Journal of Medical Internet Research, 22*(11), e1902. https://doi.org/10.2196/19002

Valmaggia, L. (2017). The use of virtual reality in psychosis research and treatment. *World Psychiatry, 16*(3), 246-247. .20443 doi:10.1002/wps

Wan, H., W, & Lam, A. (2019). The effectiveness of virtual reality-based simulation in health professions education relating to mental illness: A literature review. *Health, 11*, 646-660.

Weech, S., Kenny, S., & Barnett-Cowan, M. (2019). Presence and cybersickness in virtual reality are negatively related: A review. *Frontiers in Psychology, 10*, 158.

Weizenbaum, J. (1966). Elizala computer program for the study of natural language communication between man and machine. *Communications of the ACM, 9*(1), 36-45.

Weizenbaum, J. (1976). *Computer power and human reason: From judgment to calculation*. Academic Press.

Wongkoblap, A., Vadillo, M. A., & Curcin, V. (2017). Researching mental health disorders in the era of social media: Systematic review. *Journal of Medical Internet Research, 19*(6), e228.

Yee, N., & Bailenson, J. (2007). The proteus effect: The effect of transformed self{representation on behavior. *Human Communication Research, 33*, 271-290.

Zhang, Z., Peng, Q., & Gu, P. (2010). Improvement of user involvement in product design. In *Proceedings of the cirp design conference innovative product creation*. Elsevier.

Chapter 7
Ethical Considerations in Prosthetics and Orthotics

Jesmond Attard
University of Malta, Malta

ABSTRACT

This chapter introduces the field of advanced technology within the orthotics and prosthetics profession, a healthcare profession that combines technology and engineering science with medical and health science to produce medical devices (orthoses and prostheses) to treat medical conditions that cause physical dysfunction. The chapter sets the background to the ethical dilemmas that are encountered within the field, which technologically advanced devices cause such dilemmas and why, and then discusses the ethical dilemmas as encountered by the three stakeholders within the profession, namely the manufacturers/innovators, the prosthetic and orthotic practitioners, and the users of the devices themselves, the patients. In conclusion, the chapter looks at some solutions and recommendations to overcome or at least reduce these dilemmas.

INTRODUCTION

Orthotics and prosthetics is a field in medicine, healthcare and rehabilitation that combines knowledge of medical and health sciences with engineering and technology to treat a particular medical condition which causes physical dysfunction. The International Society for Prosthetics and Orthotics ([ISPO], n.d.) defines prosthetics and orthotics as those specialties within the field of healthcare technology concerned with the design, manufacture and application of prostheses and orthoses. Prostheses are externally applied devices used to replace, wholly or in part, absent or deficient

DOI: 10.4018/978-1-7998-7888-9.ch007

limb segments, while orthoses are externally applied devices used to modify the structural and functional characteristics of the neuromuscular and skeletal system.

Prosthetists and orthotists are those healthcare professionals (clinicians or practitioners) responsible for evaluating a patient's specific functional and cosmetic needs, designing the prosthesis/orthosis and selecting the appropriate components, taking all the necessary measurements, fabricating, fitting, including evaluating the function of the device, and educating the patient on the appropriate use and care of the device (Nielsen & Jorge, 2013).

Since orthotic and prosthetic science incorporates knowledge of both medicine and engineering science, technology plays a major role in the delivery of such services; and since technology contributes to the provision of these services, innovation is continuous, hence the ethical questions arise: who is entitled to such services? Which devices may be supplied to service users? Is this a service where only the elite will get the best that technology has to offer, or is everyone "deserving" of the most advanced technology? When designing innovative products, are principles of best practice being implemented? What impact and consequences are innovations within the prosthetic and orthotic industry having on communities?

This chapter will discuss the above questions, so that, by the end, the reader may become more aware of the ethical problems and dilemmas that technological advances within the field of orthotics and prosthetics pose to health services providers, sometimes on a daily basis. This may also prompt the reader to reflect on ways to reach out to more people who are in need of these services, giving them more opportunities to use technologically advanced devices.

The author is an orthotist/prosthetist who has been practising for 25 years; therefore, most of the statements, thoughts and opinions making up this chapter are mainly the personal experience of the author, supported, where possible, by references from the literature.

BACKGROUND

On the frontline of the orthotics and prosthetics industry are the orthotists and prosthetists; these are the healthcare professionals, allied to medicine, who, on a daily basis, are faced with patients who are in need of their services.

Prosthetists and orthotists work within the medical and health sector, but they are very much unique in how they practise their profession, as compared to other professions allied to medicine, such as physiotherapists, occupational therapists or podiatrists, in that after they perform their initial assessment of the patient, and the patient's functional and aesthetic needs have been established, prosthetists and orthotists have to prescribe and design an orthotic or prosthetic device for that patient. Such a device comes at a cost, over and above the clinician's consultation fees.

In a nutshell, funding of orthotic and prosthetic services, like all other medical and rehabilitation services, may come from one of two sources:

1. A Universal Healthcare system, where healthcare is provided free at the point of delivery to patients. This does not mean that the cost of healthcare is zero, but that the care is funded by taxpayers' contributions. The state collects the taxes and distributes some of those funds to healthcare entities so they can treat patients free of charge, including orthotic and prosthetic services.
2. A Private Healthcare system, which can be either:
    a. An Insurance-based system, where individuals take out a medical insurance which covers, fully or partially, the cost of medical care and rehabilitation depending on the premium paid by that individual; orthotic and prosthetic services can also be funded in this way, or
    b. Self-funding, when a patient who needs medical care, including rehabilitation and/or orthotic and prosthetic services, decides to pay for such services from their own private funds.

There are advantages and disadvantages for both the above systems. Light (2018) argues that waiting times within a universal healthcare system are always an issue, and they are the main reasons why people turn to the private sector; on the other hand, she goes on to argue that cost is the main reason why people prefer to use a universal healthcare system, because private medical care is very expensive. Even if one has medical insurance, the premiums are sometimes too high and unaffordable, although different countries have different insurance-based systems, some more affordable than others. Another disadvantage of private medical care is choice, where one can only get the treatment that s/he can afford, which may not necessarily be what they actually need, or what is best for them.

Thus, when prescribing and designing a particular orthotic/prosthetic device for a patient, the orthotist/prosthetist is faced with quite a few questions, depending on which healthcare system they are working in, for example:

Which device is best for the patient?
Which device can the patient afford?
Is the patient paying for the service out of their own pocket, or have they got an insurance?
How much will the insurance pay? What will the insurance pay for?

Or, if the patient is being treated as part of a Universal Healthcare System, which device can the hospital afford for this patient? Is the device that the prosthetist/orthotist is prescribing listed on the health service's or hospital's formulary?

Which components can be used to fabricate the device to satisfy this patient's needs, or which components can the patient or health service/hospital afford?

The world of orthotics and prosthetics is relatively small, when compared to the pharmaceutical world, for example; the number of people who use prosthetic and orthotic devices is small when compared to the number of people in the world who use medication. Since the market is so small, there are only a few companies that manufacture orthotic and prosthetic devices, or components that make up such devices, but the competition is intense. This may create ethical issues both at the manufacturing level of the service and also at the point of delivery by the orthotists/prosthetists.

Jack Armold (1964) defined ethics as *the study of moral values and deals primarily with a choice involving human action*; he continues to say that the key word in this definition is *"choice"*, and that *a study of ethics helps in making wise choices*. The prosthetist/orthotist is faced with such ethical choices every day of their working life; they may be faced with both professional and business choices and decisions; how do they choose which of two very similar products is best for their patient? That may depend on which model of healthcare system they are working in. These are issues that the prosthetist/orthotist, as a healthcare professional, has to face every day, and that give rise to ethical dilemmas.

Manufacturers of prosthetic/orthotic devices or their components are also faced with ethical dilemmas: how do they apply best practice? Are end users involved in the innovation of new products using advanced technology? Are the needs of civil society being considered? Are the developers of new products working in an open and transparent way?

The next section will explore all the above questions faced by the various stakeholders in the industry.

THE ETHICAL DILEMMAS

Prosthetic and Orthotic Devices

There are many different kinds of orthotic and prosthetic devices; as mentioned above, all of these come at a cost and, since the market is small, the price is relatively high. In fact, Pasquina, Carvalho and Sheehan (2015) state that *the greatest cause of prosthesis and rehabilitation-related disparities in outcomes for those who have* *had amputations is **cost***. For someone who has gone through serious trauma, and lost one or more limbs, or at least lost the function of one or more limbs, or, perhaps, lost a limb through infection or disease, or was born with a limb or limb function deficiency, the most important goal of treatment or management of their deficiency is to help that person attain the maximum function and mobility, so that they can lead a fulfilled and active life. To achieve this goal, there are two main categories of orthotic and prosthetic devices: (a) static and (b) dynamic. Static devices merely support a limb (in the case of orthotic devices) and improve aesthetic appearance of the limb and the body as a whole (in the case of prosthetic devices), while dynamic devices, whether orthotic or prosthetic, attempt to improve function and movement. Dynamic devices can also be divided into two main types: (i) mechanically controlled (body-powered) and (ii) microprocessor controlled (externally powered). In today's world of advanced technology, where research in how to use the available technology to create technologically advanced orthotic and prosthetic devices remains ongoing, the kind of devices that usually create ethical dilemmas are certainly those that are at the forefront of advances in technology, because the difference in cost between body-powered devices and technologically advanced externally-powered ones is huge. These usually include those orthotic and prosthetic devices which are microprocessor controlled, such as microprocessor controlled prosthetic lower limb prostheses, externally powered (myoelectric or bionic) prosthetic hands and upper limb prostheses, microprocessor controlled lower limb orthoses, e.g. knee-ankle-foot orthoses (KAFOs), robotic exoskeletons (for persons who suffered a spinal cord injury and live with paraplegia) and externally powered upper limb orthoses (for the weak or flail arm and hand). There are also prosthetic devices for sports and leisure activities, namely running prostheses for both transtibial (below knee) and transfemoral (above knee) amputees.

Although the market, as mentioned earlier, is relatively small, there are quite a few externally powered or microprocessor controlled products (both orthotic and prosthetic devices) that are available for use by persons with limb deficiencies, whether such deficiencies include amputations or just loss of function. The largest market is obviously that for persons living with lower limb amputation, with available products including microprocessor controlled prosthetic knees and ankles. For persons living with upper limb amputations or congenital upper limb deficiencies, there are also various externally powered prosthetic devices, including prosthetic hands and elbows. In orthotics, the number of available externally powered devices is much smaller and not as widely used, yet.

But how do such prosthetic and orthotic devices work? Why are they so important in the rehabilitation of persons with functional limb deficiencies?

The greatest advances in prosthetic/orthotic technology have, without doubt, been achieved in lower limb prosthetics, namely for persons who have had their legs amputated above the knee. Microprocessor controlled knees all feature sensors, a microprocessor, computer software, a resistance system and a battery (Otto Bock UK,). The microprocessor (an internal computer inside the prosthetic knee) controls the internal fluid, which may be air (pneumatic control) or oil (hydraulic control), and continuously monitors each phase of the gait cycle via the sensors. This control allows the microprocessor to make adjustments in the resistance of the knee so that the amputee can walk with varying speeds across different types of surfaces, up and down ramps, and ascending and descending stairs. The same sensor technology is applied in microprocessor controlled lower limb orthoses; the sensors continuously measure the flexion of the knee joint and its angular acceleration so that the brace detects the user's current walking phase, regulates the resistance and thus controls the flexion and extension of the knee joint. With regards to microprocessor controlled prosthetic ankle joints, these also work by adjusting the resistance within the joint, thus varying the speed according to the gait situation with each step, on all types of surfaces.

Technological advances bring with them measured improvements; the same can be said for advances in prosthetics and orthotics. A few advantages of a microprocessor controlled prosthetic and orthotic lower limb device include:

- Requires less energy expenditure to walk,
- Requires less cognitive input to walk, once mode of operation is learnt,
- The outcome is a more natural gait due to less effort needed to control timing – also, the device powers down safely and gracefully,
- Increased walking endurance,
- Better control on uneven surfaces and walking up and down ramps,
- Ability to go up and down stairs one step over the other, rather than one step at a time,
- Reduced risk of falling due to a stumble recovery feature,
- Knee settings can be adjusted to suit the individual's needs, by using a computer or an App on a mobile phone,
- Some knees even adjust automatically according to the load that the individual is carrying, and
- Supports weight bearing in stand to sit transition.

[Adapted from Dupes (n.d.), NZALS (n.d.) and The War Amps (n.d.)]

Various studies reported reduced levels of oxygen consumption when using a microprocessor controlled prosthetic knee, leading to a more efficient gait, increased velocity and stride length (Orendurff et al, 2006; Perry et al, 2004; Schmalz et al, 2002). In another study by Schmalz et al (2016), it was reported that persons using a microprocessor controlled Knee-Ankle-Foot Orthosis (KAFO) were more confident descending ramps and stairs, thus improving orthotic function with sustained orthotic safety.

Myoelectric (or bionic) upper limb prostheses work by picking up EMG (electromyography) signals from the amputee's muscles; these signals are then detected by electronic sensors, usually embedded in the prosthetic socket, which amplify, rectify and filter the signals, and then send these filtered signals to a motor in the prosthesis. If the filtered EMG signals that reach the motor exceed a certain threshold, the motor is activated and movement occurs in that part of the prosthesis which is being controlled by that motor, i.e. hand, fingers, wrist or elbow. The same concept applies to externally-powered upper limb orthoses, where a brace (orthosis) is fabricated to support the elbow, wrist and hand, designed to help restore the function of a weak or paralyzed upper extremity. This device picks up the faint EMG signals from muscles via sensors on the surface of the skin, amplifies them and activates the small motors to move the upper limb as the user intends. In a systematic review article, Carey et al (2015) compared myoelectric with body-powered upper limb prostheses; they reported that the literature showed both advantages and disadvantages attributed to both systems, namely that myoelectric prostheses were more comfortable and more cosmetically accepted, and people preferred to wear them when in social settings or if working in an office. They also reported a positive effect in reducing phantom limb pain, if worn for long periods. In another study, Razak et al (2014) compared patient satisfaction and the problems experienced by upper limb amputees, regarding wrist movements, of body powered prostheses versus myoelectric prostheses; their major findings were that the satisfaction with myoelectric prostheses was 12% higher, and the problems experienced were 13% higher for body-powered prostheses. Going as far back as the 1980's, in a study comparing function between myoelectric and body-powered prostheses, Stain and Walley (1983) reported that myoelectric prostheses provided the user with a higher range of motion than body-powered prostheses.

There is presently a lot of research being carried out on combining orthotics and prosthetics with robotics; examples of such devices are the robotic exoskeleton, the stride management assist device and the robotic hip disarticulation prosthesis. The robotic exoskeleton involves sensors, actuators, mechanical structures, algorithms and control strategies to acquire information and execute a motor function (Ruiz-Olaya et al, 2019). Exoskeletons are usually used by persons who suffered a spinal cord injury and can no longer stand and walk independently without expending a vast amount of energy, but can be used also with people who suffer a stroke, as well as by persons living with cerebral palsy, Parkinson's disease or poliomyelitis, who would otherwise be wheelchair bound. In a review article, Gorgey (2018) reports various benefits, apart from the advantage of community ambulation, such as reducing obesity and fat mass by decreasing sitting time and increasing physical activity. Decreasing sitting time also contributes to reducing the risk of cardiovascular disease, cancer, renal disease and other conditions that may lead to early mortality, as well as reducing the risk of lower limb flexion contractures. The stride management assist device is worn around the hips and thighs, and provides automated gait assistance; it has been used in middle aged persons (Otsuki et al, 2016) and shown to improve their gait parameters (walking distance, speed, cadence and step length) without increasing the energy cost of walking. In another study, Buesing et al (2015) reported that the stride management assist device improved the spatiotemporal parameters of gait, namely velocity, cadence, stride length, step time, stance and swing times, double support time and spatial asymmetry. This is important since gait and mobility functions tend to begin to deteriorate at around age 40, rapidly declining after age 60 (Imms and Edholm, 1981; Schrack et al, 2013, and Shumway-Cook et al, 2007). In a first report regarding the application of a robotic prosthesis for hip disarticulation amputation, Ueyama et al (2020) report that this device improved gait kinematics and symmetry, albeit that these initial experiments were carried out on a non-amputee healthy subject.

The Manufacturers/Innovators

As stated earlier in this chapter, manufacturers of prosthetic and orthotic devices are relatively few in number. Manufacturers are able to produce both complete devices as designed by prosthetists, orthotists or engineers, as well as individual components, usually designed by engineers, which are used to assemble a prosthetic or orthotic device in a prosthetic/orthotic laboratory or in a clinic. Such manufacturers, some of whom are also innovators in the field of orthotics and prosthetics, invest large amounts of money in research to come up with such devices and components, thus the retail price for such devices is relatively high. But, the price also reflects the size of the market, which is also relatively small when compared to the entire population of the world. It has been estimated that only 0.5% of any population globally requires prosthetic and orthotic devices (World Health Organization, 2017a). The World Health Organization (2017b) also states that *manufacturers and suppliers should conduct research on, develop, produce, make available and provide training in good-quality, cost–effective components and materials for the fabrication of prostheses and orthoses for the full range of treatment in various contexts*, thus recognizing the importance of innovation in the field of prosthetics and orthotics.

However, innovation means disrupting or replacing the technology that already exists (Twerenbold, 2017). Thus, is innovation good or bad? Since the beginning of humankind, there has been an instinct to make the quality of life of humans better, because humans are almost never satisfied with how things are going, so they always strive to make the world a better place (VonNostrand, 2014). Will humans ever stop being innovative, if, for example, technology is taken too far and is harmful to society?

The attraction towards being innovative may be explained by a belief in progress, driven by a belief in development towards an improved condition, towards a future that is better than the past (Fonseca, 2016). But at what cost? Are innovators foreseeing unintended impacts, maybe due to error on the part of the implementer (Unite for Sight, n.d.)? Technology has the potential to make the world a better place, but its use can also be problematic (Smart, 2019). Smart (2019) goes on to state that there is a widespread belief that innovation shapes society as if it was disassociated from it, but yet, it is a product of that same society that it helps to shape.

Engineers are always at the forefront of innovation; they are faced with making, or are asked to make, decisions, some minor and some major, on a daily basis. Therefore, ethics must always be made the main reason for major decisions (VanNostrand, 2014). Nathan (2018) states that the biggest challenges for engineers come in healthcare, where they literally need to match nature! Throughout history, since ancient Egypt, Greece and Rome, engineers have come up with innovative ideas and designs to do this, to fulfil the same function as a missing natural part of the body; wooden peg legs and strap on toes, as well as primitive attempts at jointed limbs, have been discovered by archaeologists (Nathan, 2018). Today, mankind's expectations have been raised to a very high level through science fiction: the *Six Million Dollar Man, Robocop, Star Wars*...the list is endless! These fictitious characters are always portrayed as more powerful, more efficient, faster and better at whatever they do than the most powerful, most efficient and fastest human. But none of these is a realistic reflection of what is possible in prosthetics and orthotics.

In development, innovation very often means:

1. A process – working fast and flexibly
2. Technology – incorporating the latest technology to measure everything and engage populations
3. Design – making certain that new solutions reflect the real needs of the users
4. Investing – thinking more like an incubator to create new models of shared value partnership.

(Fabian & Fabricant, 2014)

Therefore, certain ethical questions are bound to arise in the field of orthotics and prosthetics: Since technologically advanced orthotic and prosthetic devices are so expensive, do innovation and advanced technology only cater for the elite, the rich, or the affluent societies? Is there a chance that such advanced prosthetic/orthotic technology becomes freely available and accessible to all? And if so, will the main function of such devices become purely cosmetic (Sabin, 2016)? Meyer (2013) goes even further and asks *if a bionic hand let you type ten times faster and looked twice as cool as your healthy, natural hand, would you choose to amputate your hand to accommodate the new gadget?...Or a leg that lets you run faster? Would you choose to replace a healthy limb with a bionic one? Should it be allowed?*

In sport, do high tech prostheses give sportsmen an unfair advantage? Oscar Pistorius made history by becoming the first amputee athlete to compete in the Olympic Games using a pair of blade prostheses. But did his blades give Pistorius an unfair advantage over the other athletes, who were all healthy and had no physical disability? The issue resurfaced four years later at the Rio Olympics, when a bid by Paralympic athlete Markus Rehm, a unilateral amputee, to compete in the Olympic Games failed because he could not prove that the blade on the amputated side did not give him an unfair advantage (Greenemeier, 2016).

The question, thus, arises as to what and how are the manufacturers of orthotic and prosthetic devices thinking when they invest and engage in research and development? What *is* the ultimate goal of innovation? What *should be* the ultimate goal of innovation?

Orthotic and Prosthetic Practitioners

The ethical issues that arise from the role of the professionals will be discussed and explored in this section, giving examples of how different health systems and socio-economic issues may influence decisions made by individuals working at the forefront of orthotic and prosthetic provision.

Orthotic/Prosthetic practitioners are known as Orthotists and Prosthetists, and they are autonomous healthcare professionals in their own right. The Cambridge dictionary (n.d.) defines the word ***profession*** as *any type of work that needs special training or a particular skill, often one that is respected because it involves a high level of education.* The Australian Professional Standards Councils (n.d.) define a profession as *a disciplined group of individuals who adhere to ethical standards.* The British Association of Prosthetists and Orthotists, in their Ethical Code, state that *Prosthetists/Orthotists must promote and protect the interests of service users and carers, and have a duty to take reasonable care of patients whom they accept for rehabilitation* ([BAPO], 2018). Thus the orthotist/prosthetist constantly faces ethical dilemmas in their quest to treat all patients equally. However, these professionals should strive for the highest possible quality of care for all their patients.

Heitzmann (2019) reported that a patient who had been provided with a modern prosthesis consisting of the latest generation microprocessor knee and a carbon fibre foot, told his prosthetist that this prosthesis did not represent the latest state of the art technology because it did not work intuitively, like a robot, which he had seen on the internet doing a backflip! This set the prosthetist thinking that, although prosthetics and orthotics had made sizeable advances, it was still lagging behind other technologies, e.g. smartphones; this can make the clinician downhearted, that such advances in technology have not found their way into the world of prosthetics and orthotics (Heitzmann, 2019).

However, although the orthotics and prosthetics profession is a caring profession, reimbursement issues tend to present dilemmas as the realities of business finance meet with the sense of ethical obligation to help patients (Fairley, 2014). Balancing a patient's needs against reimbursement issues is a dilemma faced by orthotists and prosthetists on a daily basis. Most practitioners have a moral compass that guides them when facing ethical dilemmas to make decisions that place the patient and their needs at the very top of their ethical and moral code; but each day brings with it struggles that are related to:

- Reimbursement for the service and devices that the practitioners are providing -
    - Who is paying? Is the patient paying out of their own pocket? In which case, what can the patient afford?
    - Is it the hospital, through a Universal Healthcare Service, that is picking up the bill? If so, what is the dedicated budget?
    - Or is it the patient's medical insurance that is funding the provision of the device? What will the insurance actually pay for? If the insurance will not pay the full cost, can the patient afford to fund the rest?

Such questions may influence the prescription of the device and, as a result, the patient may not be provided with the device that addresses all his/her needs.

- Referral pressures –
    - What is the referring physician requesting?
    - What does the orthotic/prosthetic practitioner do if they do not agree with the referring physician's request?
    - Is it the referring physician or entity who's going to provide the funding for the device?
    - Does the orthotic/prosthetic practitioner need to discuss the options with the referring physician, as well as the patient?

In such situations the orthotic/prosthetic practitioner should remember that s/he is the expert on the provision of orthotic/prosthetic devices, but to be experts they must keep themselves abreast with the latest technological advances in their fields; then they can discuss with the referring physician with confidence.

- The patients' clinical and functional needs (as assessed by the orthotist/prosthetist and, where possible, the multidisciplinary team) –
    - Are the aims of treatment realistic?
    - Is the need for the latest orthotic/prosthetic technology a real need or a luxury?
    - Is the patient cognitively able to use a technologically advanced prosthesis or orthosis?

The practitioner may seek to consult with other healthcare professionals who may know the patient well enough to offer their advice.

- The patients' requests for specific devices –
    - Does the specific device that the patient is asking for meet all their functional needs?
    - Are the patient's expectations realistic?
    - Can the patient learn to use the specific device?

Gaining the patient's trust is a prerequisite to get the patient on board, so that they accept the rationale for the provision of the device that the practitioner is advising. (Adapted from Fairley,2014)

In a case that was reported by Wegmann (2014), an orthotist was faced with a patient who suffered from a rare condition that presents with the patient having a persistent desire to acquire a physical disability, and this patient requested ankle-foot orthoses; the patient described symptoms of discomfort in his legs, which dated back to his childhood, and that were aggravated by standing and walking. The orthotist carried out a physical assessment but found no abnormalities in gait, joint range of motion or muscle strength and power. What does the orthotist do in such a situation? Clinically there is no physical or functional need for ankle-foot orthoses, ever since the patient started to walk, but…will these orthoses "relieve" the symptoms? Is it ethical to give someone a type of treatment which they do not functionally need? Is it ethical, if such treatment is funded by the state, for the orthotist to use funds from what is probably a limited budget? And if the patient is paying for the orthoses privately, should the orthotist in question "give in" to the patient's request? After all, private healthcare is a profit-making business! On the other hand, what if the treatment, in this case the ankle-foot orthoses, helped alleviate the discomfort and the patient started to walk and lead a completely independent and happy life? The only thing that is clear in such a case is that there is *no* clear, easy and straightforward answer…

Another scenario that occasionally crops up, especially in a Universal Healthcare System, is when the patient is given a device, which he has not directly paid for, and they do not look after it as they should, or as instructed at the point when the device was given to them. Time and again, the patient may abuse of the device's function and perform activities that were not meant to be performed using that particular device. Is it ethical that the health service keeps on funding this device for this patient? After all it was funded by the taxpayers! Should there be a charge if the patient is judged to have abused the device, but then, is the patient not a taxpayer also? And who will be the judge who will adjudicate whether the patient has really abused the device or not?

The Service Users (The Patients)

In any business that wishes to be successful, (and every business obviously does!), the client plays the most important role. To state the obvious, no business that sells a product or service will do well if there are no clients to purchase that product or service. The same applies to prosthetics and orthotics, where the clients are the service users, those patients who need to make use of an orthotic or prosthetic device to help them in their individual rehabilitation programme, or to lead a better quality of life.

Despite the many advances in prosthetic technology, for example, there is evidence that indicates that people who have had an amputation (even those who use a prosthetic device) are still at a biomechanical disadvantage, which makes them more likely to develop musculoskeletal complications such as osteoarthritis, back pain, joint pain, and osteoporosis (Gailey et al, 2008). Some amputees even end up having to undergo hip replacement surgery, due to the biomechanical problems that arise over a period of time from having an asymmetrical gait and putting undue mechanical stress on the hip. In addition, because of the challenges with prosthetic socket or orthotic device interfaces, people who use such devices are likely to develop frequent skin complications, including eczema, irritation, skin breakdown and ulceration. (Bui et al, 2009).

As mentioned earlier, *patients* are at the centre of orthotic and prosthetic services, as they are at the centre of all medical services. But, can the patient ask for anything they like? What if a patient went to a surgeon and asked for one of their arms to be amputated, just so that they can try a bionic prosthetic arm? Sabin (2016) argues that there are two sides to such a request: i) the ethical implications of the question itself, and ii) the implications of the response. People have every right to go into a doctor's office and ask for anything they want, after all every human being strives to be the best! Whether they actually get what they want, though, is a different matter. Sabin (2016) continues to argue that in considering giving someone the surgery that they want, even though they do not need it, is actually questioning what the boundaries of medicine are. But is this not already happening in breast implant and cosmetic surgery, for example, when for the most part, implants are put in to enhance one's appearance and increase self-confidence; the analogy is not 100% accurate, however, as, in the case of breast implants, the surgeon is not removing a body part to replace it with an artificial device, but similar ethical considerations do apply.

The service users are also faced with certain issues: for instance, are they able to shop around for the best product or for the best price? Can they actually afford the best? Who will help them with funding? Who will help them to make the right choice – the sales person, or the prosthetist/orthotist? In a study carried out with Vietnam veterans in the U.S. the expected lifetime cost for a unilateral lower limb group of amputees was $1.4 million (Blough, Hubbard, McFarland, Smith, Gambel & Reiber, 2010). Is the follow-up (after sales) service good enough? Again, can the patient afford the follow-up? And in countries where there is a Universal Healthcare Service, is it ethical that some patients visit their local orthotic/prosthetic department so regularly, sometimes more than fifteen times a year, just because it's free, even for very minor complaints? This puts a strain on resources, and would they visit so often if they had to pay for every visit, as in the private sector, or would they just put up with the minor complaint?

Some patients are making their own devices using 3D printing (Amputee Coalition, 2019) because they cannot afford what is offered to them by the prosthetic/orthotic industry. A prosthetic hand could cost thousands of dollars, while a 3D printed hand would cost around $50 (Amputee Coalition, 2019). The problem for the patient is that, as yet, 3D printing materials cannot replace traditional prosthetic materials, especially the advanced technology ones, when it comes to robustness, durability, functional precision and aesthetics. But most people have no choice; if someone has an injury that results in a major disability, e.g. amputation or paraplegia, it is quite likely that that person will be out of work for an extended period of time to undergo rehabilitation. This means that that individual may lose their job and therefore their main income. The potential to work again is also diminished, and when, or if, they do go back to work it may be to a different job that does not pay as well as their previous one. Therefore, they may not be able to afford to obtain the most technologically advanced prosthetic/orthotic device, and have to revert to a 3D printed option. So, is it ethical for the orthotic and prosthetic profession, and, indeed, any health system, to leave these patients to their own devices, just because these people cannot afford to purchase a professional, state of the art prosthetic or orthotic device?

SOLUTIONS AND RECOMMENDATIONS

There are various health systems that have started to find just solutions to some of the ethical issues that the industry is facing. This final section will explore these solutions, and discuss prudent recommendations for future solutions, in the light of the importance of rehabilitating patients to their full potential so that they can form an integral part of society and contribute to the socio-economic improvement of the world as a whole.

As seen above, the biggest obstacle for people to use the most advanced technology to replace a missing limb or its function is cost. This author believes that most of the ethical issues in prosthetics and orthotics can be resolved if funding for these services was more readily available to all people who need it. It is estimated that 35-40 million people need prosthetic or orthotic services (WHO, 2017a). Therefore, any solutions to these ethical dilemmas must be found in the light of the World Health Organisation's recommendations for best practice, which will be outlined below.

As previously stated in this chapter, a few countries provide prosthetic and orthotic services under the umbrella of a Universal Health System, e.g. the United Kingdom's National Health service, for which the central government provides a budget to the health service (funds collected from taxpayers) and this in turn is distributed among all the health services and entities in the country. The advantage of having this system is that anybody who needs health and medical care will get it, irrespective of who they are, what they do, where they live or what they earn, and everyone is entitled to it. However, tax payers' money is not a bottomless pit, and the system does not necessarily provide all the medical care, including pharmaceuticals, especially the latest technology and medical advances. In other words, people, but *all* the people, who need health care, get the best that the state can afford. However, the best that the state can afford may not actually include technologically advanced devices, and this is a disadvantage in some countries using such a healthcare system; then, just like with private funding, the issue would boil down to who can afford what, since once it's not available through the health care system, one will try and source the device privately!

When medical insurances pay for medical care, it is like when one insures their car: one pays an annual premium, then when they need medical care, including orthotic and prosthetic services, the insurance pays for the care needed, dependent on the premium; the insurance will also issue the amount it is ready to pay for every single consultation and treatment that the individual can have access to. This means that people who cannot afford to pay an annual premium, will not be able to have access to any medical care, and if the insurance does not pay the full amount, the person will have to pay the rest from their own pocket.

Self-funding, much like an insurance-based system, depends solely on how rich somebody is. Even with regards to orthotic and prosthetic services, one will only be able to obtain what one can afford, rather than what one actually needs, much like buying a car when one needs their own mode of transport.

The World Health Organization (WHO) specifies the criteria that need to be adopted to determine the appropriateness of advancing technology in prosthetics and orthotics, including (among others):

- Products should be comfortable, functional, easy to put on and remove, not endanger user safety, durable, have the best possible cosmetic appearance, as lightweight as possible, be culturally appropriate, suit the climate and the local terrain, and suit local working conditions;
- Products should be affordable by the system and/or the individual;
- Products should be durable and have a long lifespan;
- Products should be easily adjusted, maintained and repaired;
- Technologies should be cost-effective and clinically effective;
- Technologies should promote sustainable development by enhancing local entrepreneurship and making use of local markets, such as locally produced components or materials;
- Technologies and working methods should be of proven, documented efficacy and safety;
- Technologies and working methods should adhere to international standards;
- Technologies should ensure biomechanically correct products that can be given proper alignment;
- Prosthetists and orthotists should have sufficient skill and knowledge to apply technologies and working methods; if this is not the case, training must be practically feasible and affordable;
- Working methods should not be hazardous to personnel;
- Materials should be easy to store.
(WHO, 2017c)

Thus, manufacturers and prosthetic/orthotic service providers will do well to keep the above WHO guidelines in mind when they are developing new, technologically advanced products or when prescribing such products. The rationale for funding orthotic and prosthetic services is a challenge for all countries, health systems and individuals. However, these services are an integral part of healthcare and rehabilitation and must be included in all health systems, including the provision of the latest advanced technological prosthetic and orthotic devices and systems.

Engineers in particular are given the immense task of making the world a better place for society (VanNostrand, 2014). Therefore, in medicine and healthcare, including the world of orthotics and prosthetics, decisions that may lead to innovation and product or system development must be made on the basis of ethics. To make the right ethical decisions one must consider some very important factors:

1. How much difference will the innovation make to improve health?
2. Will the intervention be affordable, robust and adjustable to healthcare settings in developing countries, and will it be socially, culturally and politically acceptable?
3. Will the innovation address the most pressing needs in a particular field within healthcare?
4. Can it realistically be developed and deployed in a time frame of 5–10 years?
5. Does the innovation advance healthcare by creating new knowledge?
6. Does the innovation address issues such as environmental improvement and income generation that have indirect, positive effects on health? (Unite for Sight, n.d.).

In an attempt to build an ethical framework for innovation, Fabian and Fabricant (2014) suggested nine operational principles, based on UNICEF guidelines for innovation, that need to be followed when one is involved in development and innovation; these may be used as guidelines for, and can be applied to, the development of prosthetic and orthotic technologically advanced devices:

1. Design *with* the user (not *for* the user):
    a) The innovators should get to know the people that they are designing for through meaningful conversation, observation and co-creation,
    b) They should strive to understand user characteristics, needs and challenges, and
    c) Information gathered is then used to design and re-design, build and rebuild, test and re-test the device/product, continually gathering user feedback, until it meets the users' needs.
2. Understand the existing ecosystem:
    a) Ecosystems are defined, among others, by the culture, political environment, economy, gender norms and technology infrastructure which can affect the people's ability to access and use a particular technology,
    b) An ecosystem is fluid, multi-faceted and continuously changing,
    c) Consider the particular structures and systems that already exist in countries, regions and communities, and
    d) Ensure that the developed product will be relevant and sustainable.
3. Design for scale:
    a) Achieving scale may mean different things in different contexts,

   b) Think beyond the pilot studies and make choices that will enable widespread adoption,
   c) Determine what will be affordable and usable, and
   d) Then the new initiative can be expanded more easily to other users in other countries and regions.
4. Build for sustainability:
   a) Maintains user and stakeholder support and maximises long-term impact,
   b) More likely to be embedded into policies and practices, and
   c) Leads to institutionalisation of the product.
5. Be data driven:
   a) Use data to inform decision making, and
   b) Quality information can then be available to the right people as and when they need it, to use and/or take action.
6. Use open standards, open data, open source, and open innovation:
   a) Increases collaboration in the development community,
   b) Avoids duplication of work that has already been done, and
   c) Maximises resources and impact.
7. Reuse and improve:
   a) Adapt and enhance existing products, resources and approaches where possible,
   b) Reduces the time needed for development and testing,
   c) Reduces costs, and
   d) Results in a better and more usable product.
8. Do no harm:
   a) Address privacy and security of how data is acquired, used, stored and shared,
   b) Protect identities of participants involved in the project,
   c) Protect sensitive information, and
   d) Create a post-project end-of-life policy for data collected.
9. Be collaborative:
   a) Share information, insights, strategies and resources across projects, sectors and organizations,
   b) Results in increased efficiency and impact,
   c) Brings people with a shared vision working together more closely, and
   d) Collaborating requires time, planning and dedicating resources to look for and develop new opportunities.

   (Adapted from: Fabian & Fabricant, 2014; UNICEF, n.d.)

The codes of professional and ethical conduct for orthotic and prosthetic practitioners, written by orthotics and prosthetics organizations worldwide, provide good guidelines and a foundation for making ethical decisions in one's daily work. These are targeted mainly for prosthetists and orthotists and are based on standards for best practice. Armold (1964) argues that the profession of prosthetics and orthotics is only as strong as its best practitioner and as weak as its worst one; in ethical dilemmas, prosthetists and orthotists must be free to act in accordance with their best judgement based on human values that are embraced by the profession.

In conclusion, as can be seen from this whole chapter, there is no easy answer to the ethical dilemmas in orthotic and prosthetic practice and innovation. But ethical business makes for sound business (Fairley, 2014) and a decision or a choice that is ethically wrong *may* produce a financial gain, albeit short-term; that same short-term gain may result in a long term loss. Educating one's staff members, be they engineers, designers, orthotists or prosthetists, in ethical standards will result in financial gain and sustainability. In the world of research and development, reputation is everything. Advanced technology in the field of prosthetics and orthotics is at the forefront of innovation in rehabilitation; if one works closely with the service users and stakeholders, the innovation will be a success.

And last but not least, if governments were to recognise the true value of innovation and technological advances in the field of prosthetics and orthotics, they may be more willing to aid with funding for the development of technologically advanced products, as well as subsidise the cost of such products to the users, even in societies that are not so affluent. Then, and only then, will the ethical dilemmas surrounding the industry truly diminish.

REFERENCES

Amputee Coalition. (2019). *3D printed prosthetics – where we are today*. Retrieved March 2020 from https://www.amputee-coalition.org/3d-printed-prosthetics/

Armold, J. (1964). Business and professional ethics in prosthetics and orthotics. *Orthopedic and Prosthetic Appliance Journal*, (September), 212–221.

Blough, D. K., Hubbard, S., McFarland, L. V., Smith, D. G., Gambel, J. M., & Reiber, G. E. (2010). Prosthetic cost projections for service members with major limb loss from Vietnam and OIF/OEF. *Journal of Rehabilitation Research and Development*, *47*(4), 387–402. doi:10.1682/JRRD.2009.04.0037 PMID:20803406

British Association of Prosthetists and Orthotists. (2018). Ethical code. Section 2.2. p. 4.

Buesing, C., Fisch, G., O'Donnell, M., Shahidi, I., Thomas, L., Mummidisetty, C. K., Williams, K. J., Takahashi, H., Rymer, W. Z., & Jayaraman, A. (2015). Effects of a wearable exoskeleton stride management assist system (SMA®) on spatiotemporal gait characteristics in individuals after stroke: A randomized controlled trial. *Journal of Neuroengineering and Rehabilitation*, *12*(1), 69–83. doi:10.118612984-015-0062-0 PMID:26289955

Bui, K. M., Raugi, G. J., Nguyen, V. Q., & Reiber, G. E. (2009). Skin problems in individuals with lower-limb loss: Literature review and proposed classification system. *Journal of Rehabilitation Research and Development*, *46*(9), 1085–1090. doi:10.1682/JRRD.2009.04.0052 PMID:20437314

Carey, S. L., Lura, D. J., & Highsmith, M. J. (2015). Differences in myoelectric and body-powered upper-limb prostheses: Systematic literature review. *Journal of Rehabilitation Research and Development*, *52*(3), 247–262. doi:10.1682/JRRD.2014.08.0192 PMID:26230500

Dupes, B. (n.d.). Prosthetic Knee Systems. *Amputee Coalition*. Retrieved September 2020 from https://www.amputee-coalition.org/resources/prosthetic-knee-systems/

Fabian, C., & Fabricant, R. (2014). The ethics of innovation. *Stanford Social Innovation Review*. Retrieved in March 2020 from https://ssir.org/articles/entry/the_ethics_of_innovation#

Fairley, M. (2014). Where ethics and economics meet. *The O&P Edge*. Retrieved in March 2020 from https://opedge.com/Articles/ViewArticle/2014-01-31/2014-02_01

Fonseca, M. (2016). Good and bad innovation: An overview of the ethics of innovation. *Intelligent HQ*. Retrieved in March 2020 from https://www.intelligenthq.com/good-and-bad-innovation-an-overview-on-the-ethics-of-innovation/

Gailey, R., Allen, K., Castles, J., Kucharik, J., & Roeder, M. (2008). Review of secondary physical conditions associated with lower-limb amputation and long-term prosthesis use. *Journal of Rehabilitation Research and Development*, *45*(1), 15–29. doi:10.1682/JRRD.2006.11.0147 PMID:18566923

Gorgey, A. S. (2018). Robotic exoskeletons: The current pros and cons. *World Journal of Orthopedics*, *9*(9), 112–119. doi:10.5312/wjo.v9.i9.112 PMID:30254967

Greenemeier, L. (2016). Blade runners: Do high-tech prostheses give runners an unfair advantage? *Scientific American*. Retrieved in March 2020 from https://www.scientificamerican.com/article/blade-runners-do-high-tech-prostheses-give-runners-an-unfair-advantage/

Heitzmann, D. (2019). Editorial. *Journal of Prosthetics and Orthotics*, *31*(4), 223. doi:10.1097/JPO.0000000000000276

Imms, F. J., & Edholm, O. G. (1981). Studies of gait and mobility in the elderly. *Age and Ageing*, *10*(3), 147–156. doi:10.1093/ageing/10.3.147 PMID:7270322

International Society for Prosthetics and Orthotics. (n.d.). *Prosthetic and Orthotic services*. Retrieved in March 2020 from https://www.ispoint.org/general/custom.asp?page=POservices, para 1 & 2.

Light, H. (2018). Private healthcare vs the NHS. *Star Outico – Latest News*. Retrieved in June 2021 from https://www.staroutico.com/latest-news/private-healthcare-vs-nhs

Meyer, B. (2013). Bertolt Meyer: 'Ethical questions are looming for prosthetics'. *Wired*. Retrieved in March 2020 from https://www.wired.co.uk/article/now-we-need-to-talk-about-our-bionic-future

Nathan, S. (2018). Future prosthetic: towards the bionic human. *The Engineer*. Retrieved in March 2020 from https://www.theengineer.co.uk/future-prosthetic/

Nielsen, C. C., & Jorge, M. (2013). Orthotics and prosthetics in rehabilitation: multidisciplinary approach. In M. Lusardi, M. Jorge, & C. Nielsen (Eds.), *Orthotics & Prosthetics in Rehabilitation* (p. 2). Elsevier Saunders. doi:10.1016/B978-1-4377-1936-9.00001-1

Orendurff, M. S., Segal, A. D., Klute, G. K., McDowell, M. L., Pecoraro, J. A., & Czerniecki, J. M. (2006). Gait efficiency using the C-Leg. *Journal of Rehabilitation Research and Development*, *43*(2), 239–246. doi:10.1682/JRRD.2005.06.0095 PMID:16847790

Otto Bock, U. K. (n.d.). *Microprocessor controlled knees – How do they work?* Retrieved in September 2020 from https://www.ottobock.co.uk/prosthetics/info_for_new_amputees/prosthetic-technology-explained/computer_controlled_knees/

Pasquina, P. F., Carvalho, A. J., & Sheehan, T. P. (2015). Ethics in rehabilitation: Access to prosthetics and quality care following amputation. *American Medical Association Journal*, *17*(6), 535–546. PMID:26075981

Profession. (n.d.) In *Cambridge Dictionary online*. Retrieved in March 2020 from https://dictionary.cambridge.org/dictionary/english/profession

Professional Standards Councils. (n.d.). *What is a Profession*? Retrieved in March 2020 from https://www.psc.gov.au/what-is-a-profession

Razak, A., Osman, A., Kamyab, M., Abas, W., & Gholizadeh, H. (2014). Satisfaction and problems experienced with wrist movements. *American Journal of Physical Medicine & Rehabilitation*, *93*(5), 437–444. doi:10.1097/PHM.0b013e3182a51fc2 PMID:24429510

Ruiz-Olaya, A. F., Lopez-Delis, A., & Rocha, A. F. (2019). Upper and lower extremity exoskeletons. In J. Segil (Ed.), Handbook of Biomechanics (pp. 283–317). Academic Press.

Sabin, D. (2016). Do we have a right to bionic arms? *Inverse*. Retrieved in March 2020 from https://www.inverse.com/article/18220-robot-arms-cyborgs-advanced-prosthetics-and-medical-ethics

Schmalz, T., Blumentritt, S., & Jarasch, R. (2002). Energy expenditure and biomechanical characteristics of lower limb amputee gait: The influence of prosthetic alignment and different prosthetic components. *Gait & Posture*, *16*(3), 255–263. doi:10.1016/S0966-6362(02)00008-5 PMID:12443950

Schmalz, T., Pröbsting, E., Auberger, R., & Siewert, G. (2016). A functional comparison of conventional knee–ankle–foot orthoses and a microprocessor-controlled leg orthosis system based on biomechanical parameters. *Prosthetics and Orthotics International*, *40*(2), 277–286. doi:10.1177/0309364614546524 PMID:25249381

Schrack, J. A., Simonsick, E. M., & Ferrucci, L. (2013). The relationship of the energetic cost of slow walking and peak energy expenditure to gait speed in mid-to-late life. *American Journal of Physical Medicine & Rehabilitation*, *92*(1), 28–35. doi:10.1097/PHM.0b013e3182644165 PMID:22854908

Shumway-Cook, A., Guralnik, J. M., Phillips, C. L., Coppin, A. K., Ciol, M. A., Bandinelli, S., & Ferrucci, L. (2007). Age-associated declines in complex walking task performance: The Walking InCHIANTI toolkit. *Journal of the American Geriatrics Association*, *55*(1), 58–65. doi:10.1111/j.1532-5415.2006.00962.x PMID:17233686

Smart, Z. (2019). Bringing the ethics into innovation. *IEC e-tech*. Retrieved in March 2020 from https://iecetech.org/issue/2019-01/Bringing-the-ethics-into-innovation

The War Amps. (n.d.). *Prosthetic Knees for Adults*. Retrieved September 2020 from https://www.waramps.ca/pdf/english-site/ways-we-help/artificial-limbs-and-devices/lower-limb/knees-for-adults.pdf

Twerenbold, R. (2017). *The good, the bad and the innovative: Understanding the darker side of innovation for development.* United Nations Research Institute for Social Development (UNRISD). Retrieved in March 2020 from http://www.unrisd.org/80256B3C005BE6B5/(httpNews)/9CD705AC73D6E013C12580D7004F285C?OpenDocument&newstype=viewpoint

UNICEF. (n.d.). *What we do*. Retrieved September 2020 from https://www.unicef.org/innovation/what-we-do-new

Unite for Sight. (n.d.). *Ethics of Innovation*. Retrieved in March 2020 from http://www.uniteforsight.org/global-health-university/ethics-of-innovation

VanNostrand, C. (2014). Prosthetics: The ethical issues surrounding them. *Semantic Scholar*. Retrieved in March 2020 from https://pdfs.semanticscholar.org/3b16/4b5c1f072d95551b4e770476eeb9d9116d65.pdf?_ga=2.127456843.791674419.1585559520-1453370591.1585559520

Waihanga. (n.d.). *Knee Joints*. Retrieved September 2020 from https://www.nzals.co.nz/products/categories/knee-joints

Wegmann, M. (2014). Orthotic Intervention for those without physical limitations: An ethical perspective. *The O&P Edge*. Retrieved in March 2020 from https://opedge.com/Articles/ViewArticle/2014-01-31/2014-02_02

World Health Organization. (2017a). Standards for Prosthetics and Orthotics: Part 1 – Standards, p. xxvi.

World Health Organization. (2017b). Standards for Prosthetics and Orthotics: Part 2 – Implementation Manual, p. 5.

World Health Organization. (2017c). Standards for Prosthetics and Orthotics: Part 2 – Implementation Manual, p. 34.

ADDITIONAL READING

Fenton, J. (1983). Canons of ethics and professionalism. *Clinical Prosthetics & Orthotics*, *7*(3), 1.

Harman, J. H. (1983). Canons of ethical conduct and the law. *Clinical Prosthetics & Orthotics*, *7*(3), 1–2.

Chapter 8
Prediction of Skin Diseases Using Machine Learning

Siddhartha Kumar Arjaria
Maulana Azad National Institute of Technology, India

Priyanshu Shrivastava
Rajkiye Engineering College, Banda, India

Vikas Raj
Rajkiye Engineering College, Banda, India

Monu Kumar
Rajkiye Engineering College, Banda, India

Sunil Kumar
Rajkiye Engineering College, Banda, India

Jincy S. Cherian
The Bhopal School of Social Sciences, Bhopal, India

ABSTRACT

Skin disease rates have been increasing over the past few decades. It has led to both fatal and non-fatal disabilities all around the world, especially in those areas where medical resources are not good enough. Early diagnosis of skin diseases increases the chances of cure significantly. Therefore, this work is comparing six machine learning algorithms, namely KNN, random forest, neural network, naïve bayes, logistic regression, and SVM, for the prediction of the skin diseases. The information gain, gain ratio, gini decrease, chi-square, and relieff are used to rank the features. This work comprises the introduction, literature review, and proposed methodology parts. In this research paper, a new method of analyzing skin disease has been proposed in which six different data mining techniques are used to develop an ensemble method that integrates all the six data mining techniques as a single one. The ensemble method used on the dermatology dataset gives improved result with 94% accuracy in comparison to other classifier algorithms and hence is more effective in this area.

DOI: 10.4018/978-1-7998-7888-9.ch008

INTRODUCTION

Skin disease is one of the most important and gradually increasing disease in the world. Most of the skin diseases cases increases just my touching or getting in contact with the affected person. These types of diseases causes heavy financial, psychological and emotional burden on patients and on their families. As a result people in the world specially those who belongs to poor resources region, are unable to fight against these challenges.

Some of the common causes of skin disease includes: weakened immune system, parasites, fungus or some other microorganisms residing on the skin, many viruses, genetic factors of person, getting in get in touch with allergens, irritants, or other person's infected skin, some bacteria those are confined in skin pores and hair follicles, diseases related to thyroid, kidneys are some important causes of dermatology diseases. Climate change may also cause skin disease but it differs from one region to another region.

Despite the fact that dermatology diseases are characterized by large range of diseases, bulk of skin diseases belong to less than ten categories as suggested by many prevalence surveys. These results are very useful in spreading information and provide preventive programs on health, which is very essential. These diseases are also categorized as infectious (that spreads from person to person) or non-infectious.

There are a variety of symptoms of skin diseases. Some of the symptoms that seem to be due to common problem, might not be every time caused due to any skin disorder. Such type of common skin problems are sores from new shoes or roughness from tight pants. Typical indications of a skin disorder include: too much flushing, raised up bumps which have red or white color, a loss of skin pigment, a rash, which might be hurting or itchy, changes in mole color or size, scaly or rough skin, bumps that are fleshy, warts, or other skin growths, ulcers, peeling skin, discolored patches of skin, open sores or lesions and cracked skin.

Many skin diseases are not avoidable, which occurs due to some genetic conditions or any other ailments. These diseases are also categorized as infectious (that spreads from person to person) or non-infectious. However, it is possible to avert the spread of skin diseases.

Some tips to prevent these types of skin conditions are:

- Regularly washing hands with soap and water
- Taking nutritious diet
- Avoiding sharing utensils and drinking glasses with others
- Getting proper vaccines to prevent some skin disorders, like chickenpox
- Avoiding direct contact with people who have skin infections
- Avoiding excessive emotional or physical stress

- Cleaning stuffs in public spaces before using them such as gym equipment
- Avoid sharing of personal things like blankets, hairbrushes, or swimsuits
- Drinking plenty of water
- Sleeping for at least seven hours each night.

LITERATURE REVIEW

We live in an era where data is new oil. Medical data of a large number of people are collected and analyzed for medical research. Automatic diagnosis helps doctors to precisely predict the diseases. Elngar (1998) used Naïve Bayesian theorem to obtain data patterns. It helps to find the chance of happening of different dermatology diseases and the percentage of the disease has occurred.

Bapko (2011) used (Artificial Neural Networks) ANN for analysis and diagnosis of many skin infections and they attained an accuracy of 90%.

Ahmed (2013) took preprocessed data clusters, using k-means algorithms to differentiate both unrelated and associated data into skin disorders. The patterns with similarity were analysed using the MAFIA algorithm. AprioriTid and Decision tree algorithms then applied to find out frequent patterns from the clustered data sets. Based on the input symptoms data mining algorithm can classify the disease. For this six dermatology disease is taken into consideration and accuracy is measured with some algorithm, Random forest had 97.80%, K Nearest Neighbors 94.44%, SVM had 94.35%.Linear regression had an accuracy of 81% respectively.

Sharma (2013) have used a confidential weighted voting scheme and combined two data mining methods namely SVM and ANN, to classify 6 types of erythema-squamous diseases (ESDs). In this process they managed to achieve the accuracy of 98.99%.

Vijaya (2015) have used support vector machines (SVM) to study skin cancer and its types, to accurately predict different disease types. In pre-processed training data sets, chrominance and texture features are excluded. The accuracy achieved in this way is around 97%.

S.Reena Parvin (2017) Images are gathered from different database and computerized analyses are done to predict the disease. Image preprocessing is done using the Gaussian Filter technique, segmentation using k means clustering algorithm. Keeping health records is very necessary nowadays for proper diagnosis of patients. For this purpose electronic health record is kept which is simple, enable quality recording and analytical processing. It also helps in achieving good relation between academics and healthcare.

Qusay Kanaan Kadhim (2017) finds Digital image processing is widely used to determine skin disease but when it is used analyzed along with decision tree more accurate results are generated. Preprocessing is performed on data and MATLAB is used to design and implement the system.

Shrinidhi (2017) concluded that MATLAB process is used for preprocessing and processing of skin image from the given data sets. Histogram is used to calculate tolerance value which helps in highlighting the unaffected area.

Mishra (2019) used Deep learning for classification of images to detect the type of skin disease. Color, shape, and texture are used to identify the disease conditions. It helps people who doesn't have access to skin specialist. It has the accuracy of around 80%.

Verma (2019) said machine learning is used in various fields including dermatology. When machine learning techniques are applied on skin disease prediction very high disease prediction is achieved.

Gound (2018) taken image processing and data mining technique in order to predict the dermatology related disorders. Images are captured through the smartphone. Preprocessing, segmentation and feature extraction is performed on the type of dermatology disease. General feature is extracted and compared with training data set.

Isaac (2019) used web based skin disease detection system is a way in which online users can detect skin disease and advises possible medical actions in the shortest period of time. Disease identification accuracy are 88%, 85%, 84.7% for Atopic dermatitis, Acne vulgaris and Scabies respectively

Materials and Methods

Machine Learning data mining techniques are very helpful in creation of new algorithms, which enables the computers to learn from previously stored information and data. In our work we have included the demonstration of different methods namely (a) Neural Network, (b) Support Vector Machines (SVM), (c) Logistic regression, (d) Random Forest (RF), (e) naïve Bayesian, (f) K- nearest neighbor (k-NN). The Technique used in this paper is totally data driven and has number of advantages on previously used approaches.

Neural Network

Neural network is a series of algorithms that is arranged in such a way that it works same as human brain functions. It can adapt to any changes given as input and produce best possible result. It does not requires the need to create output criteria.

Support Vector Machine (SVM)

The Support Vector Machines (SVM) is a supervised machine learning technique. It is helpful in classification problems, but it can be used for both classification and regression. In this the given data is plotted in form of points in an n-dimensional space. Here specific coordinate denotes the value of each feature. Then classification is carried out by locating a hyper-plane which can very well differentiate the two classes.

Logistic Regression

The Logistic regression is also a supervised learning algorithm. It is used to predict the dependent variable and the probability of target variable. It is called binary logistic regression, when the dependent variable has two types. The nature of dependent variable is dichotomous, which means that there could be only two possible classes. It is an ordinal logistic regression as the dependent variable category is to be ranked. Logistic regression is of three types on the basis of number of categories.

1. Binary and Binomial
2. Multinomial
3. Ordinal

Random Forest (RF)

Random forest is also a supervised learning algorithm. Just like Support Vector Machines, it can also be used for both classification and the regression problems. But it is mainly used for classification problems. Random forest classifier can handle the missing data. This classifier would not over fit the model, when we have more trees in the forest. It creates decision trees for the given data samples and then gets the prediction from each of the samples and in the last it selects the best solution by voting process.

Naïve Bayesian

Naïve Bayesian uses probabilistic technique which is used for constructing classifiers. Naive Bayes classifier's characteristic assumption is to consider the given class variable, the value of any feature is independent from the values of rest of the features. This is a model of conditional probability. Any given problem instance which is to be classified is symbolized by a vector Y = (y1... yn) it represents n features which are not dependent on other variables, it gives instance probabilities for each of the K possible outcomes.

K-Nearest Neighbor (K-NN)

K-nearest-neighbor algorithm (K-NN), is a data mining technique to classify data on the basis of likelihood. It estimates that how a data point can belong to a particular group. In other words it is depending on which group nearest, data point to it are there. K-NN is also called lazy learner algorithm as it is not able to build a model until query on the data is performed.

Dataset Analysis

The dataset used in this study contains 34 variables that are compared and ranked on 6 different formats. Ten attributes are clinical and rest 24 attributes are Histopathological. Table 1 list out the name of six classes which refer to 6 types of skin disease and 34 attributes.

Some of the 34 variables are itching, age, family history, acanthosis, scaling, hyperkeratosis, perifollicular parakeratosis, follicular papules, follicular horn plug etc. 6 formats on which these variables are compared are information gain, gain ratio, Gini decrease, Chi-square, relief and FCBF. Then we have ranked these 6 formats to above mentioned data mining techniques. The rank had been taken from 3 to 7 of 5 different ranks.

Data Preprocessing

In this research paper, data preprocessing is the first step of the methodology proposed. It is performed on number of steps that are:

1. Selection of patient record and then eliminating those variables which is not required for the analysis process. It is done by data driven method.
2. The cleaning process is performed as this data may have noise, inconsistent, incorrect and missing values.
3. In this step still the data is not ready for technical mining as they may be in different formats and can't be used directly. Now this data is converted into format which is suitable for mining process. Aggregation, normalization, smoothing, etc. are used to perform the transformation.

Table 1. Skin Disease Dataset taken from UCI Knowledge Discovery in Databases Archive provided by Guvenir (1998)

Classes	Clinical Attributes	Histopathological Attributes
Y1 – psoriasis Y2 - seboreic dermatitis Y3- lichen planus Y4 - pityriasis rosea Y5 - chronic dermatitis Y6 - pityriasis rubra pilaris.	Xl: scaling X2: erythema X3: definite borders X4: polygonal papules X5:koebner phenomenon X6: itching X7: follicular papules X8: scalp involvement X9: knee and elbow X10: oral mucosal X11: family history	X12:melanin incontinence X13: fibrosis of the papillary dermis X14: PNL infiltrate X15: eosinophils in the infiltrate X16: exocytosis X17: parakeratosis X18: hyperkeratosis X19: acanthosis X20: clubbing of the rete ridges involvement X21: spongiform pustule X22: thinning of the suprapapillary epidermis X23: elongation of the rete ridges X24: munromicroabscess X25: vacuolization and damage of basal layer X26: disappearance of the granular layer X27: focal hypergranulosis X28: spongiosis X29: perifollicular parakeratosis X30: follicular horn plug X31: saw-tooth appearance of rete ridges X32: inflammatory mononuclear infiltrate X33: age X34: band-like infiltrate

Ensemble Method

In this study, we have evaluated an ensemble method called stacking to predict the types of skin disease. Stacking is known to be one of the best ensemble method which helps in improving the classification accuracy. In the proposed methodology as mentioned in Figure 1, the predictions of 5 different classification methods are combined into one single model called the meta-classifier. In the first level the predictions from K-nearest neighbor, Support vector machine, Neural network, Naïve bayes, and Random forest is calculated. Then in the next level, the meta-classifier is trained with the help of the predictions made by other base classifiers. Here logistic regression is used as the meta classifier. Each classifier is tested with 10-fold cross validation.

RESULT ANALYSIS

After completing the preprocessing, the dataset has no missing values and the dataset is now used to find out the best ranked features. This is done with the help of some

Figure 1. Methodological Approach used

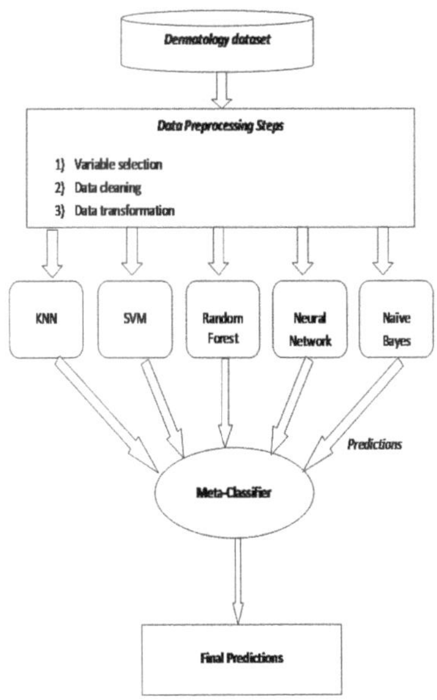

feature selection algorithms namely information gain, gini decrease, relief, gain ratio and chi-square. These selected features are then applied to above stated data mining algorithms individually and their results are compared. This same dataset with minimal features is also set as input for the ensemble method. Finally the results of classification is compared with the help of their accuracy obtained.

Result Analysis With Information Gain

Table 2 shows the list of scores obtained by different attribute. These score are arranged in descending order according to their scores.

The best 3,4,5,6 and 7 ranking features are selected and the different data mining algorithms are compared along with the ensemble method. The results are listed in Table 3. It is observed in Figure 2 that ensemble method with best 4 and best 7 features is able to give an accuracy of 94.3% which is more than the other data mining algorithms.

Result Analysis With Gain Ratio

The list of scores obtained by different attribute is listed in Table 4. These score are arranged in descending order according to their scores.

Table 2. Feature ranking with information gain

Features	Information gain
Elongation of rete ridges	0.863
Clubbing of the rete ridges	0.794
Thinning of the suprapapillary Epidermis	0.789
Band-like infiltrate	0.702
Saw tooth appearances of Rete	0.688
Vacuolisation and damage of basal layer	0.685
Melanin incontinence	0.668
Focalhypergranulosis	0.685
Polygonal papules	0.649
Exocytosis	0.620
Oral mucosal involvement	0.615
Spongiosis	0.605
Knee and elbow involvement	0.590
Fibrosis of the papillary Dermis	0.575
Scalp involvement	0.498
Munro Microabcess	0.458
PNL infiltrate	0.450
Koebner phenomenon	0.404
Disappearance of the granular layer	0.374
Definite borders	0.360
Parakeratosis	0.311
Perifollicular parakeratosis	0.304
Follicular papules	0.301
Itching	0.294
Spongiform pustule	0.281
Scaling	0.270
Follicular horn plug	0.262
Age	0.162
Family history	0.159
Erythema	0.141
Hyperkeratosis	0.132
Acanthosis	0.127
Inflammatory monoluclear infiltrate	0.093

Figure 2. Comparison of data mining methods using Information Gain

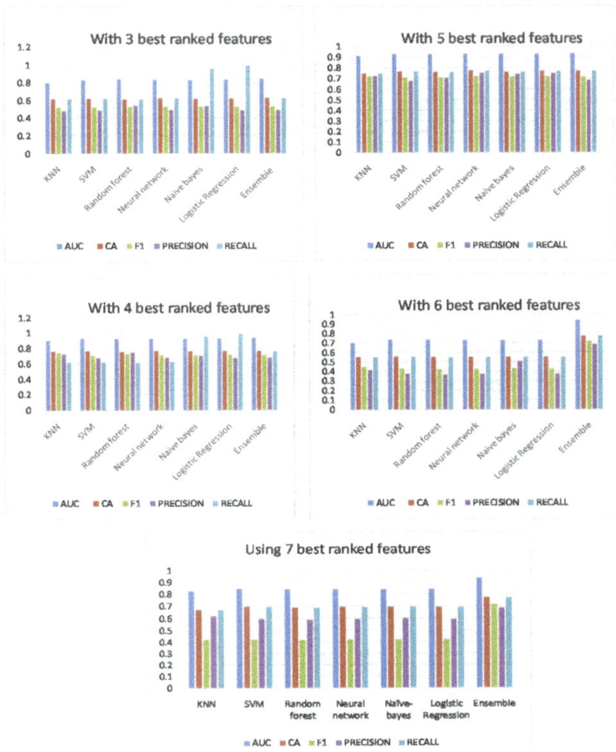

The best 3,4,5,6 and 7 ranking features are selected and the different data mining algorithms are compared along with the ensemble method. The results are listed in Table 5. The ensemble method with 7 best ranked feature is giving an accuracy of 85.4% accuracy. The results are compared in chart as shown in Figure 3.

Result Analysis With Gini Decrease

The list of scores obtained by different attribute is listed in Table 6. These score are arranged in descending order according to their scores.

The best 3,4,5,6 and 7 ranking features are selected and the different data mining algorithms are compared along with the ensemble method. The results are listed in Table 7.The ensemble method is giving an accuracy of 94.3% accuracy with 7 best ranked features. The results are compared in chart as shown in Figure 4.

Table 3. Result analysis with information gain

MODEL	AUC	CA	F1	PRECISION	RECALL
With 3 best ranked features					
KNN	0.803	0.620	0.525	0.487	0.620
SVM	0.837	0.623	0.528	0.492	0.623
Random forest	0.844	0.617	0.530	0.547	0.617
Neural network	0.842	0.628	0.532	0.494	0.628
Naïve bayes	0.836	0.620	0.529	0.543	0.961
Logistic Reg.	0.841	0.626	0.529	0.491	0.993
ensemble	0.851	0.628	0.532	0.494	0.628
With 4 best ranked features					
KNN	0.908	0.765	0.748	0.733	0.620
SVM	0.937	0.768	0.711	0.680	0.623
Random forest	0.931	0.760	0.730	0.751	0.617
Neural network	0.935	0.773	0.717	0.687	0.628
Naïve bayes	0.935	0.765	0.715	0.710	0.961
Logistic Reg.	0.935	0.770	0.713	0.681	0.993
ensemble	0.943	0.770	0.714	0.684	0.770
With 5 best ranked features					
KNN	0.916	0.751	0.723	0.727	0.751
SVM	0.935	0.768	0.713	0.684	0.768
Random forest	0.933	0.765	0.713	0.707	0.765
Neural network	0.936	0.776	0.723	0.755	0.776
Naïve bayes	0.935	0.765	0.720	0.746	0.765
Logistic Reg.	0.935	0.773	0.721	0.752	0.773
ensemble	0.941	0.773	0.717	0.687	0.773
With 6 best ranked features					
KNN	0.706	0.554	0.447	0.413	0.554
SVM	0.740	0.555	0.427	0.374	0.555
Random forest	0.739	0.549	0.422	0.367	0.549
Neural network	0.734	0.552	0.426	0.373	0.552
Naïve bayes	0.732	0.552	0.430	0.507	0.552
Logistic Reg.	0.732	0.552	0.426	0.373	0.552
ensemble	0.942	0.773	0.717	0.687	0.773
With 7 best ranked features					
KNN	0.831	0.675	0.424	0.624	0.675
SVM	0.851	0.699	0.424	0.598	0.699
Random forest	0.847	0.691	0.420	0.590	0.691
Neural network	0.848	0.697	0.423	0.597	0.697
Naïve bayes	0.845	0.697	0.423	0.600	0.697
Logistic Reg.	0.848	0.694	0.424	0.594	0.694
ensemble	0.943	0.773	0.717	0.687	0.773

Table 4. Feature ranking with Gain ratio

Features	Gain Ratio
Elongation of rete ridges	0.530
Clubbing of the rete ridges	0.592
Thinning of the suprapapillary epidermis	0.601
Band-like infiltrate	0.724
Saw tooth appearances of rete	0.711
Vacuolisation and damage of basal layer	0.725
Melanin incontinence	0.709
Focal hypergranulosis	0.663
Polygonal papules	0.722
Exocytosis	0.325
Oral mucosal involvement	0.674
Spongiosis	0.371
Knee and elbow involvement	0.439
Fibrosis of the papillary dermis	0.702
Scalp involvement	0.399
Munro microabcess	0.429
PNL infiltrate	0.325
Koebner phenomenon	0.267
Disappearance of the granular layer	0.317
Definite borders	0.198
Parakeratosis	0.169
Perifollicular parakeratosis	0.771
Follicular papules	0.527
Itching	0.149
Spongiform pustule	0.294
Scaling	0.177
Follicular horn plug	0.628
Age	0.082
Family history	0.291
Erythema	0.098
hyperkeratosis	0.096
Acanthosis	0.083
Inflammatory monoluclear infiltrate	0.060

Figure 3. Comparison of data mining methods using Gain Ratio

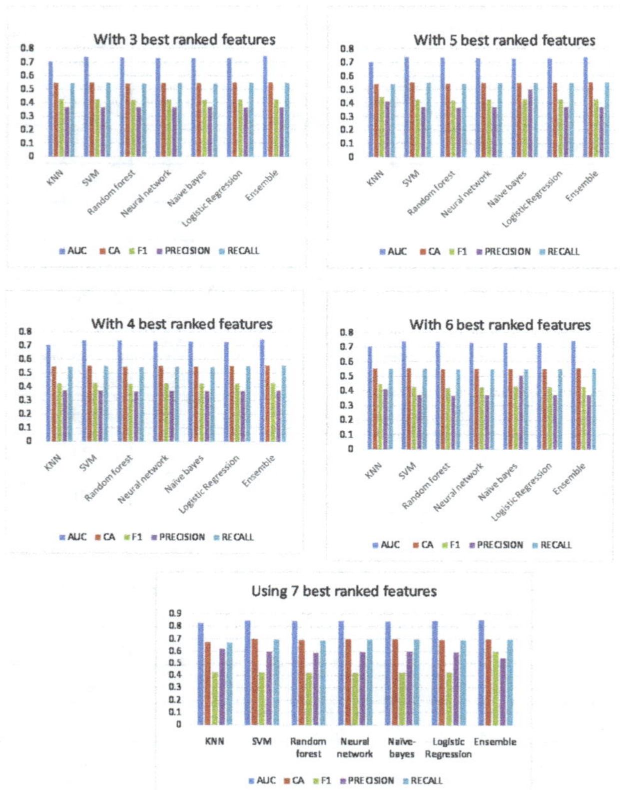

Result Analysis With Chi-Square X²

The list of scores obtained by different attribute is listed in Table 8. These score are arranged in descending order according to their scores.

The best 3,4,5,6 and 7 ranking features are selected and the different data mining algorithms are compared along with the ensemble method. The results are listed in Table 9. The accuracy of 85.7% is achieved with ensemble method when only best 4 features were used. It can be also be observed in Figure 5.

Result Analysis With Relieff

The list of scores obtained by different attribute is listed in Table 10. These score are arranged in descending order according to their scores.

Table 5. Result analysis with Gain ratio

MODEL	AUC	CA	F1	PRECISION	RECALL
With 3 best ranked features					
KNN	0.803	0.620	0.525	0.487	0.620
SVM	0.837	0.623	0.528	0.492	0.623
Random forest	0.844	0.617	0.530	0.547	0.617
Neural network	0.842	0.628	0.532	0.494	0.628
Naïve bayes	0.836	0.620	0.529	0.543	0.961
Logistic Reg.	0.841	0.626	0.529	0.491	0.993
ensemble	0.851	0.628	0.532	0.494	0.628
With 4 best ranked features					
KNN	0.908	0.765	0.748	0.733	0.620
SVM	0.937	0.768	0.711	0.680	0.623
Random forest	0.931	0.760	0.730	0.751	0.617
Neural network	0.935	0.773	0.717	0.687	0.628
Naïve bayes	0.935	0.765	0.715	0.710	0.961
Logistic Reg.	0.935	0.770	0.713	0.681	0.993
ensemble	0.943	0.770	0.714	0.684	0.770
With 5 best ranked features					
KNN	0.916	0.751	0.723	0.727	0.751
SVM	0.935	0.768	0.713	0.684	0.768
Random forest	0.933	0.765	0.713	0.707	0.765
Neural network	0.936	0.776	0.723	0.755	0.776
Naïve bayes	0.935	0.765	0.720	0.746	0.765
Logistic Reg.	0.935	0.773	0.721	0.752	0.773
ensemble	0.941	0.773	0.717	0.687	0.773
With 6 best ranked features					
KNN	0.706	0.554	0.447	0.413	0.554
SVM	0.740	0.555	0.427	0.374	0.555
Random forest	0.739	0.549	0.422	0.367	0.549
Neural network	0.734	0.552	0.426	0.373	0.552
Naïve bayes	0.732	0.552	0.430	0.507	0.552
Logistic Reg.	0.732	0.552	0.426	0.373	0.552
ensemble	0.942	0.773	0.717	0.687	0.773
With 7 best ranked features					
KNN	0.831	0.675	0.424	0.624	0.675
SVM	0.851	0.699	0.424	0.598	0.699
Random forest	0.847	0.691	0.420	0.590	0.691
Neural network	0.848	0.697	0.423	0.597	0.697
Naïve bayes	0.845	0.697	0.423	0.600	0.697
Logistic Reg.	0.848	0.694	0.424	0.594	0.694
ensemble	0.943	0.773	0.717	0.687	0.773

Table 6. Feature ranking with Gini Decrease

Features	Gini Decrease
Elongation of rete ridges	0.197
Clubbing of the rete ridges	0.239
Thinning of the suprapapillary epidermis	0.241
Band-like infiltrate	0.193
Saw tooth appearances of rete	0.193
Vacuolisation and damage of basal layer	0.192
Melanin incontinence	0.191
Focal hypergranulosis	0.189
Polygonal papules	0.188
Exocytosis	0.175
Oral mucosal involvement	0.181
Spongiosis	0.141
Knee and elbow involvement	0.153
Fibrosis of the papillary dermis	0.146
Scalp involvement	0.159
Munro microabcess	0.154
PNL infiltrate	0.104
Koebner phenomenon	0.703
Disappearance of the granular layer	0.108
Definite borders	0.083
Parakeratosis	0.084
Perifollicular parakeratosis	0.061
Follicular papules	0.057
Itching	0.067
Spongiform pustule	0.092
Scaling	0.069
Follicular horn plug	0.054
Age	0.022
Family history	0.037
Erythema	0.037
hyperkeratosis	0.030
Acanthosis	0.023
Inflammatory monoluclear infiltrate	0.021

Figure 4. Comparison of data mining methods using Gini Decrease

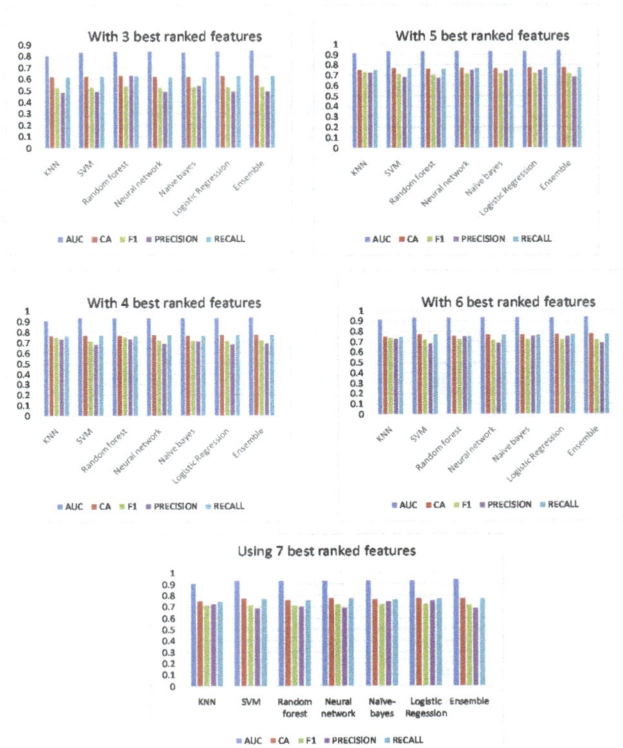

The best 3,4,5,6 and 7 ranking features are selected and the different data mining algorithms are compared along with the ensemble method. The results are listed in Table 11. An accuracy of 93.8% is achieved with ensemble method when only 5,6 and 7 features were used for classification. It is also depicted in Figure 6.

CONCLUSION

The main term which helps in finding out the feasibility of particular classifier is its accuracy. The accuracy shows process's efficiency. In this study the accuracy of different classifiers are compared using only best ranked features. In spite of use of limited features, the classifier is still able to give good classification accuracy. If we talk about the accuracy of the used methodology, this technique shows the prediction of diseases with 94% of accuracy. Hence this study gave a conclusion that in case

Table 7. Result analysis with Gini decrease

MODEL	AUC	CA	F1	PRECISION	RECALL
With 3 best ranked features					
KNN	0.803	0.620	0.525	0.487	0.620
SVM	0.835	0.623	0.528	0.492	0.623
Random forest	0.842	0.628	0.539	0.631	0.628
Neural network	0.843	0.620	0.526	0.491	0.620
Naïve bayes	0.836	0.620	0.529	0.543	0.620
Logistic Reg.	0.841	0.626	0.529	0.491	0.626
ensemble	0.851	0.628	0.532	0.492	0.628
With 4 best ranked features					
KNN	0.908	0.765	0.748	0.733	0.765
SVM	0.938	0.768	0.711	0.680	0.768
Random forest	0.935	0.762	0.747	0.732	0.762
Neural network	0.935	0.773	0.717	0.687	0.773
Naïve bayes	0.935	0.765	0.715	0.710	0.765
Logistic Reg.	0.935	0.770	0.713	0.681	0.770
ensemble	0.941	0.773	0.717	0.687	0.773
With 5 best ranked features					
KNN	0.916	0.751	0.730	0.727	0.751
SVM	0.934	0.768	0.713	0.684	0.768
Random forest	0.934	0.760	0.705	0.676	0.760
Neural network	0.935	0.770	0.719	0.753	0.770
Naïve bayes	0.935	0.765	0.720	0.746	0.765
Logistic Reg.	0.935	0.773	0.721	0.752	0.773
ensemble	0.941	0.773	0.717	0.687	0.773
With 6 best ranked features					
KNN	0.917	0.751	0.738	0.730	0.751
SVM	0.938	0.773	0.717	0.687	0.773
Random forest	0.936	0.757	0.727	0.752	0.757
Neural network	0.937	0.768	0.715	0.688	0.768
Naïve bayes	0.935	0.768	0.722	0.757	0.768
Logistic Reg.	0.935	0.773	0.721	0.752	0.773
ensemble	0.942	0.776	0.720	0.690	0.776
With 7 best ranked features					
KNN	0.908	0.751	0.713	0.725	0.751
SVM	0.935	0.773	0.717	0.687	0.773
Random forest	0.931	0.760	0.712	0.702	0.760
Neural network	0.933	0.776	0.720	0.691	0.776
Naïve bayes	0.935	0.765	0.720	0.748	0.765
Logistic Reg.	0.935	0.773	0.723	0.756	0.773
ensemble	0.943	0.773	0.717	0.687	0.773

of a dataset with large number of features, selecting the highly ranked features with

Table 8. Feature ranking with Chi-Square

Features	X^2
Elongation of rete ridges	401.375
Clubbing of the rete ridges	513.124
Thinning of the suprapapillary epidermis	513.814
Band-like infiltrate	759.365
Saw tooth appearances of rete	667.742
Vacuolisation and damage of basal layer	671.800
Melanin incontinence	604.333
Focal hypergranulosis	577.996
Polygonal papules	669.667
Exocytosis	198.654
Oral mucosal involvement	563.500
Spongiosis	275.436
Knee and elbow involvement	356.051
Fibrosis of the papillary dermis	688.000
Scalp involvement	324.209
Munro microabcess	276.275
PNL infiltrate	188.149
Koebner phenomenon	161.801
Disappearance of the granular layer	199.666
Definite borders	73.882
parakeratosis	71.246
Perifollicular parakeratosis	690.579
Follicular papules	537.371
Itching	111.247
Spongiform pustule	176.647
Scaling	28.571
Follicular horn plug	552.411
Age	41.884
Family history	67.812
Erythema	12.683
hyperkeratosis	47.426
Acanthosis	12,810
Inflammatory monoluclear infiltrate	8.905

Figure 5. Comparison of data mining methods using Chi-square

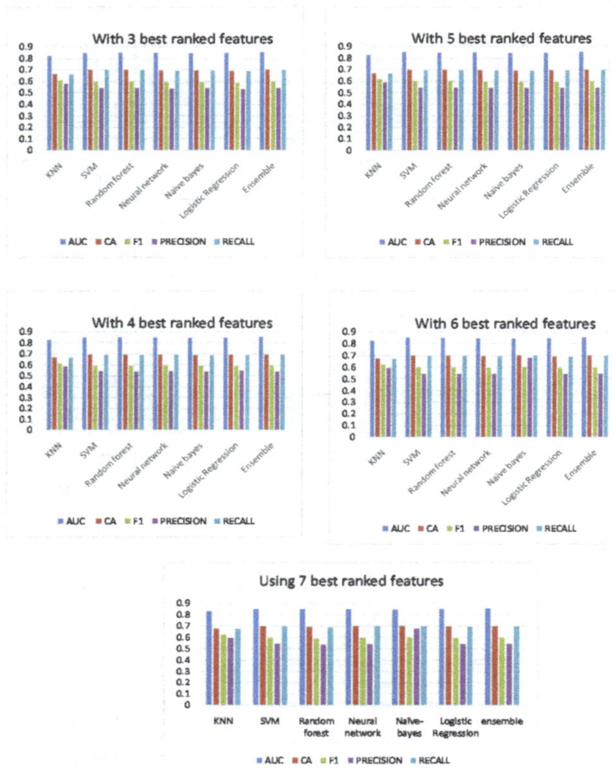

ensemble data mining techniques can help to provide better classification accuracy.

ACKNOWLEDGMENT

The authors wish to thank the Rajkiya engineering college Banda for all the support. The present study was done in fulfillment of requirements for B.tech degree.

Table 9. Result analysis with Chi-Square

MODEL	AUC	CA	F1	PRECISION	RECALL
With 3 best ranked features					
KNN	0.823	0.661	0.610	0.579	0.661
SVM	0.848	0.697	0.595	0.541	0.697
Random forest	0.850	0.697	0.595	0.541	0.697
Neural network	0.850	0.691	0.591	0.537	0.691
Naïve bayes	0.847	0.694	0.593	0.540	0.694
Logistic Reg.	0.848	0.689	0.587	0.532	0.689
ensemble	0.856	0.697	0.595	0.541	0.697
With 4 best ranked features					
KNN	0.827	0.667	0.616	0.586	0.667
SVM	0.851	0.694	0.594	0.543	0.694
Random forest	0.852	0.691	0.590	0.536	0.691
Neural network	0.851	0.694	0.594	0.543	0.694
Naïve bayes	0.845	0.689	0.592	0.539	0.689
Logistic Reg.	0.848	0.691	0.591	0.551	0.691
ensemble	0.857	0.694	0.593	0.540	0.694
With 5 best ranked features					
KNN	0.829	0.667	0.618	0.589	0.667
SVM	0.855	0.697	0.597	0.545	0.697
Random forest	0.848	0.697	0.597	0.545	0.697
Neural network	0.851	0.691	0.593	0.542	0.691
Naïve bayes	0.844	0.689	0.592	0.541	0.689
Logistic Reg.	0.847	0.691	0.593	0.542	0.691
ensemble	0.856	0.697	0.595	0.543	0.697
With 6 best ranked features					
KNN	0.828	0.672	0.623	0.593	0.672
SVM	0.851	0.697	0.597	0.545	0.697
Random forest	0.850	0.697	0.597	0.545	0.697
Neural network	0.848	0.694	0.596	0.545	0.694
Naïve bayes	0.845	0.699	0.603	0.680	0.699
Logistic Reg.	0.848	0.691	0.593	0.542	0.691
ensemble	0.855	0.699	0.598	0.546	0.699
With 7 best ranked features					
KNN	0.831	0.675	0.624	0.595	0.675
SVM	0.851	0.699	0.598	0.546	0.699
Random forest	0.849	0.691	0.591	0.539	0.691
Neural network	0.849	0.697	0.595	0.543	0.697
Naïve bayes	0.845	0.697	0.600	0.677	0.697
Logistic Reg.	0.848	0.694	0.594	0.543	0.694
ensemble	0.854	0.699	0.598	0.546	0.699

Table 10. Feature ranking with Relieff

Features	Relieff
Elongation of rete ridges	0.324
Clubbing of the rete ridges	0.217
Thinning of the suprapapillary epidermis	0.215
Band-like infiltrate	0.298
Saw tooth appearances of rete	0.224
Vacuolisation and damage of basal layer	0.223
Melanin incontinence	0.207
Focal hypergranulosis	0.190
Polygonal papules	0.227
Exocytosis	0.210
Oral mucosal involvement	0.132
Spongiosis	0.238
Knee and elbow involvement	0.140
Fibrosis of the papillary dermis	0.289
Scalp involvement	0.084
Munro microabcess	0.068
PNL infiltrate	0.161
Koebner phenomenon	0.117
Disappearance of the granular layer	0.110
Definite borders	0.085
Parakeratosis	0.067
Perifollicular parakeratosis	0.053
Follicular papules	0.067
Itching	0.121
Spongiform pustule	0.038
Scaling	0.070
Follicular horn plug	0.030
Age	0.032
Family history	0.055
Erythema	0.045
hyperkeratosis	0.032
Acanthosis	0.033
Inflammatory monoluclear infiltrate	0.018

Figure 6. Comparison of data mining methods with Relieff

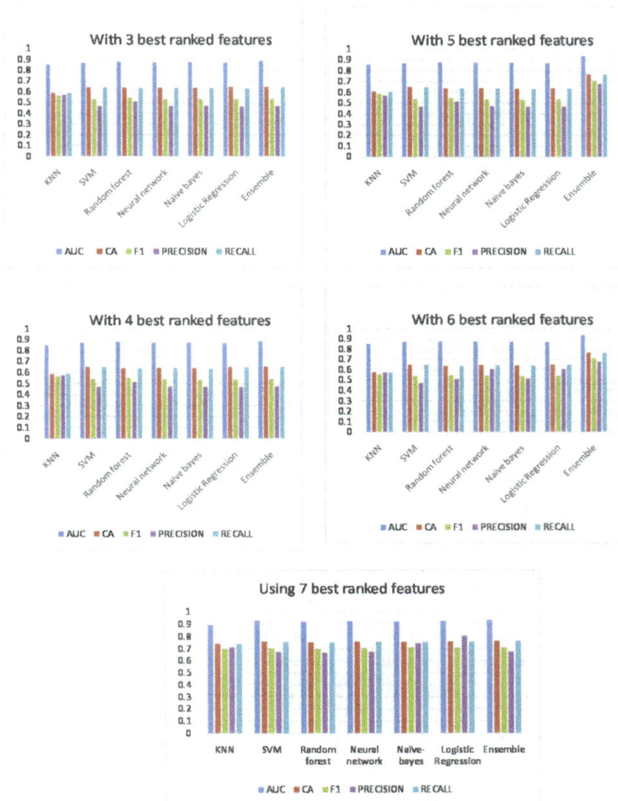

Table 11. Result analysis with Relieff

MODEL	AUC	CA	F1	PRECISION	RECALL
With 3 best ranked features					
KNN	0.853	0.590	0.566	0.574	0.590
SVM	0.871	0.642	0.532	0.468	0.642
Random forest	0.881	0.639	0.547	0.512	0.639
Neural network	0.878	0.639	0.532	0.468	0.639
Naïve bayes	0.877	0.637	0.532	0.471	0.637
Logistic Reg.	0.873	0.645	0.533	0.465	0.635
ensemble	0.891	0.648	0.535	0.469	0.648
With 4 best ranked features					
KNN	0.851	0.587	0.565	0.574	0.587
SVM	0.871	0.648	0.537	0.471	0.648
Random forest	0.881	0.639	0.550	0.516	0.639
Neural network	0.876	0.642	0.537	0.474	0.642
Naïve bayes	0.877	0.639	0.534	0.471	0.639
Logistic Reg.	0.872	0.648	0.535	0.469	0.648
ensemble	0.889	0.650	0.538	0.472	0.650
With 5 best ranked features					
KNN	0.860	0.609	0.585	0.573	0.609
SVM	0.871	0.650	0.538	0.472	0.650
Random forest	0.881	0.639	0.549	0.517	0.639
Neural network	0.877	0.639	0.535	0.473	0.639
Naïve bayes	0.877	0.637	0.532	0.471	0.637
Logistic Reg.	0.872	0.638	0.537	0.471	0.638
ensemble	0.938	0.765	0.710	0.681	0.765
With 6 best ranked features					
KNN	0.855	0.574	0.556	0.574	0.574
SVM	0.877	0.650	0.538	0.472	0.650
Random forest	0.880	0.637	0.548	0.512	0.637
Neural network	0.878	0.645	0.542	0.608	0.645
Naïve bayes	0.877	0.642	0.539	0.516	0.642
Logistic Reg.	0.873	0.650	0.542	0.606	0.650
ensemble	0.938	0.765	0.710	0.681	0.765
With 7 best ranked features					
KNN	0.899	0.743	0.703	0.716	0.743
SVM	0.934	0.762	0.707	0.678	0.762
Random forest	0.925	0.754	0.700	0.671	0.754
Neural network	0.929	0.762	0.706	0.677	0.762
Naïve bayes	0.926	0.760	0.713	0.748	0.760
Logistic Reg.	0.929	0.762	0.710	0.809	0.762
ensemble	0.938	0.765	0.710	0.681	0.765

REFERENCES

Elngar, Ahmed A., & Kumar, Rishabh, A Hayat and P Churi. (1998). Intelligent System for Skin Disease Prediction using Machine Learning. *Journal of Physics: Conference Series.*

Ahmed, Jesmin, & Rahman. (2013). Early Prevention and Detection of Skin Cancer Risk using Data Mining. *International Journal of Computer Applications, 62*(4), 1-6. DOI: doi:10.5120/10065-4662.2013

Bakpo, F. S., & Kabari, L. G. (2011). Diagnosing skin diseases using an Artificial Neural Network. In *Artificial Neural Networks*. Methodological Advances and Biomedical Applications.

Gound, Gadre, Gaikwad, & Wagh. (2018). Skin Disease Diagnosis System using Image Processing and Data Mining. *International Journal of Computer Applications, 179*(16).

Kadhim. (2017). Classification of Human Skin Diseases using Data Mining. *International Journal of Advanced Engineering Research and Science, 4*(1).

Mishra, Imaizumi, & Yamasaki. (2019). Interpreting Fine-Grained Dermatological Classification by Deep Learning. *IEEE Explore*.

Nti, Akyeramfo-Sam, Philip, Yeboah, & Nancy. (2019). A Web-Based Skin Disease Detection System. *American Journal of Computer Science and Information Technology, 7*.

Reena Parvin, S., & Mohamed Jafar, O. A. (2017, July). Prediction of skin disease using data mining techniques. *International Journal of Innovative Research in Computer and Communication Engineering*, *6*(7).

Sharma & Hota. (2013). Data mining techniques for prediction of different categories of dermatology diseases. *Academy of Information and Management Sciences Journal, 16*(2).

Shrinidhi Gindhi, E. (2017, July). An innovative Approach For Skin Disease Detection Using Image Processing and Data Mining. *International Journal of Innovative Research in Computer and Communication Engineering*, *5*(4).

UCI KDD Archive. (1998). http:/kdd.ics.uci.edu

Verma, Pal, & Kumar. (2019). *Classification of Skin Disease Using Ensembles Data Mining Techniques*. doi:10.31557/APJCP.2019.20.6.1887

Vijaya, M. S. (2015). Categorization of Non-Melanoma Skin Lesion Diseases Using Support Vector Machine and Its Variants. *International Journal of Medical Imaging*.

Compilation of References

Bakas, S. (2015, October). GLISTRboost: combining multimodal MRI segmentation, registration, and biophysical tumor growth modeling with gradient boosting machines for glioma segmentation. In *BrainLes 2015* (pp. 144–155). Springer.

Gaonkar, B., Beckett, J., Villaroman, M. H. S. D., Ahn, B. S. C., Edwards, B. S. M., Moran, S., Attiah, M., Babayan, D., Ames, C., Villablanca, J. P., Salamon, N., Bui, A., & Macyszyn, L. (2019). Quantitative analysis of neural foramina in the lumbar spine: An imaging informatics and machine learning study. *Radiology. Artificial Intelligence*, *1*(2), 180037. doi:10.1148/ryai.2019180037 PMID:33937788

Attiah, M., Gaonkar, B., Alkhalid, Y., Villaroman, D., Medina, R., Ahn, C., Niu, T., Beckett, J., Ames, C., & Macyszyn, L. (2019). Natural history of the aging spine: A cross-sectional analysis of spinopelvic parameters in the asymptomatic population. *Journal of Neurosurgery. Spine*, *32*(1), 63–68. doi:10.3171/2019.7.SPINE181164 PMID:31561232

Macyszyn, L., Akbari, H., Pisapia, J. M., Da, X., Attiah, M., Pigrish, V., Bi, Y., Pal, S., Davuluri, R. V., Roccograndi, L., Dahmane, N., Martinez-Lage, M., Biros, G., Wolf, R. L., Bilello, M., O'Rourke, D. M., & Davatzikos, C. (2015). Imaging patterns predict patient survival and molecular subtype in glioblastoma via machine learning techniques. *Neuro-Oncology*, *18*(3), 417–425. doi:10.1093/neuonc/nov127 PMID:26188015

Davenport, T., & Kalakota, R. (2019). The potential for artificial intelligence in healthcare. *Future Healthcare Journal*, *6*(2), 94–98. doi:10.7861/futurehosp.6-2-94 PMID:31363513

Sotiras, A. (2016). Machine learning as a means toward precision diagnostics and prognostics. In *Machine learning and medical imaging* (pp. 299–334). Academic Press. doi:10.1016/B978-0-12-804076-8.00010-4

Matheny, M. E., Whicher, D., & Israni, S. T. (2020). Artificial Intelligence in health Care: A report from the National Academy of Medicine. *Journal of the American Medical Association*, *323*(6), 509–510. doi:10.1001/jama.2019.21579 PMID:31845963

Office, U. (2020, January 21). *Artificial Intelligence in Health Care: Benefits and Challenges of Machine Learning in Drug Development* [Reissued with revisions on Jan. 31, 2020]. https://www.gao.gov/products/GAO-20-215SP

Schwartz, W. B. (1970). Medicine and the computer: the promise and problems of change. In *Use and Impact of Computers in Clinical Medicine* (pp. 321–335). Springer. doi:10.1007/978-1-4613-8674-2_20

Lori, K. (n.d.). Putting the AI in Radiology. *Radiology Today, 19*(1), 10.

Lakhani, P., Prater, A. B., Hutson, R. K., Andriole, K. P., Dreyer, K. J., Morey, J., Prevedello, L. M., Clark, T. J., Geis, J. R., Itri, J. N., & Hawkins, C. M. (2018). Machine learning in radiology: Applications beyond image interpretation. *Journal of the American College of Radiology*, *15*(2), 350–359. doi:10.1016/j.jacr.2017.09.044 PMID:29158061

Esteva, A., Kuprel, B., Novoa, R. A., Ko, J., Swetter, S. M., Blau, H. M., & Thrun, S. (2017). Dermatologist-level classification of skin cancer with deep neural networks. *Nature*, *542*(7639), 115–118. doi:10.1038/nature21056 PMID:28117445

Liu, Y., Gadepalli, K., & Norouzi, M. (2017). *Detecting cancer metastases on gigapixel pathology images*. https://arxiv.org/pdf/1703.02442.pdf

He, K., Zhang, X., & Ren, S. (2017). *Delving deep into rectifiers: surpassing human-level performance on imageNet classification*. https://arxiv.org/pdf/1502.01852.pdf

Oram, A. (2001). *Peer-to-peer. Harnessing the power of disruptive technologies*. O'Reilly & Associates.

Kohli, M., Prevedello, L. M., Filice, R. W., & Geis, J. R. (2017). Implementing machine learning in radiology practice and research. *AJR. American Journal of Roentgenology*, *208*(4), 754–760. doi:10.2214/AJR.16.17224 PMID:28125274

Kaggle Data Science Bowl. (2017). https://www.kaggle.com/c/data-science-bowl-2017

Prevedello, L. M., Erdal, B. S., Ryu, J. L., Little, K. J., Demirer, M., Qian, S., & White, R. D. (2017, July 3). Automated critical test findings identification and online notification system using artificial intelligence in imaging. *Radiology*, *285*(3), 162664. Advance online publication. doi:10.1148/radiol.2017162664 PMID:28678669

Jha, S., & Topol, E. J. (2016). Adapting to artificial intelligence: Radiologists and pathologists as information specialists. *Journal of the American Medical Association*, *316*(22), 2353–2354. doi:10.1001/jama.2016.17438 PMID:27898975

Gaonkar, B., Kim, K., & Macyszyn, L. (2020). Ethical issues arising due to bias in Training A.I. algorithms in healthcare and data sharing as a potential solution. *AI Ethics Journal*, *1*(1), 1–9. doi:10.47289/AIEJ20200916

Gianfrancesco, M. A., Tamang, S., Yazdany, J., & Schmajuk, G. (2018). Potential biases in machine learning algorithms using electronic health record data. *JAMA Internal Medicine*, *178*(11), 1544–1547. doi:10.1001/jamainternmed.2018.3763 PMID:30128552

Russell, S., & Bohannon, J. (2015). Artificial intelligence. Fears of an AI pioneer. *Science*, *349*(6245), 252. doi:10.1126cience.349.6245.252 PMID:26185241

Wong, J., Horwitz, M. M., Zhou, L., & Toh, S. (2018). Using machine learning to identify health outcomes from electronic health record data. *Current Epidemiology Reports*, *5*(4), 331–342. doi:10.100740471-018-0165-9 PMID:30555773

Wei, W. Q., Teixeira, P. L., Mo, H., Cronin, R. M., Warner, J. L., & Denny, J. C. (2016). Combining billing codes, clinical notes, and medications from electronic health records provides superior phenotyping performance. *Journal of the American Medical Informatics Association: JAMIA*, *23*(1), 20–27. doi:10.1093/jamia/ocv130 PMID:26338219

Shivade, C., Raghavan, P., Fosler-Lussier, E., Embi, P. J., Elhadad, N., Johnson, S. B., & Lai, A. M. (2014). A review of approaches to identifying patient phenotype cohorts using electronic health records. *Journal of the American Medical Informatics Association: JAMIA*, *21*(2), 221–230. doi:10.1136/amiajnl-2013-001935 PMID:24201027

Ford, E., Carroll, J. A., Smith, H. E., Scott, D., & Cassell, J. A. (2016). Extracting information from the text of electronic medical records to improve case detection: A systematic review. *Journal of the American Medical Informatics Association: JAMIA*, *23*(5), 1007–1015. doi:10.1093/jamia/ocv180 PMID:26911811

Araujo, T., Aresta, G., Castro, E., Rouco, J., Aguiar, P., Eloy, C., Polónia, A., & Campilho, A. (2017). Classification of breast cancer histology images using convolutional neural networks. *PLoS One*, *12*(6), e0177544. doi:10.1371/journal.pone.0177544 PMID:28570557

Halevy, A., Norvig, P., & Pereira, F. (2009). The unreasonable effectiveness of data. *IEEE Intelligent Systems*, *24*(2), 8–12. doi:10.1109/MIS.2009.36

Arpey, N. C., Gaglioti, A. H., & Rosenbaum, M. E. (2017). How socioeconomic status affects patient perceptions of health care: A qualitative study. *Journal of Primary Care & Community Health*, *8*(3), 169–175. doi:10.1177/2150131917697439 PMID:28606031

Bond, R. R., Novotny, T., Andrsova, I., Koc, L., Sisakova, M., Finlay, D., Guldenring, D., McLaughlin, J., Peace, A., McGilligan, V., Leslie, S. J., Wang, H., & Malik, M. (2018). Automation bias in medicine: The influence of automated diagnoses on interpreter accuracy and uncertainty when reading electrocardiograms. *Journal of Electrocardiology*, *51*(6), S6–S11. doi:10.1016/j.jelectrocard.2018.08.007 PMID:30122457

Goddard, K., Roudsari, A., & Wyatt, J. C. (2012). Automation bias: A systematic review of frequency, effect mediators, and mitigators. *Journal of the American Medical Informatics Association: JAMIA*, *19*(1), 121–127. doi:10.1136/amiajnl-2011-000089 PMID:21685142

Parasuraman, R., Molloy, R., & Singh, I. L. (1993). Performance consequences of automation-induced 'complacency'. *The International Journal of Aviation Psychology*, *3*(1), 1–23. doi:10.120715327108ijap0301_1

Chartrand, G., Cheng, P. M., Vorontsov, E., Drozdzal, M., Turcotte, S., Pal, C. J., Kadoury, S., & Tang, A. (2017). Deep learning: A primer for radiologists. *Radiographics*, *37*(7), 2113–2131. doi:10.1148/rg.2017170077 PMID:29131760

Lease, M. (2011). On quality control and machine learning in crowdsourcing. *Human Computation (Fairfax, Va.)*, *11*(11).

Mason, W., Vaughan, J. W., & Wallach, H. (2014). Computational social science and social computing. *Machine Learning*, *95*(3), 257–260. doi:10.100710994-013-5426-8

Goodfellow, I., Bengio, Y., & Courville, A. (2016). *Deep learning*. MIT Press.

Samuel, A. L. (1959). Some studies in machine learning using the game of checkers. *IBM Journal of Research and Development*, *3*(3), 210–229. doi:10.1147/rd.33.0210

Lee, J. G., Jun, S., Cho, Y. W., Lee, H., Kim, G. B., Seo, J. B., & Kim, N. (2017). Deep learning in medical imaging: A general overview. *Korean Journal of Radiology*, *18*(4), 570–584. doi:10.3348/kjr.2017.18.4.570 PMID:28670152

Tripathi, S. (2021). *Artificial Intelligence: A Brief Review*. Analyzing Future Applications of AI, Sensors, and Robotics in Society.

Gaonkar, B., Shinohara, R. T., & Davatzikos, C. (2015). Interpreting support vector machine models for multivariate group wise analysis in neuroimaging. *Medical Image Analysis*, *24*(1), 190–204. doi:10.1016/j.media.2015.06.008 PMID:26210913

Gaonkar, B., & Davatzikos, C. (2013). Analytic estimation of statistical significance maps for support vector machine based multivariate image analysis and classification. *NeuroImage*, *78*, 270–283. doi:10.1016/j.neuroimage.2013.03.066 PMID:23583748

Acosta Calderon, C. A., Mohan, E. R., & Ng, B. S. (2015). Development of a hospital mobile platform for logistics tasks. *Digital Communications and Networks*, *1*(2), 102–111. doi:10.1016/j.dcan.2015.03.001

Ahmad, O. F., Stoyanov, D., & Lovat, L. B. (2020). Barriers and pitfalls for artificial intelligence in gastroenterology: Ethical and regulatory issues. *Techniques and Innovations in Gastrointestinal Endoscopy*, *22*(2), 80–84. doi:10.1016/j.tgie.2019.150636

Ahmed, Jesmin, & Rahman. (2013). Early Prevention and Detection of Skin Cancer Risk using Data Mining. *International Journal of Computer Applications, 62*(4), 1-6. Doi:10.5120/10065-4662.2013

Akinloye, F. O., Obe, O., & Boyinbode, O. (2020). Development of an affective-based e-healthcare system for autistic children. *Scientific American*, *9*, e00514.

Akremi, L. (2014). Stichprobenziehung in der qualitativen Sozialforschung [Sampling in qualitative social research]. In N. Baur & J. Blasius (Eds.), *Handbuch Methoden der empirischen Sozialforschung*. Springer Fachmedien Wiesbaden. doi:10.1007/978-3-531-18939-0_17

Alaya, F. (2020). Healthcare difficulties in the post-GDPR era. *Trinity Student Medical Journal*, *20*, 8–12.

Alimadadi, A., Aryal, S., Manandhar, I., Munroe, P. B., Joe, B., & Cheng, X. (2020). Artificial intelligence and machine learning to fight COVID-19. *Physiological Genomics*, *52*(4), 200–202. doi:10.1152/physiolgenomics.00029.2020 PMID:32216577

Al-Jefri, M., Evans, R., Uchyigit, G., & Ghezzi, P. (2018). What is health information quality? Ethical dimension and perception by users. *Frontiers in Medicine*, *5*, 260. doi:10.3389/fmed.2018.00260 PMID:30294599

Amputee Coalition. (2019). *3D printed prosthetics – where we are today*. Retrieved March 2020 from https://www.amputee-coalition.org/3d-printed-prosthetics/

Annan, K. (2003). *Universal Values - Peace, Freedom, Social Progress, Equal Rights, HUman Dignity - Acutely Needed*. SG/SM 9076. https://www.un.org/press/en/2003/sgsm9076.doc.htm

Armold, J. (1964). Business and professional ethics in prosthetics and orthotics. *Orthopedic and Prosthetic Appliance Journal*, (September), 212–221.

Awad, E., Dsouza, S., Kim, R., Schulz, J., Henrich, J., Shariff, A., Bonnefon, J.-F., & Rahwan, I. (2018). The Moral Machine experiment. *Nature*, *563*(7729), 59–64. doi:10.103841586-018-0637-6 PMID:30356211

Bakpo, F. S., & Kabari, L. G. (2011). Diagnosing skin diseases using an Artificial Neural Network. In *Artificial Neural Networks*. Methodological Advances and Biomedical Applications.

Banks, J., Ericksson, G., Burrage, K., Yellowlees, P., Ivermee, S., & Tichon, J. (2004). Constructing the hallucinations of psychosis in virtual reality. *Journal of Network and Computer Applications, 27*(1), 1-11. doi:10.1016/S1084-8045(03)00031-6

Becker, H. (Ed.). (2013). Robotik in Betreuung und Gesundheitsversorgung. Zürich: vdf Hochschulverl. doi:10.14512/tatup.22.1.62

Bedaf, S., Gelderblom, G. J., & de Witte, L. (2015). Overview and categorization of robots supporting independent living of elderly people: What activities do they support and how far have they developed. *Assistive Technology*, *27*(2), 88–100. doi:10.1080/10400435.2014.978916 PMID:26132353

Bedi, G., Carrillo, F., Cecchi, G. A., Slezak, D. F., Sigman, M., Mota, N. B., Ribeiro, S., Javitt, D. C., Copelli, M., & Corcoran, C. M. (2015). Au-tomated analysis of free speech predicts psychosis onset in high-risk youths. *NPJ Schizophrenia, 1*, 15030.

Behr, K., Nosper, A., Klimmt, C., & Hartmann, T. (2005). Some practical considerations of ethical issues in vr research. *Presence, 14*(6), 668- 676.

Bellon, J., & Nähr-Wagener, S. (2020). Interdisziplinarität, ELSI und Integrierte Forschung – aus Einem Vieles und aus Vielem Eines? In B. Gransche & A. Manzeschke (Eds.), *Das geteilte Ganze* (pp. 37–52). Springer Fachmedien Wiesbaden. doi:10.1007/978-3-658-26342-3_2

Bemelmans, R., Gelderblom, G. J., Jonker, P., & de Witte, L. (2012). Socially assistive robots in elderly care: A systematic review into effects and effectiveness. *Journal of the American Medical Directors Association*, *13*(2), 114–120.e1. doi:10.1016/j.jamda.2010.10.002 PMID:21450215

Berlin, L., Sosna, J., & Halevy, D. (2017). Radiologist found liable for malpractice in Israel for causing a patient's suicide by sending a "bad news" report: Can this happen in the United States? *AJR. American Journal of Roentgenology*, *208*(2), 241–244. doi:10.2214/AJR.16.16804 PMID:27809563

Bertino, E., Kundu, A., & Sura, Z. (2019). Data transparency with blockchain and AI ethics. *ACM Journal of Data and Information Quality*, *11*(4), 16. doi:10.1145/3312750

Blough, D. K., Hubbard, S., McFarland, L. V., Smith, D. G., Gambel, J. M., & Reiber, G. E. (2010). Prosthetic cost projections for service members with major limb loss from Vietnam and OIF/OEF. *Journal of Rehabilitation Research and Development*, *47*(4), 387–402. doi:10.1682/JRRD.2009.04.0037 PMID:20803406

Borangíu, T., & Purcarea, V. (2008). The future of healthcare-Information based medicine. *Journal of Medicine and Life*, *1*, 233–237. PMID:20108471

British Association of Prosthetists and Orthotists. (2018). Ethical code. Section 2.2. p. 4.

Broekens, J., Heerink, M., & Rosendal, H. (2009). Assistive social robots in elderly care: A review. *Gerontechnology (Valkenswaard)*, *8*(2), 94–103. doi:10.4017/gt.2009.08.02.002.00

Broussard, M. (2018). *Artificial Unintelligence. How Computers Misunderstand the World*. The MIT Press. doi:10.7551/mitpress/11022.001.0001

Bučková, B., Brunovský, M., Bareš, M., & Hlinka, J. (2020). Predicting sex from EEG: Validity and generalizability of deep-learning-based interpretable classifier. *Frontiers in Neuroscience*, *14*, 589303. doi:10.3389/fnins.2020.589303 PMID:33192274

Buesing, C., Fisch, G., O'Donnell, M., Shahidi, I., Thomas, L., Mummidisetty, C. K., Williams, K. J., Takahashi, H., Rymer, W. Z., & Jayaraman, A. (2015). Effects of a wearable exoskeleton stride management assist system (SMA®) on spatiotemporal gait characteristics in individuals after stroke: A randomized controlled trial. *Journal of Neuroengineering and Rehabilitation*, *12*(1), 69–83. doi:10.118612984-015-0062-0 PMID:26289955

Bui, K. M., Raugi, G. J., Nguyen, V. Q., & Reiber, G. E. (2009). Skin problems in individuals with lower-limb loss: Literature review and proposed classification system. *Journal of Rehabilitation Research and Development*, *46*(9), 1085–1090. doi:10.1682/JRRD.2009.04.0052 PMID:20437314

Burr, C., Morley, J., Taddeo, M., & Floridi, L. (2020). Digital psychiatry: Risks and opportunities for public health and wellbeing. *IEEE Transactions on Technology and Society*, *1*(1), 21–33. doi:10.1109/TTS.2020.2977059

Calvo, R. A., & D'Mello, S. (2010). Affect detection: An interdisciplinary review of models, methods, and their applications. *IEEE Transactions on Affective Computing*, *1*(1), 18–37. doi:10.1109/T-AFFC.2010.1

Camilleri, J., Scicluna, D., Bria, V., Camiller, V., Dingli, A., & Montebello, M. (2016). *If you aren't experiencing it, you're not understanding it! using virtual reality to understand migrants*. Academic Press.

Camilleri, V., Haddod, F., Montebello, M., Camilleri, J. C., Dingli, A., & Bria, V. (2019). Virtual reality (vr) applications in learning: living autism. In *Cases on immersive virtual reality techniques*. IGI Global.

Camilleri, V., Montebello, M., Dingli, A., & Bria, V. (2017). Walking in small shoes: Investigating the power of vr on empathising with children's dificulties, In *2017 23rd international conference on virtual system & multimedia (vsmm)*. IEEE.

Canca, C. (2020). *Why 'Mandatory Privacy-Preserving Digital Contact Tracing' is the Ethical Measure against COVID-19*. https://medium.com/@cansucanca/why-mandatory-privacy-preserving-digital-contact-tracing-is-the-ethical-measure-against-covid-19-a0d143b7c3b6

Carey, S. L., Lura, D. J., & Highsmith, M. J. (2015). Differences in myoelectric and body-powered upper-limb prostheses: Systematic literature review. *Journal of Rehabilitation Research and Development*, *52*(3), 247–262. doi:10.1682/JRRD.2014.08.0192 PMID:26230500

Castellanos, S. (2020). Pandemic-Related Disruptions Hurt Reliability of Some AI Models. *Wall Street Journal*. https://www.wsj.com/articles/pandemic-related-disruptions-hurt-reliability-of-some-ai-models-11591781402

Charles, D., Mcneill, M., McAlister, M., Black, M., Moore, A., Stringer, K., ... Kerr, A. (2005). *Player-centred game design: Player modelling and adaptive digital games*. Academic Press.

Chirico, A., Maiorano, P., Indovina, P., Milanese, C., Giordano, G. G., Alivernini, F., Iodice, G., Gallo, L., De Pietro, G., Lucidi, F., Botti, G., De Laurentiis, M., & Giordano, A. (2020). Virtual reality and music therapy as distraction interventions to alleviate anxiety and improve mood states in breast cancer patients during chemotherapy. *Journal of Cellular Physiology*, *235*(6), 5353–5362. doi:10.1002/jcp.29422 PMID:31957873

Chrunch, T. (2018). *Facebook rolls out ai to detect suicidal posts before they're reported*. https://newsroom.intel.com/news- releases/u- s- healthcare- leaders-expect-widespread-adoption-arti cial-intelligence-2023/

Clarke, D., McGregor, G., Rubin, B., Stanford, J., & Graham, T. (2016). Ar-caid:addressing situation awareness and simulator sickness in a virtual reality pac-man game. *Proceedings of the 2016 Annual Symposium on Computer-Human Interaction in Play Companion Extended Abstracts*, 39-45.

Combs, C., & Combs, F. (2019). Emerging roles of virtual patients in the age of ai. *AMA Journal of Ethics, 21*(2), 153. amajethics.2019.153 doi:10.1001/

Corcoran, C. M., Carrillo, F., Fernandez-Slezak, D., Bedi, G., Klim, C., Javitt, D. C., Bearden, C. E., & Cecchi, G. A. (2018). Prediction of psychosis across protocols and risk cohorts using automated language analysis. *World Psychiatry, 17*(1), 67-75.

Corporation, I. (2018). *Us healthcare leaders expect widespread adoption of ai by 2023*. Accessed on 22nd May 2020. https://newsroom.intel.com/news- releases/u- s- healthcare- leaders-expect-widespread-adoption-arti cial-intelligence-2023/

Ćosić, K., Povović, S., Šarlija, M., & Kesedžić, I. (2020). Impact of human disasters and COVID-19 pandemic on mental health: Potential of digital psychiatry. *Psychiatria Danubina*, *32*(1), 25–31. doi:10.24869/psyd.2020.25 PMID:32303026

Csikszentmihalyi, M. (2014). Play and intrinsic rewards. In *Flow and the foundations of positive psychology* (pp. 135–153). Springer.

Cullen, W., Gulati, G., & Kelly, B. (2020). Mental health in the covid-19 pandemic. *QJM: An International Journal of Medicine, 113*(5), 311-312.

Currie, G., Hawk, K. E., & Rohren, E. M. (2020). Ethical principles for the application of artificial intelligence (AI) in nuclear medicine. *European Journal of Nuclear Medicine and Molecular Imaging*, *47*(4), 748–752. doi:10.100700259-020-04678-1 PMID:31927637

D'Ignazio, C., & Klein, L. F. (2020). *Data Feminism*. The MIT Press. doi:10.7551/mitpress/11805.001.0001

D'Lima, D., Crawford, M. J., Darzi, A., & Archer, S. (2017). Patient safety and quality of care in mental health: A world of its own? *BJPsych Bulletin*, *41*(5), 241–243. doi:10.1192/pb.bp.116.055327 PMID:29018546

Davis, K. D., Flor, H., Greely, H. T., Iannetti, G. D., Mackey, S., Ploner, M., Pustilnik, A., Tracey, I., Treede, R. D., & Wager, T. D. (2017). Brain imaging tests for chronic pain: Medical, legal and ethical issues and recommendations. *Nature Reviews. Neurology*, *13*(10), 624–638. doi:10.1038/nrneurol.2017.122 PMID:28884750

De la Pena, N., Weil, P., Llobera, J., Giannopoulos, E., Pomes, A., Spanlang, B., Friedman, D., Sanchez-Vives, M., & Slater, M. (2010). Immersive journalism: Immersive virtual reality for the rst-person experience of news. *Presence: Teleoperators and Virtual Environments, 19*(4), 291-301.

Deibert, R. (2020). *Burning Data*. CBC Massey Lecture #5. https://www.cbc.ca/radio/ideas/reset-reclaiming-the-internet-for-civil-society-1.5795345

Demkow, U., & Wolanczyk, T. (2017). Genetic tests in major psychiatric disorders–Integrating molecular medicine with clinical psychiatry–why is it so difficult? *Translational Psychiatry*, *7*(6), e1151. doi:10.1038/tp.2017.106 PMID:28608853

Dhieb, N., Ghazzai, H., Besbes, H., & Massoud, Y. (2020). A secure AI-driven architecture for automated insurance systems: Fraud detection and risk measurement. *IEEE Access: Practical Innovations, Open Solutions*, *8*, 58546–58558. doi:10.1109/ACCESS.2020.2983300

Ding, J. (2018). Deciphering China's AI Dream The context, components, capabilities, and consequences of China's strategy to lead the world in AI. Centre for the Governance of AI, Future of Humanity Institute, University of Oxford.

Dolic, Z., Castro, R., & Moarcas, A. (2019). *Robots in healthcare: A solution or a problem? Workshop proceedings*. Brussels. https://www.europarl.europa.eu/RegData/etudes/IDAN/2019/638391/IPOL_IDA(2019)638391_EN.pdf

Dubner, R. (Ed.). (2013). *The neural basis of oral and facial function*. Springer Science & Business Media.

Dupes, B. (n.d.). Prosthetic Knee Systems. *Amputee Coalition*. Retrieved September 2020 from https://www.amputee-coalition.org/resources/prosthetic-knee-systems/

Egan, D., Brennan, S., Barrett, J., Qiao, Y., Timmerer, C., & Murray, N. (2016). An evaluation of heart rate and electrodermal activity as an objec- tive qoe evaluation method for immersive virtual reality environments. *Eighth International Conference on Quality of Multimedia Experience (QoMEX)*, 1-6.

Ekman, P. (1992). An argument for basic emotions. *Cognition and Emotion*, *6*(3-4), 169–200. doi:10.1080/02699939208411068

Elngar, Ahmed A., & Kumar, Rishabh, A Hayat and P Churi. (1998). Intelligent System for Skin Disease Prediction using Machine Learning. *Journal of Physics: Conference Series*.

Emma, B., Baylor, E., Hersch, F., Iurchenko, A., Wilcox, L., Ruamviboonsuk, P., & Vardoulakis L. (2020). A Human-Centered Evaluation of a Deep Learning System Deployed in Clinics for the Detection of Diabetic Retinopathy. *CHI '20: Proceedings of the 2020 CHI Conference on Human Factors in Computing Systems*. 10.1145/3313831.3376718

Eubanks, V. (2019). *Automating Inequality. How High-Tech Tools Profile, Police, and Punish the Poor.* Picador Editions.

European Commission. (2019). *Shaping Europe's digital future - Ethics guidelines for trustworthy AI*. https://ec.europa.eu/digital-single-market/en/news/ethics-guidelines-trustworthy-ai

Ewbank, M. P., Cummins, R., Tablan, V., Bateup, S., Catarino, A., Mar-tin, A. J., & Blackwell, A. D. (2020). Quantifying the association be-tween psychotherapy content and clinical outcomes using deep learning. *JAMA Psychiatry, 77*(1), 35-43.

Fabian, C., & Fabricant, R. (2014). The ethics of innovation. *Stanford Social Innovation Review*. Retrieved in March 2020 from https://ssir.org/articles/entry/the_ethics_of_innovation#

Fabiano, D., Canavan, S., Agazzi, H., Hinduja, S., & Goldgof, D. (2020). Gaze-based classi cation of autism spectrum disorder. *Pattern Recognition Letters*.

Fairley, M. (2014). Where ethics and economics meet. *The O&P Edge*. Retrieved in March 2020 from https://opedge.com/Articles/ViewArticle/2014-01-31/2014-02_01

Fellbaum, K.-R. (1982). *Telekommunikation von A – Z* [Telecommunication from A to Z]. VDE-Verl.

Firmani, D., Tanca, L., & Torlone, R. (2019). Ethical dimensions for data quality. *ACM Journal of Data and Information Quality*, *12*, 2.

Fiske, A., Henningsen, P., & Buyx, A. (2019). Your robot therapist will see you now: Ethical implications of embodied artificial intelligence in psychiatry, psychology, and psychotherapy. *Journal of Medical Internet Research, 21*(5), e13216. doi:10.2196/13216 PMID:31094356

Fitzpatrick, K. K., Darcy, A., & Vierhile, M. (2017). Delivering cognitive behavior therapy to young adults with symptoms of depression and anxiety using a fully automated conversational agent (woebot): A randomized controlled trial. *JMIR Mental Health, 4*(2), e19.

Flandorfer, P. (2012). Population ageing and socially assistive robots for elderly persons: The importance of sociodemographic factors for user acceptance. *International Journal of Population Research, 2012*, 1–13. doi:10.1155/2012/829835

Fonseca, M. (2016). Good and bad innovation: An overview of the ethics of innovation. *Intelligent HQ*. Retrieved in March 2020 from https://www.intelligenthq.com/good-and-bad-innovation-an-overview-on-the-ethics-of-innovation/

Ford, P. (2001). A further analysis of the ethics of representation in virtual reality: Multi-user environments. *Ethics and Information Technology, 3*, 113-121.

Ford, M. (2015). *Rise of the Robots. Technology and the Threat of a Jobless Future*. Basic Books.

Freeman, D., Reeve, S., Robinson, A., Ehlers, A., Clark, D., Spanlang, B., & Slater, M. (2017). Virtual reality in the assessment, understanding, and treatment of mental health disorders. *Psychological Medicine, 47*, 2393-2400. doi:10.1017/S003329171700040X

Freeman, D., Lister, R., Waite, F., Yu, L.-M., Slater, M., Dunn, G., & Clark, D. (2019). Automated psychological therapy using virtual reality (vr) for patients with persecutory delusions: Study protocol for a single-blind parallel-group randomised controlled trial (thrive). *Trials, 20*(1). https://doi.org/10.1186/s13063-019-3198-6

Frennert, S., & Östlund, B. (2014). Review: Seven matters of concern of social robots and older people. *International Journal of Social Robotics, 6*(2), 299–310. doi:10.100712369-013-0225-8

Friedersdorf, C. (2019). Mass Surveillance Is Coming to a City Near You. A tech entrepreneur wants to track the residents of a high-crime American community. *The Atlantic*. https://www.theatlantic.com/ideas/archive/2019/06/mass-surveillance-tech/592117/

Gailey, R., Allen, K., Castles, J., Kucharik, J., & Roeder, M. (2008). Review of secondary physical conditions associated with lower-limb amputation and long-term prosthesis use. *Journal of Rehabilitation Research and Development, 45*(1), 15–29. doi:10.1682/JRRD.2006.11.0147 PMID:18566923

Galison, P. (2019). Algorists Dream of Objectivity. In Possible Minds. 25 Ways of Looking at AI. New York: Penguin Press.

Garland, E. L. (2012). Pain processing in the human nervous system: A selective review of nociceptive and biobehavioral pathways. *Primary Care: Clinics in Office Practice, 39*(3), 561–571. doi:10.1016/j.pop.2012.06.013 PMID:22958566

Gattupalli, S., Ebert, D., Papakostas, M., Makedon, F., & Athitsos, V. (2017). Cognilearn: A deep learning-based interface for cognitive behavior as-sessment. *Proceedings of the 22nd international conference on intelligent user interfaces.*

Giroux, M., Barra, J., Gra, C., & Guerraz, M. (2019). Illusory perception of one's own movements in virtual reality. *Neurophysiologie Clinique*, *49*(6), 437.

Goldscheider, A. (1894). *Ueber den schmerz in physiologischer und klinischer hinsicht: nach einem vortrage in der Berliner militärärztlichen gesellschaft am 22. januar 1894*. Hirschwald.

Gonzalez-Franco, M., & Lanier, J. (2017). *Model of illusions and virtual reality*. Academic Press.

Gopichandran, V., Subramaniam, S., & Kalsingh, M. J. (2020). COVID-19 pandemic: A litmus test of trust in the health system. *Asian Bioethics Review*, *12*(2), 213–221. doi:10.100741649-020-00122-6 PMID:32837551

Gorgey, A. S. (2018). Robotic exoskeletons: The current pros and cons. *World Journal of Orthopedics*, *9*(9), 112–119. doi:10.5312/wjo.v9.i9.112 PMID:30254967

Gound, Gadre, Gaikwad, & Wagh. (2018). Skin Disease Diagnosis System using Image Processing and Data Mining. *International Journal of Computer Applications, 179*(16).

Graf, B. (2020). Assistenzroboter für die Pflege: Verfügbare Produkte und Forschungsfelder. *Zeitschrift für Gerontologie und Geriatrie*, *53*(7), 608–614. doi:10.100700391-020-01782-7 PMID:32986162

Greenemeier, L. (2016). Blade runners: Do high-tech prostheses give runners an unfair advantage? *Scientific American*. Retrieved in March 2020 from https://www.scientificamerican.com/article/blade-runners-do-high-tech-prostheses-give-runners-an-unfair-advantage/

Gregg, L., & Tarrier, N. (2007). Virtual reality in mental health: A review of the literature. *Social Psychiatry and Psychiatric Epidemiology, 42*, 343-354.

Gruber, J., Prinstein, M. J., Clark, L. A., Rottenberg, J., Abramowitz, J. S., Albano, A. M., Aldao, A., Borelli, J. L., Chung, T., & Davila, J. (2020). Mental health and clinical psychological science in the time of covid-19: Challenges, opportunities, and a call to action. *American Psychologist*.

Guan, J. (2019). Artificial intelligence in healthcare and medicine: Promises, ethical challenges and governance. *Chinese Medical Sciences Journal*, *34*, 76–83. PMID:31315747

Hamet, P., & Tremblay, J. (2017). Artificial intelligence in medicine. *Metabolism, 69*, S36-S40.

Haney, C., Banks, W., & Zimbardo, P. (1973). Study of prisoners and guards in a simulated prison. *Naval Research Reviews, 9*, 1-17.

Heaven. (2020). Our weird behavior during the pandemic is messing with AI models. *MIT Technology Review*. https://www.technologyreview.com/2020/05/11/1001563/covid-pandemic-broken-ai-machine-learning-amazon-retail-fraud-humans-in-the-loop/

Heim, E., Rötger, A., Lorenz, N., & Maercker, A. (2018). Working alliance with an avatar: How far can we go with internet interventions? *Internet Interventions: the Application of Information Technology in Mental and Behavioural Health*, *11*, 41–46. doi:10.1016/j.invent.2018.01.005 PMID:30135758

Heitzmann, D. (2019). Editorial. *Journal of Prosthetics and Orthotics*, *31*(4), 223. doi:10.1097/JPO.0000000000000276

Herreros, B., Gella, P., & de Asua, D. R. (2020). Triage during the COVID-19 epidemic in Spain: Better and worse ethical arguments. *Journal of Medical Ethics*, *46*(7), 455–458. doi:10.1136/medethics-2020-106352 PMID:32424063

Hershfield, H., Goldstein, D., Sharpe, W., Fox, J., Yeykelis, L., & Carstensen, L. (2011). Increasing saving behavior through age-progressed renderings of the future self. *Journal of Marketing Research, 48*, S23-S37.

Hicks, M. (2018). *Programmed Inequality. How Britain Discarded Women Technologists and Lost Its Edge on Computing*. MIT Press.

Hlinka, J., Paluš, M., Vejmelka, M., Mantini, D., & Corbetta, M. (2011). Functional connectivity in resting-state fMRI: Is linear correlation sufficient? *NeuroImage*, *54*(3), 2218–2225. doi:10.1016/j.neuroimage.2010.08.042 PMID:20800096

Ho, A. (2019). Deep ethical learning: Taking the interplay of human and artificial intelligence seriously. *The Hastings Center Report*, *49*(1), 36–39. doi:10.1002/hast.977 PMID:30790317

Hoffman, H. G., Seibel, E. J., Richards, T. L., Furness, T. A., Patterson, D. R., & Sharar, S. R. (2006). Virtual reality helmet display quality influences the magnitude of virtual reality analgesia. *The Journal of Pain*, *7*(11), 843–850. doi:10.1016/j.jpain.2006.04.006 PMID:17074626

Hong, S.-H. (2020). *Technologies of Speculation. The Limits of Knowledge in a Data-Driven Society*. New York University Press. doi:10.18574/nyu/9781479860234.001.0001

Hynek, M., Kalina, J., Zvárová, J., & Long, J. D. (2018). Statistical methods for constructing gestational age-related charts for fetal size and pregnancy dating using longitudinal data. *Biocybernetics and Biomedical Engineering*, *38*(4), 992–1003. doi:10.1016/j.bbe.2018.09.001

Hynek, M., Zvárová, J., Smetanová, D., Stejskal, D., & Kalina, J. (2021). Real-time quality control of nuchal translucency measurements using the exponentially weighted moving average chart. *Taiwanese Journal of Obstetrics & Gynecology*, *60*(1), 84–89. doi:10.1016/j.tjog.2020.11.012 PMID:33495014

Imms, F. J., & Edholm, O. G. (1981). Studies of gait and mobility in the elderly. *Age and Ageing*, *10*(3), 147–156. doi:10.1093/ageing/10.3.147 PMID:7270322

International Society for Prosthetics and Orthotics. (n.d.). *Prosthetic and Orthotic services*. Retrieved in March 2020 from https://www.ispoint.org/general/custom.asp?page=POservices, para 1 & 2.

Jacobson, N. J., Bentley, K. H., Walton, A., Wang, S. B., Fortgang, R. G., Millner, A. J., Coombs, G. III, Rodman, A. M., & Coppersmith, D. D. L. (2020). Ethical dilemmas posed by mobile health and machine learning in psychiatry research. *Bulletin of the World Health Organization*, *98*(4), 270–276. doi:10.2471/BLT.19.237107 PMID:32284651

James, S., Rao, S. V., & Granger, C. B. (2015). Registry-based randomized clinical trials–A new clinical trial paradigm. *Nature Reviews. Cardiology*, *12*(5), 312–316. doi:10.1038/nrcardio.2015.33 PMID:25781411

Jiang, F., Jiang, Y., Zhi, H., Dong, Y., Li, H., Ma, S., Wang, Y., Dong, Q., Shen, H., & Wang, Y. (2017). Artificial intelligence in healthcare: Past, present and future. *Stroke and Vascular Neurology*, *2*(4), e000101. doi:10.1136vn-2017-000101 PMID:29507784

Johansson-Pajala, R.-M., & Gustafsson, C. (2020). Significant challenges when introducing care robots in Swedish elder care. *Disability and Rehabilitation. Assistive Technology*, 1–11. doi:10.1080/17483107.2020.1773549 PMID:32538206

Johnson, M. H. (2005). How does distraction work in the management of pain? *Current Pain and Headache Reports*, *9*(2), 90–95. doi:10.100711916-005-0044-1 PMID:15745617

Just, M. A., Pan, L., Cherkassky, V. L., McMakin, D. L., Cha, C., Nock, M. K., & Brent, D. (2017). Machine learning of neural representations of sui-cide and emotion concepts identi es suicidal youth. *Nature human Behaviour, 1*(12), 911-919.

Kachouie, R., Sedighadeli, S., Khosla, R., & Chu, M.-T. (2014). Socially assistive robots in elderly care: A mixed-method systematic literature review. *International Journal of Human-Computer Interaction*, *30*(5), 369–393. doi:10.1080/10447318.2013.873278

Kadhim. (2017). Classification of Human Skin Diseases using Data Mining. *International Journal of Advanced Engineering Research and Science, 4*(1).

Kahneman, D. (1973). *Attention and effort* (Vol. 1063). Prentice-Hall.

Kalina, J., Neoral, A., & Vidnerová, P. (2021). Effective automatic method selection for nonlinear regression modeling. *International Journal of Neural Systems*. doi:10.1142/S0129065721500209

Kalina, J. (2012). Highly robust statistical methods in medical image analysis. *Biocybernetics and Biomedical Engineering*, *32*(2), 3–16. doi:10.1016/S0208-5216(12)70033-5

Kalina, J. (2015). Statistical challenges of Big Data analysis in medicine. *International Journal on Biomedicine and Healthcare, 3*, 24–27.

Kalina, J. (2021). Mental health clinical decision support exploiting Big Data. In *Research Anthology on Mental Health Stigma, Education, and Treatment* (pp. 341–359). IGI Global. doi:10.4018/978-1-7998-8544-3.ch020

Kalina, J., & Hlinka, J. (2017). Implicitly weighted robust classification applied to brain activity research. In A. Fred & H. Gamboa (Eds.), *Biomedical Engineering Systems and Technologies. Communications in Computer and Information Science, 690, 87-107.* doi:10.1007/978-3-319-54717-6_6

Kalina, J., & Matonoha, C. (2020). A sparse pair-preserving centroid-based supervised learning method for high-dimensional biomedical data or images. *Biocybernetics and Biomedical Engineering*, *40*(2), 774–786. doi:10.1016/j.bbe.2020.03.008

Kalina, J., & Schlenker, A. (2018). Dimensionality reduction methods for biomedical data. *Clinician and Technology*, *48*, 29–35.

Katchapakirin, K., Wongpatikaseree, K., Yomaboot, P., & Kaewpitakkun, Y. (2018). Facebook social media for depression detection in the Thai community. In *2018 15th international joint conference on computer science and software engineering (JCSSE).* IEEE.

Kehl, C. (2018). *Robotik und assistive Neurotechnologien in der Pflege - gesellschaftliche Herausforderungen*, Berlin: Büro für Technikfolgen-Abschätzung beim Deutschen Bundestag (TAB). https://www.tab-beim-bundestag.de/de/pdf/publikationen/berichte/TAB-Arbeitsbericht-ab177.pdf

Keim-Malpass, J., & Moorman, L. P. (2021). Nursing and precision predictive analytics monitoring in the acute and intensive care setting: An emerging role for responding to COVID-19 and beyond. *International Journal of Nursing Studies*, *3*, 100019. doi:10.1016/j.ijnsa.2021.100019 PMID:33426534

Keizer, A., Van Elburg, A., Helms, R., & Dijkerman, H. (2016). a virtual reality full body illusion improves body image disturbance in anorexia nervosa. *PLoS One*, *11*, e0163921.

Kilbride, M. K., & Joffe, S. (2018). The new age of patient autonomy. Implications for the patient-physician relationship. *Journal of the American Medical Association*, *320*(19), 1973–1974. doi:10.1001/jama.2018.14382 PMID:30326026

Kim, H. K., Park, J., Choi, Y., & Choe, M. (2018). Virtual reality sickness questionnaire (vrsq): Motion sickness measurement index in a virtual reality environment. *Applied Ergonomics, 69*, 66-73.

Klebbe, R., & Eicher, C. (2020). Wer sind eigentlich diese Nutzer? Zur Rolle älterer und pflegebedürftiger Erwachsener in der Entwicklung robotischer Assistenzsysteme [Who are exactly these users? The role of older adults and people in need of care in the development of robotic systems]. In J. Hergesell, A. Maibaum, & M. Meister (Eds.), *Genese und Folgen der Pflegerobotik - Die Konstitution eines interdisziplinären Forschungsfeldes* (1st ed.). Beltz Juventa in der Verlagsgruppe Beltz.

Kohli, A., & Jha, S. (2018). Why CAD failed in mammography. *Journal of the American College of Radiology*, *15*(3), 535–537. doi:10.1016/j.jacr.2017.12.029 PMID:29398499

Konečný, J., McMahan, H. B., Ramage, D., & Richtárik, P. (2016). *Federated optimisation: Distributed machine learning for on-device intelligence*. arXiv preprint arXiv:1610.02527.

Lambert, V., Boylan, P., Boran, L., Hicks, P., Kirubakaran, R., Devane, D., & Matthews, A. (2020). Virtual reality distraction for acute pain in children. *Cochrane Database of Systematic Reviews*, 10. PMID:33089901

Lanier, J. (1992). An insider's view of the future of virtual reality. *Journal of Communication, 42*, 150-172.

Lanier, J. (2017). *Dawn of the new everything: Encounters with reality and virtual reality*. Henry Holt, Co., Inc.

LaViola, J. (2000). A discussion of cybersickness in virtual environments. *SIGCHI Bulletin, 32*, 47-56.

Law, M., Sutherland, C., Ahn, H. S., MacDonald, B. A., Peri, K., Johanson, D. L., Vajsakovic, D.-S., Kerse, N., & Broadbent, E. (2019). Developing assistive robots for people with mild cognitive impairment and mild dementia: A qualitative study with older adults and experts in aged care. *BMJ Open*, *9*(9), 1–9. doi:10.1136/bmjopen-2019-031937 PMID:31551392

Light, H. (2018). Private healthcare vs the NHS. *Star Outico – Latest News*. Retrieved in June 2021 from https://www.staroutico.com/latest-news/private-healthcare-vs-nhs

Li, L., Li, Y., Wang, Y., & Yan, L. (2021). Intelligent medical diagnosis and misoprostol medical abortion nursing based on embedded system. *Microprocessors and Microsystems*, *81*, 103770. doi:10.1016/j.micpro.2020.103770

Lin, L. & Hou, Z. (2020). Combat COVID-19 with artificial intelligence and big data. *Journal of Travel Medicine*. doi:10.1093/jtm/taaa080

Liutsko, L. (2014). Differential effects of two virtual reality interventions: Distraction versus pain control. *Cyberpsychology, Behavior, and Social Networking*, *17*(6), 353–358. doi:10.1089/cyber.2014.0057 PMID:24892197

Lup, K., Trub, L., & Rosenthal, L. (2015). Instagram# instasad? Exploring associations among instagram use, depressive symptoms, negative social comparison, and strangers followed. *Cyberpsychology, Behavior, and Social Networking, 18*(5), 247-252.

Madary, M., & Metzinger, T. (2016). Real virtuality: A code of ethical conduct. recommendations or good scientific practice and the consumers of vr-technology. *Frontiers in Robotics and AI, 3*. frobt.2016.00003 doi:10.3389/

Madrigal, A. C. (2012). I'm Being Followed: How Google—and 104 Other Companies—Are Tracking Me on the Web. *The Atlantic*. https://www.theatlantic.com/technology/archive/2012/02/im-being-followed-how-google-151-and-104-other-companies-151-are-tracking-me-on-the-web/253758/

Maguire, M., & Bevan, N. (2002). User requirements analysis. In J. Hammond, T. Gross, & J. Wesson (Eds.), Usability: Gaining a competitive edge. Springer US. doi:10.1007/978-0-387-35610-5_9

Malgaroli, M., & Schultebraucks, K. (2021). Artificial Intelligence and Posttraumatic Stress Disorder (PTSD). *European Psychologist.*

Masic, I., & Mihalas, G. (Eds.). (2014). *History of medical informatics*. Avicena.

Mayring, P. (2015). *Qualitative Inhaltsanalyse: Grundlagen und Techniken (Qualitative content analysis: Principles and techniques)* (12 überarbeitete Auflage). Beltz Verlag.

McGreevey, J. D. III, Hanson, W. III, & Koppel, R. (2020). Clinical, legal, and ethical aspects of artificial intelligence-assisted conversational agents in health care. *Journal of the American Medical Association*, *324*(6), 552–553. doi:10.1001/jama.2020.2724 PMID:32706386

McKernan, L. C., Clayton, E. W., & Walsh, C. G. (2018). Protecting life while preserving liberty: Ethical recommendations for suicide prevention with artificial intelligence. *Frontiers in Psychiatry*, *9*, 650. doi:10.3389/fpsyt.2018.00650 PMID:30559686

Meltzo, J. (2005). *Ethics in research*. Academic Press.

Melzack, R., & Wall, P. D. (1965). Pain mechanisms: A new theory. *Science*, *150*(3699), 971–979. doi:10.1126cience.150.3699.971 PMID:5320816

Meyer, B. (2013). Bertolt Meyer: 'Ethical questions are looming for prosthetics'. *Wired*. Retrieved in March 2020 from https://www.wired.co.uk/article/now-we-need-to-talk-about-our-bionic-future

Mian, A., & Khan, S. (2020). Coronavirus: The spread of misinformation. *BMC Medicine*, *18*(1), 89. doi:10.118612916-020-01556-3 PMID:32188445

Milgram, S. (1974). *Obedience to authority. an experimental view*. Tavi-stock.

Milk, C. (2015). *How virtual reality can create the ultimate empathy machine* [TED Talk]. https://www.ted.com/talks/chris milk how virtual reality can create the ultimate empathy machine

Mishra, Imaizumi, & Yamasaki. (2019). Interpreting Fine-Grained Dermatological Classification by Deep Learning. *IEEE Explore*.

Moayedi, M., & Davis, K. D. (2013). Theories of pain: From specificity to gate control. *Journal of Neurophysiology*, *109*(1), 5–12. doi:10.1152/jn.00457.2012 PMID:23034364

Montemayor, C., Halpern, J., & Fairweather, A. (2021). In principle obstacles for empathic AI: Why we can't replace human empathy in healthcare. *AI & Society*. . doi:10.1007/s00146-021-01230-z

Moreau, N. (2020). The paradox of overspecialization: Can't see the forest for the trees. *Journal of Oral Medical Surgery*, *26*(1), E1. doi:10.1051/mbcb/2020005

Morgan, A., Reavley, N., Ross, A., Too, L., & Jorm, A. (2018). Interventions to reduce stigma towards people with severe mental illness: Systematic review and meta-analysis. *Journal of Psychiatric Research, 130*, 120-133.

Mosadeghi, S., Reid, M., Martinez, B., Rosen, B., & Spiegel, B. (2016). Feasibility of an immersive virtual reality intervention for hospitalized patients: An observational cohort study. *JMIR Mental Health, 3*, 1-10.

Mostert, M., Koomen, B. M., van Delden, J. J. M., & Bredenoord, A. L. (2018). Privacy in Big Data psychiatric and behavioural research: A multiple-case study. *International Journal of Law and Psychiatry*, *60*, 40–44. doi:10.1016/j.ijlp.2018.07.002 PMID:30217329

Mouchabac, S., Adrien, V., Falala-Séchet, C., Bonnot, O., Maatoug, R., Millet, B., Peretti, C.-S., Bourla, A., & Ferreri, F. (2021). Psychiatric advance directives and artificial intelligence: A conceptual framework for theoretical and ethical principles. *Frontiers in Psychiatry*, *11*, 622506. doi:10.3389/fpsyt.2020.622506 PMID:33551883

Musen, M. A., Middleton, B., & Greenes, R. A. (2014). Clinical Decision-Support Systems. In *Biomedical Informatics* (pp. 643–674). Springer. doi:10.1007/978-1-4471-4474-8_22

Nagao, K. (2019). *Artificial intelligence accelerates human learning. Discussion data analytics*. Springer. doi:10.1007/978-981-13-6175-3

Nathan, S. (2018). Future prosthetic: towards the bionic human. *The Engineer*. Retrieved in March 2020 from https://www.theengineer.co.uk/future-prosthetic/

Nielsen, C. C., & Jorge, M. (2013). Orthotics and prosthetics in rehabilitation: multidisciplinary approach. In M. Lusardi, M. Jorge, & C. Nielsen (Eds.), *Orthotics & Prosthetics in Rehabilitation* (p. 2). Elsevier Saunders. doi:10.1016/B978-1-4377-1936-9.00001-1

Nielsen, L. (2013). *Personas - User Focused Design*. Springer London. doi:10.1007/978-1-4471-4084-9

Noble, S. U. (2018). *Algorithms of Oppression. How Search Engines Reinforce Racism*. New York University Press. doi:10.2307/j.ctt1pwt9w5

Nti, Akyeramfo-Sam, Philip, Yeboah, & Nancy. (2019). A Web-Based Skin Disease Detection System. *American Journal of Computer Science and Information Technology, 7*.

O'Hear, S. (2017, Jan. 4). Babylon health partners with uk's nhs to replace telephone helpline with ai-powered chatbot. *TechCrunch*.

O'Neil, C. (2019). *Weapons of Math Destruction. How Big Data Increase Inequality and Threatens Democracy*. Broadway Books.

Obermeyer, Powers, Vogeli, & Mullainathan. (2019). Dissecting racial bias in an algorithm used to manage the health of populations. *Science, 366*(6464), 447-453. doi:10.1126/science.aax2342

Orendurff, M. S., Segal, A. D., Klute, G. K., McDowell, M. L., Pecoraro, J. A., & Czerniecki, J. M. (2006). Gait efficiency using the C-Leg. *Journal of Rehabilitation Research and Development*, *43*(2), 239–246. doi:10.1682/JRRD.2005.06.0095 PMID:16847790

Osterweis, M., Kleinman, A., & Mechanic, D. (1987). Measuring pain and dysfunction. In *Pain and Disability: Clinical, Behavioral, and Public Policy Perspectives*. National Academies Press.

Otto Bock, U. K. (n.d.). *Microprocessor controlled knees – How do they work?* Retrieved in September 2020 from https://www.ottobock.co.uk/prosthetics/info_for_new_amputees/prosthetic-technology-explained/computer_controlled_knees/

Palinkas, L. A., & Zatzick, D. (2019). Rapid Assessment Procedure Informed Clinical Ethnography (RAPICE) in Pragmatic Clinical Trials of Mental Health Services Implementation: Methods and Applied Case Study. *Administration and Policy in Mental Health*, *46*(2), 255–270. doi:10.100710488-018-0909-3 PMID:30488143

Park, K., Ku, J., Choi, S., Jang, H., Park, J., Kim, S., & Kim, J. (2011). A virtual reality application in role-plays of social skills training for schizophrenia: A randomized, controlled trial. *Psychiatry Research, 189*, 166-172.

Park, Kuo, Barbarin, Kaziunas, Chow, Singh, Wilcox, & Lasecki. (2019). *Identifying Challenges and Opportunities in Human-AI Collaboration in Healthcare*. Academic Press.

Parsons, T., & Rizzo, A. (2008). Affective outcomes of virtual reality exposure therapy for anxiety and specific phobias: A meta-analysis. *Journal of Behavior Therapy and Experimental Psychiatry, 39*, 250-261.

Pasquina, P. F., Carvalho, A. J., & Sheehan, T. P. (2015). Ethics in rehabilitation: Access to prosthetics and quality care following amputation. *American Medical Association Journal*, *17*(6), 535–546. PMID:26075981

Patel, B. N., Rosenberg, L., Willcox, G., Baltaxe, D., Lyons, M., Irvin, J., Rajpurkar, P., Amrhein, T., Gupta, R., Halabi, S., Langlotz, C., Lo, E., Mammarappallil, J., Mariano, A. J., Riley, G., Seekins, J., Shen, L., Zucker, E., & Lungren, M. P. (2019). Human-machine partnership with artificial intelligence for chest radiograph diagnosis. *NPJ Digital Medicine*, *2*(1), 111. doi:10.103841746-019-0189-7 PMID:31754637

Pearce, S. (1983). A review of cognitive-behavioural methods for the treatment of chronic pain. *Journal of Psychosomatic Research*, *27*(5), 431–440. doi:10.1016/0022-3999(83)90082-X PMID:6366219

Perreira, C. (2019). Consumed by Disease. Medical Archives, Latino Fictions, and Carceral Health Imaginaries. In Captivating Technology. Race, Carceral Technoscience, and Liberatory Imagination in Everyday Life (pp. 50-66). Duke University Press

Peter, J. P., & Olson, J. C. (2010). *Consumer behavior & marketing strategy* (9th ed.). McGraw-Hill Irwin.

Peters, B. S., Armijo, P. R., Krause, C., Choudhury, S. A., & Oleynikov, D. (2018). Review of emerging surgical robotic technology. *Surgical Endoscopy*, *32*(4), 1636–1655. doi:10.100700464-018-6079-2 PMID:29442240

Piano, S. L. (2020). Ethical principles in machine learning and artificial intelligence: Cases from the field and possible ways forward. *Humanities and Social Sciences Communications*, *7*(1), 9. doi:10.105741599-020-0501-9

Picard, R. W. (2000). *Affective Computing*. MIT Press. doi:10.7551/mitpress/1140.001.0001

Pinals, D. A. (2019). Liability and patient suicide. *Focus (San Francisco, Calif.)*, *17*, 349–354. PMID:32047380

Pontefract, Coleman, Vallance, Hirsch, Shah, Marriot, & Redwood. (2018). The impact of computerized physician order entry and clinical decision support on pharmacist-physician communication in the hospital setting: A qualitative study. *PloS One, 13*(11), e0207450.

Profession. (n.d.) In *Cambridge Dictionary online*. Retrieved in March 2020 from https://dictionary.cambridge.org/dictionary/english/profession

Professional Standards Councils. (n.d.). *What is a Profession*? Retrieved in March 2020 from https://www.psc.gov.au/what-is-a-profession

Rammert, W. (2010). Die Innovationen der Gesellschaft [The innovations of society]. In J. Howaldt & H. Jacobsen (Eds.), *Soziale Innovation: Auf dem Weg zu einem postindustriellen Innovationsparadigma*. VS Verlag für Sozialwissenschaften. doi:10.1007/978-3-531-92469-4_2

Razak, A., Osman, A., Kamyab, M., Abas, W., & Gholizadeh, H. (2014). Satisfaction and problems experienced with wrist movements. *American Journal of Physical Medicine & Rehabilitation*, *93*(5), 437–444. doi:10.1097/PHM.0b013e3182a51fc2 PMID:24429510

Reena Parvin, S., & Mohamed Jafar, O. A. (2017, July). Prediction of skin disease using data mining techniques. *International Journal of Innovative Research in Computer and Communication Engineering*, *6*(7).

Rezaii, N., Walker, E., & Wol, P. (2019). A machine learning approach to predicting psychosis using semantic density and latent content analysis. *NPJ Schizophrenia, 5*(1), 1-12.

Rigby, M. J. (2019). Ethical dimensions of using artificial intelligence in health care. *AMA Journal of Ethics*, *21*(2), E121–E124. doi:10.1001/amajethics.2019.121

Rosenfeld, L., Torous, J., & Vahia, I. V. (2017). Data security and privacy in apps for dementia: An analysis of existing privacy policies. *The American Journal of Geriatric Psychiatry*, *25*(8), 873–877. doi:10.1016/j.jagp.2017.04.009 PMID:28645535

Röß, A., & Warnke, P. (2020). Organisationale Rahmenbedingungen für Integrierte Forschung: Perspektiven aus einer angewandten Forschungsorganisation. In B. Gransche & A. Manzeschke (Eds.), *Das geteilte Ganze* (pp. 119–132). Springer Fachmedien Wiesbaden. doi:10.1007/978-3-658-26342-3_6

Rubin, J., & Chisnell, D. (2008). *Handbook of usability testing: How to plan, design, and conduct effective tests* (2nd ed.). Wiley Pub.

Ruiz-Olaya, A. F., Lopez-Delis, A., & Rocha, A. F. (2019). Upper and lower extremity exoskeletons. In J. Segil (Ed.), Handbook of Biomechanics (pp. 283–317). Academic Press.

Rus-Calafell, M., Garety, P., Sason, E., Craig, T. J. K., & Valmaggia, L. R. (2018). Virtual reality in the assessment and treatment of psychosis: A systematic review of its utility, acceptability and effectiveness. *Psychological Medicine, 48*(3), 362-391.

Russell, J. A., & Mehrabian, A. (1977). Evidence for a three-factor theory of emotions. *Journal of Research in Personality, 11*(3), 273–294. doi:10.1016/0092-6566(77)90037-X

Sabin, D. (2016). Do we have a right to bionic arms? *Inverse*. Retrieved in March 2020 from https://www.inverse.com/article/18220-robot-arms-cyborgs-advanced-prosthetics-and-medical-ethics

Safdar, N. M., Banja, J. D., & Meltzer, C. C. (2020). Ethical considerations in artificial intelligence. *European Journal of Radiology, 122*, 108768. doi:10.1016/j.ejrad.2019.108768 PMID:31786504

Santana, M., Manalili, K., Lu, M., Jolley, R., & Zelinsky, S. (2018). How to practice person-centred care: A conceptual framework. *Health Expectations: An International Journal of Public Participation in Health Care and Health Policy, 21*(2), 429. .1111/hex.12640 doi:https://doi.org/https://doi.org/10

Sato, K., Fukumori, S., Matsusaki, T., Maruo, T., Ishikawa, S., Nishie, H., Takata, K., Mizuhara, H., Mizobuchi, S., Nakatsuka, H., Matsumi, M., Gofuku, A., Yokoyama, M., & Morita, K. (2010). Nonimmersive virtual reality mirror visual feedback therapy and its application for the treatment of complex regional pain syndrome: An open-label pilot study. *Pain Medicine, 11*(4), 622–629. doi:10.1111/j.1526-4637.2010.00819.x PMID:20202141

Sayed, S. I., Tsiakas, K., Bell, M., Athitsos, V., & Makedon, F. (2019). Cognitive assessment in children through motion capture and computer vision: The cross-your-body task. *Proceedings of the 6th international workshop on sensor-based activity recognition and interaction.*

Schmalz, T., Blumentritt, S., & Jarasch, R. (2002). Energy expenditure and biomechanical characteristics of lower limb amputee gait: The influence of prosthetic alignment and different prosthetic components. *Gait & Posture, 16*(3), 255–263. doi:10.1016/S0966-6362(02)00008-5 PMID:12443950

Schmalz, T., Pröbsting, E., Auberger, R., & Siewert, G. (2016). A functional comparison of conventional knee–ankle–foot orthoses and a microprocessor-controlled leg orthosis system based on biomechanical parameters. *Prosthetics and Orthotics International, 40*(2), 277–286. doi:10.1177/0309364614546524 PMID:25249381

Scholten, M. R., Kelders, S. M., & Van Gemert-Pijnen, J. E. W. C. (2017). Self-guided web-based interventions: Scoping review on user needs and the potential of embodied conversational agents to address them. *Journal of Medical Internet Research, 19*(11), e383. doi:10.2196/jmir.7351 PMID:29146567

Schrack, J. A., Simonsick, E. M., & Ferrucci, L. (2013). The relationship of the energetic cost of slow walking and peak energy expenditure to gait speed in mid-to-late life. *American Journal of Physical Medicine & Rehabilitation*, *92*(1), 28–35. doi:10.1097/PHM.0b013e3182644165 PMID:22854908

Senders, J. T., Harary, M., Stopa, B. M., Staples, P., Broekman, M. L. D., Smith, T. R., Gormley, W. B., & Arnaout, O. (2018). Information-based medicine in glioma patients: A clinical perspective. *Computational and Mathematical Methods in Medicine*, *2018*, 8572058. doi:10.1155/2018/8572058 PMID:30008798

Servaty, R., Kersten, A., Brukamp, K., Möhler, R., & Mueller, M. (2020). Implementation of robotic devices in nursing care. Barriers and facilitators: An integrative review. *BMJ Open*, *10*(9), e038650. doi:10.1136/bmjopen-2020-038650 PMID:32958491

Shaffer, F., & Ginsberg, J. P. (2017). An overview of heart rate variability metrics and norms. *Frontiers in Public Health*, *5*, 258. doi:10.3389/fpubh.2017.00258 PMID:29034226

Sharma & Hota. (2013). Data mining techniques for prediction of different categories of dermatology diseases. *Academy of Information and Management Sciences Journal, 16*(2).

Sharma, N., & Gedeon, T. (2012). Objective measures, sensors and computational techniques for stress recognition and classification: A survey. *Computer Methods and Programs in Biomedicine*, *108*(3), 1287–1301. doi:10.1016/j.cmpb.2012.07.003 PMID:22921417

Shrinidhi Gindhi, E. (2017, July). An innovative Approach For Skin Disease Detection Using Image Processing and Data Mining. *International Journal of Innovative Research in Computer and Communication Engineering*, *5*(4).

Shumway-Cook, A., Guralnik, J. M., Phillips, C. L., Coppin, A. K., Ciol, M. A., Bandinelli, S., & Ferrucci, L. (2007). Age-associated declines in complex walking task performance: The Walking InCHIANTI toolkit. *Journal of the American Geriatrics Association*, *55*(1), 58–65. doi:10.1111/j.1532-5415.2006.00962.x PMID:17233686

Siegele, D. S. (1974). The gate control theory. *AJN The American Journal of Nursing*, *74*(3), 498. PMID:4361027

Sigurdsson, E. L., Blondal, A. B., Jonsson, J. S., Tomasdottir, M. O., Hrafnkelsson, H., Linnet, K., & Sigurdsson, J. A. (2020). How prirmary healthcare in Iceland swiftly changed its strategy in response to the COVID-19 pandemic. *BMJ Open*, *10*(12), e043151. doi:10.1136/bmjopen-2020-043151 PMID:33293329

Simon, J. C., & Gutsell, J. N. (2021). Recognizing humanity: Dehumanization predicts neural mirroring and empathic accuracy in face-to-face interactions. *Social Cognitive and Affective Neuroscience*, *2021*(5), 463–473. doi:10.1093can/nsab014 PMID:33515023

Slater, M. (2018). Immersion and the illusion of presence in virtual reality. *British Journal of Psychology, 109*(3), 431-433.

Slawomirski, L., Auraaen, A., & Klazinga, N. (2017). *The economics ofpatient safety: Strengthening a value-based approach to reducing patient harm at national level.* OECD Health Working Papers, No. 96, OECD Publishing.

Smart, Z. (2019). Bringing the ethics into innovation. *IEC e-tech*. Retrieved in March 2020 from https://iecetech.org/issue/2019-01/Bringing-the-ethics-into-innovation

Soltan, A. A. S., Kouchaki, S., Zhu, T., Kiyasseh, D., Taylor, T., Hussain, Z. B., Peto, T., Brent, A. J., Eyre, D. W., & Clifton, D. A. (2021). Rapid triage for COVID-19 using routine clinical data for patients attending hospital: Development and prospective validation of an artificial intelligence screening test. *The Lancet. Digital Health*, *3*(2), 78–87. doi:10.1016/S2589-7500(20)30274-0 PMID:33509388

Song, D. Y., Kim, S. Y., Bong, G., Kim, J. M., & Yoo, H. J. (2019). The use of artificial intelligence in screening and diagnosis of autism spectrum disorder: A literature review. *Journal of the Korean Academy of Child and Adolescent Psychiatry*, *30*(4), 145–152. doi:10.5765/jkacap.190027 PMID:32595335

Spiegel, J. (2018). The ethics of virtual reality technology: Social hazards and public policy recommendations. *Science and Engineering Ethics, 24*, 1537-1550.

Spindler, M., Booz, S., Gieseler, H., Runschke, S., Wydra, S., & Zinsmaier, J. (2020). How to achieve integration?: Methodological concepts and challenges for the integration of ethical, legal, social and economic aspects into technological development. In B. Gransche & A. Manzeschke (Eds.), *Das geteilte Ganze* (pp. 213–239). Springer Fachmedien Wiesbaden. doi:10.1007/978-3-658-26342-3_11

Starke, G., De Clercq, E., Borgwardt, S., & Elger, B. S. (2020). Computing schizophrenia: Ethical challenges for machine learning in psychiatry. *Psychological Medicine*, *1*(3), 1–7. PMID:32536358

Stein, M. B., & Smoller, J. W. (2018). Precision Psychiatry: Will genomic medicine lead the way? *JAMA Psychiatry*, *75*(7), 663–664. doi:10.1001/jamapsychiatry.2018.0375 PMID:29800947

Straus, S., Glasziou, P., Richardson, W. S., & Haynes, R. B. (2018). *Evidence-based medicine: How to practice and teach EBM* (5th ed.). Elsevier.

Stubbe, J. (2020). Sechs Thesen für gelingende Integrierte Forschung. In B. Gransche & A. Manzeschke (Eds.), *Das geteilte Ganze* (pp. 197–211). Springer Fachmedien Wiesbaden. doi:10.1007/978-3-658-26342-3_10

Tao, J., & Tan, T. (2005, October). Affective Computing: A review. In *International Conference on Affective Computing and intelligent interaction* (pp. 981-995). Springer. 10.1007/11573548_125

The Shock Wave of COVID-19. (2020). In *The New Yorker Radio Hour* [podcast]. https://www.newyorker.com/podcast/the-new-yorker-radio-hour/the-shock-wave-of-covid-19

The War Amps. (n.d.). *Prosthetic Knees for Adults*. Retrieved September 2020 from https://www.waramps.ca/pdf/english-site/ways-we-help/artificial-limbs-and-devices/lower-limb/knees-for-adults.pdf

Torales, J., O'Higgins, M., Castaldelli-Maia, J. M., & Ventriglio, A. (2020). The outbreak of covid-19 coronavirus and its impact on global mental health. *The International Journal of Social Psychiatry*.

Tripathi, S. (2021). Artificial intelligence: A brief review. In T. H. Musiolik & A. D. Cheok (Eds.), *Analyzing future applications of AI, sensors, and robotics in society* (pp. 1–16). IGI Global. doi:10.4018/978-1-7998-3499-1.ch001

TsamadosA.AggarwalN.CowlsJ.MorleyJ.RobertsH.TaddeoM.FloridiL. (2021). The ethics of algorithms: Key problems and solutions. AI & Society. Online first. doi:10.2139/ssrn.3662302

Tsang, M., & Mann, D. (2013). A virtual reality-based vocational training system (vrvts) for people with schizophrenia in vocational rehabilitation. *Schizophrenia Research, 144*, 51-62.

Tsung-Yi, L., Huang, C., Hsu, H., Liao, J., Cheng, V., Wang, S., & Guo, J. (2020). Effects of a combination of three-dimensional virtual reality and hands-on horticultural therapy on institutionalized older adults' physical and mental health: Quasi-experimental design. *Journal of Medical Internet Research, 22*(11), e1902. https://doi.org/10.2196/19002

Twerenbold, R. (2017). *The good, the bad and the innovative: Understanding the darker side of innovation for development.* United Nations Research Institute for Social Development (UNRISD). Retrieved in March 2020 from http://www.unrisd.org/80256B3C005BE6B5/(httpNews)/9CD705AC73D6E013C12580D7004F285C?OpenDocument&newstype=viewpoint

UCI KDD Archive. (1998). http:/kdd.ics.uci.edu

UNICEF. (n.d.). *What we do.* Retrieved September 2020 from https://www.unicef.org/innovation/what-we-do-new

Unite for Sight. (n.d.). *Ethics of Innovation.* Retrieved in March 2020 from http://www.uniteforsight.org/global-health-university/ethics-of-innovation

Valmaggia, L. (2017). The use of virtual reality in psychosis research and treatment. *World Psychiatry, 16*(3), 246-247. .20443 doi:10.1002/wps

VanNostrand, C. (2014). Prosthetics: The ethical issues surrounding them. *Semantic Scholar.* Retrieved in March 2020 from https://pdfs.semanticscholar.org/3b16/4b5c1f072d95551b4e770476eeb9d9116d65.pdf?_ga=2.127456843.791674419.1585559520-1453370591.1585559520

Verma, Pal, & Kumar. (2019). *Classification of Skin Disease Using Ensembles Data Mining Techniques.* doi:10.31557/APJCP.2019.20.6.1887

Vijaya, M. S. (2015). Categorization of Non-Melanoma Skin Lesion Diseases Using Support Vector Machine and Its Variants. *International Journal of Medical Imaging.*

Vollmer Dahlke, D., Lee, S., Smith, M. L., Shubert, T., Popovich, S., & Ory, M. G. (2021). Attitudes Toward Technology and Use of Fall Alert Wearables in Caregiving: Survey Study. *JMIR Aging, 4*(1), e23381. doi:10.2196/23381 PMID:33502320

Wachter, R. M., & Gupta, K. (2018). *Understanding patient safety* (3rd ed.). McGraw-Hill Education.

Waihanga. (n.d.). *Knee Joints*. Retrieved September 2020 from https://www.nzals.co.nz/products/categories/knee-joints

Walsh, C. G., Chaudhry, B., Dua, P., Goodman, K. W., Kaplan, B., Kavuluru, R., Solomonides, A., & Subbian, V. (2020). Stigma, biomarkers, and algorithmic bias: Recommendations for precision behavioral health with artificial intelligence. *JAMIA Open*, *3*(1), 9–15. doi:10.1093/jamiaopen/ooz054 PMID:32607482

Wan, H., W, & Lam, A. (2019). The effectiveness of virtual reality-based simulation in health professions education relating to mental illness: A literature review. *Health, 11*, 646-660.

Waterson. (1990). "Calvin and Hobbes", January 9, 10, 11. In *The Complete Calvin and Hobbes, Book Three 1990-1992*. Adrew McMeel Publishing.

Weech, S., Kenny, S., & Barnett-Cowan, M. (2019). Presence and cybersickness in virtual reality are negatively related: A review. *Frontiers in Psychology*, *10*, 158.

Wegmann, M. (2014). Orthotic Intervention for those without physical limitations: An ethical perspective. *The O&P Edge*. Retrieved in March 2020 from https://opedge.com/Articles/ViewArticle/2014-01-31/2014-02_02

Weizenbaum, J. (1966). Eliza|a computer program for the study of natural language communication between man and machine. *Communications of the ACM, 9*(1), 36-45.

Weizenbaum, J. (1976). *Computer power and human reason: From judgment to calculation.* Academic Press.

Wiech, K., & Tracey, I. (2009). The influence of negative emotions on pain: Behavioral effects and neural mechanisms. *NeuroImage*, *47*(3), 987–994. doi:10.1016/j.neuroimage.2009.05.059 PMID:19481610

Wiederhold, B. K., Gao, K., Sulea, C., & Wiederhold, M. D. (2014). Virtual reality as a distraction technique in chronic pain patients. *Cyberpsychology, Behavior, and Social Networking*, *17*(6), 346–352. doi:10.1089/cyber.2014.0207 PMID:24892196

Wittenberg-Cox, A. (2020). What Do Countries With The Best Coronavirus Responses Have In Common? Women Leaders. *Forbes*. https://www.forbes.com/sites/avivahwittenbergcox/2020/04/13/what-do-countries-with-the-best-coronavirus-reponses-have-in-common-women-leaders/#36f031293dec

Wongkoblap, A., Vadillo, M. A., & Curcin, V. (2017). Researching mental health disorders in the era of social media: Systematic review. *Journal of Medical Internet Research*, *19*(6), e228.

Woods, P. J., Griffith, B. A., Page, R. P., & Rodier, P. M. (1967). Human responses to various conditions of water temperature. *Perception & Psychophysics*, *2*(4), 157–160. doi:10.3758/BF03210311

World Health Organization. (2017a). Standards for Prosthetics and Orthotics: Part 1 – Standards, p. xxvi.

World Health Organization. (2017b). Standards for Prosthetics and Orthotics: Part 2 – Implementation Manual, p. 5.

World Health Organization. (2017c). Standards for Prosthetics and Orthotics: Part 2 – Implementation Manual, p. 34.

Yannakakis, G. N. (2018). Enhancing health care via affective. *Computing*.

Ye, J., Feng, C., & Xue, Y. (2020). *Contact tracing – the privacy vs urgency dilemma for governments in the fight against Covid-19*. South China Morning Press. https://www.scmp.com/tech/big-tech/article/3087325/contact-tracing-privacy-versus-urgency-dilemma-governments-fight

Yee, N., & Bailenson, J. (2007). The proteus effect: The effect of transformed self{representation on behavior. *Human Communication Research, 33*, 271-290.

Zhang, Z., Peng, Q., & Gu, P. (2010). Improvement of user involvement in product design. In *Proceedings of the cirp design conference innovative product creation*. Elsevier.

Zvárová, J., & Zvára, K. (2011). e3Health: Three main features of modern healthcare. In E-health systems quality and reliability: Models and standards. IGI Global.

Related References

To continue our tradition of advancing information science and technology research, we have compiled a list of recommended IGI Global readings. These references will provide additional information and guidance to further enrich your knowledge and assist you with your own research and future publications.

Abu Seman, S. A., & Ramayah, T. (2017). Are We Ready to App?: A Study on mHealth Apps, Its Future, and Trends in Malaysia Context. In J. Pelet (Ed.), *Mobile Platforms, Design, and Apps for Social Commerce* (pp. 69–83). Hershey, PA: IGI Global. doi:10.4018/978-1-5225-2469-4.ch005

Aggarwal, S., & Azad, V. (2017). A Hybrid System Based on FMM and MLP to Diagnose Heart Disease. In S. Bhattacharyya, S. De, I. Pan, & P. Dutta (Eds.), *Intelligent Multidimensional Data Clustering and Analysis* (pp. 293–325). Hershey, PA: IGI Global. doi:10.4018/978-1-5225-1776-4.ch011

Akaichi, J., & Mhadhbi, L. (2016). A Clinical Decision Support System: Ontology-Driven Approach for Effective Emergency Management. In J. Moon & M. Galea (Eds.), *Improving Health Management through Clinical Decision Support Systems* (pp. 270–294). Hershey, PA: IGI Global. doi:10.4018/978-1-4666-9432-3.ch013

Akerkar, R. (2016). Towards an Intelligent Integrated Approach for Clinical Decision Support. In A. Aggarwal (Ed.), *Managing Big Data Integration in the Public Sector* (pp. 187–205). Hershey, PA: IGI Global. doi:10.4018/978-1-4666-9649-5.ch011

Al-Busaidi, S. S. (2018). Interdisciplinary Relationships Between Medicine and Social Sciences. In M. Al-Suqri, A. Al-Kindi, S. AlKindi, & N. Saleem (Eds.), *Promoting Interdisciplinarity in Knowledge Generation and Problem Solving* (pp. 124–137). Hershey, PA: IGI Global. doi:10.4018/978-1-5225-3878-3.ch009

Al Kareh, T., & Thoumy, M. (2018). The Impact of Health Information Digitization on the Physiotherapist-Patient Relationship: A Pilot Study of the Lebanese Community. *International Journal of Healthcare Information Systems and Informatics, 13*(2), 29–53. doi:10.4018/IJHISI.2018040103

Alenzuela, R. (2017). Research, Leadership, and Resource-Sharing Initiatives: The Role of Local Library Consortia in Access to Medical Information. In S. Ram (Ed.), *Library and Information Services for Bioinformatics Education and Research* (pp. 199–211). Hershey, PA: IGI Global. doi:10.4018/978-1-5225-1871-6.ch012

Ameri, H., Alizadeh, S., & Noughabi, E. A. (2017). Application of Data Mining Techniques in Clinical Decision Making: A Literature Review and Classification. In E. Noughabi, B. Raahemi, A. Albadvi, & B. Far (Eds.), *Handbook of Research on Data Science for Effective Healthcare Practice and Administration* (pp. 257–295). Hershey, PA: IGI Global. doi:10.4018/978-1-5225-2515-8.ch012

Anand, S. (2017). Medical Image Enhancement Using Edge Information-Based Methods. In B. Singh (Ed.), *Computational Tools and Techniques for Biomedical Signal Processing* (pp. 123–148). Hershey, PA: IGI Global. doi:10.4018/978-1-5225-0660-7.ch006

Angjellari-Dajci, F., Sapienza, C., Lawless, W. F., & Kavanagh, K. (2016). Human Capital Accumulation in Medical Simulated Learning Environments: A Framework for Economic Evaluation. In M. Russ (Ed.), *Quantitative Multidisciplinary Approaches in Human Capital and Asset Management* (pp. 65–88). Hershey, PA: IGI Global. doi:10.4018/978-1-4666-9652-5.ch004

Anil, M., Ayyildiz-Tamis, D., Tasdemir, S., Sendemir-Urkmez, A., & Gulce-Iz, S. (2016). Bioinspired Materials and Biocompatibility. In M. Bououdina (Ed.), *Emerging Research on Bioinspired Materials Engineering* (pp. 294–322). Hershey, PA: IGI Global. doi:10.4018/978-1-4666-9811-6.ch011

Anton, J. L., Soriano, J. V., Martinez, M. I., & Garcia, F. B. (2018). Comprehensive E-Learning Appraisal System. In M. Khosrow-Pour, D.B.A. (Ed.), Encyclopedia of Information Science and Technology, Fourth Edition (pp. 5787-5799). Hershey, PA: IGI Global. doi:10.4018/978-1-5225-2255-3.ch503

Arabi, M. (2016). Redesigning the Organizational Structure to Reach Efficiency: The Case of Ministry of Health and Medical Education of Iran. In R. Gholipour & K. Rouzbehani (Eds.), *Social, Economic, and Political Perspectives on Public Health Policy-Making* (pp. 257–294). Hershey, PA: IGI Global. doi:10.4018/978-1-4666-9944-1.ch012

Assis-Hassid, S., Heart, T., Reychav, I., & Pliskin, J. S. (2016). Modelling Factors Affecting Patient-Doctor-Computer Communication in Primary Care. *International Journal of Reliable and Quality E-Healthcare*, *5*(1), 1–17. doi:10.4018/IJRQEH.2016010101

Atzori, B., Hoffman, H. G., Vagnoli, L., Messeri, A., & Grotto, R. L. (2018). Virtual Reality as Distraction Technique for Pain Management in Children and Adolescents. In M. Khosrow-Pour, D.B.A. (Ed.), Encyclopedia of Information Science and Technology, Fourth Edition (pp. 5955-5965). Hershey, PA: IGI Global. doi:10.4018/978-1-5225-2255-3.ch518

Audibert, M., Mathonnat, J., Pélissier, A., & Huang, X. X. (2018). The Impact of the New Rural Cooperative Medical Scheme on Township Hospitals' Utilization and Income Structure in Weifang Prefecture, China. In I. Management Association (Ed.), Health Economics and Healthcare Reform: Breakthroughs in Research and Practice (pp. 109-121). Hershey, PA: IGI Global. doi:10.4018/978-1-5225-3168-5.ch007

Ayyachamy, S. (2016). Analysis and Comparison of Developed 2D Medical Image Database Design using Registration Scheme, Retrieval Scheme, and Bag-of-Visual-Words. In N. Dey & A. Ashour (Eds.), *Classification and Clustering in Biomedical Signal Processing* (pp. 149–168). Hershey, PA: IGI Global. doi:10.4018/978-1-5225-0140-4.ch007

Babalola, A. C. (2016). Literacy and Decision Making on Health Issues among Married Women in Southwest Nigeria. In V. Wang (Ed.), *Handbook of Research on Advancing Health Education through Technology* (pp. 191–212). Hershey, PA: IGI Global. doi:10.4018/978-1-4666-9494-1.ch009

Babu, A., & Ayyappan, S. (2017). A Methodological Evaluation of Crypto-Watermarking System for Medical Images. In C. Bhatt & S. Peddoju (Eds.), *Cloud Computing Systems and Applications in Healthcare* (pp. 189–217). Hershey, PA: IGI Global. doi:10.4018/978-1-5225-1002-4.ch010

Bakke, A. (2017). Ethos in E-Health: From Informational to Interactive Websites. In M. Folk & S. Apostel (Eds.), *Establishing and Evaluating Digital Ethos and Online Credibility* (pp. 85–103). Hershey, PA: IGI Global. doi:10.4018/978-1-5225-1072-7.ch005

Bali, S. (2018). Enhancing the Reach of Health Care Through Telemedicine: Status and New Possibilities in Developing Countries. In U. Pandey & V. Indrakanti (Eds.), *Open and Distance Learning Initiatives for Sustainable Development* (pp. 339–354). Hershey, PA: IGI Global. doi:10.4018/978-1-5225-2621-6.ch019

Barrett, T. E. (2018). Essentials for Education and Training for Tomorrow's Physicians. In C. Smith (Ed.), *Exploring the Pressures of Medical Education From a Mental Health and Wellness Perspective* (pp. 230–252). Hershey, PA: IGI Global. doi:10.4018/978-1-5225-2811-1.ch010

Barrett, T. J. (2016). Knowledge in Action: Fostering Health Education through Technology. In V. Wang (Ed.), *Handbook of Research on Advancing Health Education through Technology* (pp. 39–62). Hershey, PA: IGI Global. doi:10.4018/978-1-4666-9494-1.ch003

Berrahal, S., & Boudriga, N. (2017). The Risks of Wearable Technologies to Individuals and Organizations. In A. Marrington, D. Kerr, & J. Gammack (Eds.), *Managing Security Issues and the Hidden Dangers of Wearable Technologies* (pp. 18–46). Hershey, PA: IGI Global. doi:10.4018/978-1-5225-1016-1.ch002

Bhagat, A. P., & Atique, M. (2016). Medical Image Mining Using Fuzzy Connectedness Image Segmentation: Efficient Retrieval of Patients' Stored Images. In W. Karâa & N. Dey (Eds.), *Biomedical Image Analysis and Mining Techniques for Improved Health Outcomes* (pp. 184–209). Hershey, PA: IGI Global. doi:10.4018/978-1-4666-8811-7.ch009

Bhargava, P. (2018). Blended Learning: An Effective Application to Clinical Teaching. In S. Tang & C. Lim (Eds.), *Preparing the Next Generation of Teachers for 21st Century Education* (pp. 302–320). Hershey, PA: IGI Global. doi:10.4018/978-1-5225-4080-9.ch018

Binh, N. T., & Tuyet, V. T. (2016). The Combination of Adaptive Filters to Improve the Quality of Medical Images in New Wavelet Domain. In N. Dey & A. Ashour (Eds.), *Classification and Clustering in Biomedical Signal Processing* (pp. 46–76). Hershey, PA: IGI Global. doi:10.4018/978-1-5225-0140-4.ch003

Bird, J. L. (2017). Writing Healing Narratives. In V. Bryan & J. Bird (Eds.), *Healthcare Community Synergism between Patients, Practitioners, and Researchers* (pp. 1–28). Hershey, PA: IGI Global. doi:10.4018/978-1-5225-0640-9.ch001

Bottrighi, A., Leonardi, G., Piovesan, L., & Terenziani, P. (2016). Knowledge-Based Support to the Treatment of Exceptions in Computer Interpretable Clinical Guidelines. *International Journal of Knowledge-Based Organizations*, *6*(3), 1–27. doi:10.4018/IJKBO.2016070101

Bougoulias, K., Kouris, I., Prasinos, M., Giokas, K., & Koutsouris, D. (2017). Ob/Gyn EMR Software: A Solution for Obstetricians and Gynecologists. In A. Moumtzoglou (Ed.), *Design, Development, and Integration of Reliable Electronic Healthcare Platforms* (pp. 101–111). Hershey, PA: IGI Global. doi:10.4018/978-1-5225-1724-5.ch006

Bouslimi, R., Ayadi, M. G., & Akaichi, J. (2018). Medical Image Retrieval in Healthcare Social Networks. *International Journal of Healthcare Information Systems and Informatics, 13*(2), 13–28. doi:10.4018/IJHISI.2018040102

Bouzaabia, O., Bouzaabia, R., & Mejri, K. (2017). Role of Internet in the Development of Medical Tourism Service in Tunisia. In A. Capatina & E. Rancati (Eds.), *Key Challenges and Opportunities in Web Entrepreneurship* (pp. 211–241). Hershey, PA: IGI Global. doi:10.4018/978-1-5225-2466-3.ch009

Briz-Ponce, L., Juanes-Méndez, J. A., & García-Peñalvo, F. J. (2016). The Role of Gender in Technology Acceptance for Medical Education. In M. Cruz-Cunha, I. Miranda, R. Martinho, & R. Rijo (Eds.), *Encyclopedia of E-Health and Telemedicine* (pp. 1013–1027). Hershey, PA: IGI Global. doi:10.4018/978-1-4666-9978-6.ch079

Briz-Ponce, L., Juanes-Méndez, J. A., & García-Peñalvo, F. J. (2016). A Research Contribution to the Analysis of Mobile Devices in Higher Education from Medical Students' Point of View. In L. Briz-Ponce, J. Juanes-Méndez, & F. García-Peñalvo (Eds.), *Handbook of Research on Mobile Devices and Applications in Higher Education Settings* (pp. 196–221). Hershey, PA: IGI Global. doi:10.4018/978-1-5225-0256-2.ch009

Brown-Jackson, K. L. (2018). Telemedicine and Telehealth: Academics Engaging the Community in a Call to Action. In S. Burton (Ed.), *Engaged Scholarship and Civic Responsibility in Higher Education* (pp. 166–193). Hershey, PA: IGI Global. doi:10.4018/978-1-5225-3649-9.ch008

Bwalya, K. J. (2017). Next Wave of Tele-Medicine: Virtual Presence of Medical Personnel. In K. Moahi, K. Bwalya, & P. Sebina (Eds.), *Health Information Systems and the Advancement of Medical Practice in Developing Countries* (pp. 168–180). Hershey, PA: IGI Global. doi:10.4018/978-1-5225-2262-1.ch010

Carlton, E. L., Holsinger, J. W. Jr, & Anunobi, N. (2016). Physician Engagement with Health Information Technology: Implications for Practice and Professionalism. *International Journal of Computers in Clinical Practice, 1*(2), 51–73. doi:10.4018/IJCCP.2016070103

Castillo-Page, L., Eliason, J., Conrad, S. S., & Nivet, M. A. (2016). Diversity in Undergraduate Medical Education: An Examination of Organizational Culture and Climate in Medical Schools. In C. Scott & J. Sims (Eds.), *Developing Workforce Diversity Programs, Curriculum, and Degrees in Higher Education* (pp. 304–326). Hershey, PA: IGI Global. doi:10.4018/978-1-5225-0209-8.ch016

Cebeci, H. I., & Hiziroglu, A. (2016). Review of Business Intelligence and Intelligent Systems in Healthcare Domain. In N. Celebi (Ed.), *Intelligent Techniques for Data Analysis in Diverse Settings* (pp. 192–206). Hershey, PA: IGI Global. doi:10.4018/978-1-5225-0075-9.ch009

Celik, G. (2018). Determining Headache Diseases With Genetic Algorithm. In U. Kose, G. Guraksin, & O. Deperlioglu (Eds.), *Nature-Inspired Intelligent Techniques for Solving Biomedical Engineering Problems* (pp. 249–262). Hershey, PA: IGI Global. doi:10.4018/978-1-5225-4769-3.ch012

Chakraborty, C., Gupta, B., & Ghosh, S. K. (2016). Mobile Telemedicine Systems for Remote Patient's Chronic Wound Monitoring. In A. Moumtzoglou (Ed.), *M-Health Innovations for Patient-Centered Care* (pp. 213–239). Hershey, PA: IGI Global. doi:10.4018/978-1-4666-9861-1.ch011

Chakraborty, S., Chatterjee, S., Ashour, A. S., Mali, K., & Dey, N. (2018). Intelligent Computing in Medical Imaging: A Study. In N. Dey (Ed.), *Advancements in Applied Metaheuristic Computing* (pp. 143–163). Hershey, PA: IGI Global. doi:10.4018/978-1-5225-4151-6.ch006

Chavez, A., & Kovarik, C. (2017). Open Source Technology for Medical Practice in Developing Countries. In K. Moahi, K. Bwalya, & P. Sebina (Eds.), *Health Information Systems and the Advancement of Medical Practice in Developing Countries* (pp. 33–59). Hershey, PA: IGI Global. doi:10.4018/978-1-5225-2262-1.ch003

Chen, E. T. (2016). Examining the Influence of Information Technology on Modern Health Care. In P. Manolitzas, E. Grigoroudis, N. Matsatsinis, & D. Yannacopoulos (Eds.), *Effective Methods for Modern Healthcare Service Quality and Evaluation* (pp. 110–136). Hershey, PA: IGI Global. doi:10.4018/978-1-4666-9961-8.ch006

Chin, S. (2016). Surviving Sandy: Recovering Collections after a Natural Disaster. In E. Decker & J. Townes (Eds.), *Handbook of Research on Disaster Management and Contingency Planning in Modern Libraries* (pp. 366–388). Hershey, PA: IGI Global. doi:10.4018/978-1-4666-8624-3.ch016

Chojnacki, M., & Wöjcik, A. (2016). Security and the Role of New Technologies and Innovation in Medical Ethics. In A. Rosiek & K. Leksowski (Eds.), *Organizational Culture and Ethics in Modern Medicine* (pp. 52–77). Hershey, PA: IGI Global. doi:10.4018/978-1-4666-9658-7.ch003

Cılız, N., Yıldırım, H., & Temizel, Ş. (2016). Structure Development for Effective Medical Waste and Hazardous Waste Management System. In U. Akkucuk (Ed.), *Handbook of Research on Waste Management Techniques for Sustainability* (pp. 303–327). Hershey, PA: IGI Global. doi:10.4018/978-1-4666-9723-2.ch016

Ciufudean, C. (2018). Innovative Formalism for Biological Data Analysis. In M. Khosrow-Pour, D.B.A. (Ed.), Encyclopedia of Information Science and Technology, Fourth Edition (pp. 1814-1824). Hershey, PA: IGI Global. doi:10.4018/978-1-5225-2255-3.ch158

Ciufudean, C., & Ciufudean, O. (2016). Tele-Monitoring for Medical Diagnosis Availability. In M. Cruz-Cunha, I. Miranda, R. Martinho, & R. Rijo (Eds.), *Encyclopedia of E-Health and Telemedicine* (pp. 401–411). Hershey, PA: IGI Global. doi:10.4018/978-1-4666-9978-6.ch032

Colaguori, R., & Danesi, M. (2017). Medical Semiotics: A Revisitation and an Exhortation. *International Journal of Semiotics and Visual Rhetoric*, *1*(1), 11–18. doi:10.4018/IJSVR.2017010102

Cole, A. W., & Salek, T. A. (2017). Adopting a Parasocial Connection to Overcome Professional Kakoethos in Online Health Information. In M. Folk & S. Apostel (Eds.), *Establishing and Evaluating Digital Ethos and Online Credibility* (pp. 104–120). Hershey, PA: IGI Global. doi:10.4018/978-1-5225-1072-7.ch006

Contreras, E. C., & Puente, G. J. (2016). How to Identify Rheumatic Diseases by General Physicians. In T. Gasmelseid (Ed.), *Advancing Pharmaceutical Processes and Tools for Improved Health Outcomes* (pp. 136–166). Hershey, PA: IGI Global. doi:10.4018/978-1-5225-0248-7.ch006

D'Andrea, A., Ferri, F., & Grifoni, P. (2016). RFID Technologies in Healthcare Setting: Applications and Future Perspectives. *International Journal of Computers in Clinical Practice*, *1*(1), 15–27. doi:10.4018/IJCCP.2016010102

Damianakis, A., Kallonis, P., Loudos, G., Tsatsos, D., & Tsoukalis, A. (2016). Exploiting 3D Medical Equipment Simulations to Support Biomedical Engineering Academic Courses: Design Methodology and Implementation in a Small Scale National Project. In B. Khan (Ed.), *Revolutionizing Modern Education through Meaningful E-Learning Implementation* (pp. 277–295). Hershey, PA: IGI Global. doi:10.4018/978-1-5225-0466-5.ch015

Demiroz, E. (2016). Principles of Instructional Design for E-Learning and Online Learning Practices: Implications for Medical Education. In V. Wang (Ed.), *Handbook of Research on Advancing Health Education through Technology* (pp. 419–451). Hershey, PA: IGI Global. doi:10.4018/978-1-4666-9494-1.ch018

Deperlioglu, O. (2018). Intelligent Techniques Inspired by Nature and Used in Biomedical Engineering. In U. Kose, G. Guraksin, & O. Deperlioglu (Eds.), *Nature-Inspired Intelligent Techniques for Solving Biomedical Engineering Problems* (pp. 51–77). Hershey, PA: IGI Global. doi:10.4018/978-1-5225-4769-3.ch003

Dey, N., & Ashour, A. S. (2018). Meta-Heuristic Algorithms in Medical Image Segmentation: A Review. In N. Dey (Ed.), *Advancements in Applied Metaheuristic Computing* (pp. 185–203). Hershey, PA: IGI Global. doi:10.4018/978-1-5225-4151-6.ch008

Dey, N., Ashour, A. S., & Althoupety, A. S. (2017). Thermal Imaging in Medical Science. In V. Santhi (Ed.), *Recent Advances in Applied Thermal Imaging for Industrial Applications* (pp. 87–117). Hershey, PA: IGI Global. doi:10.4018/978-1-5225-2423-6.ch004

Di Virgilio, F., Camillo, A. A., & Camillo, I. C. (2017). The Impact of Social Network on Italian Users' Behavioural Intention for the Choice of a Medical Tourist Destination. *International Journal of Tourism and Hospitality Management in the Digital Age*, *1*(1), 36–49. doi:10.4018/IJTHMDA.2017010103

Dias, C. M., Ribeiro, A. G., & Furtado, S. F. (2016). An Overview about the Use of Healthcare Applications on Mobile Devices. In M. Cruz-Cunha, I. Miranda, R. Martinho, & R. Rijo (Eds.), *Encyclopedia of E-Health and Telemedicine* (pp. 285–298). Hershey, PA: IGI Global. doi:10.4018/978-1-4666-9978-6.ch024

Dogra, A. K., & Dogra, P. (2017). The Medical Tourism Industry in the BRIC Nations: An Indian Analysis. In M. Dhiman (Ed.), *Opportunities and Challenges for Tourism and Hospitality in the BRIC Nations* (pp. 320–336). Hershey, PA: IGI Global. doi:10.4018/978-1-5225-0708-6.ch020

Drowos, J. L., & Wood, S. K. (2017). Preparing Future Physicians to Adapt to the Changing Health Care System: Promoting Humanism through Curricular Design. In V. Bryan & J. Bird (Eds.), *Healthcare Community Synergism between Patients, Practitioners, and Researchers* (pp. 106–125). Hershey, PA: IGI Global. doi:10.4018/978-1-5225-0640-9.ch006

Dulam, K. (2017). Medical Patents and Impact on Availability and Affordability of Essential Medicines in India. In R. Aggarwal & R. Kaur (Eds.), *Patent Law and Intellectual Property in the Medical Field* (pp. 41–57). Hershey, PA: IGI Global. doi:10.4018/978-1-5225-2414-4.ch003

Dutta, P. (2017). Decision Making in Medical Diagnosis via Distance Measures on Interval Valued Fuzzy Sets. *International Journal of System Dynamics Applications*, *6*(4), 63–83. doi:10.4018/IJSDA.2017100104

Edoh, T. O., Pawar, P. A., Brügge, B., & Teege, G. (2016). A Multidisciplinary Remote Healthcare Delivery System to Increase Health Care Access, Pathology Screening, and Treatment in Developing Countries: The Case of Benin. *International Journal of Healthcare Information Systems and Informatics*, *11*(4), 1–31. doi:10.4018/IJHISI.2016100101

El Guemhioui, K., & Demurjian, S. A. (2017). Semantic Reconciliation of Electronic Health Records Using Semantic Web Technologies. *International Journal of Information Technology and Web Engineering*, *12*(2), 26–48. doi:10.4018/IJITWE.2017040102

Ellouze, N., Rekhis, S., & Boudriga, N. (2016). Forensic Investigation of Digital Crimes in Healthcare Applications. In O. Isafiade & A. Bagula (Eds.), *Data Mining Trends and Applications in Criminal Science and Investigations* (pp. 169–210). Hershey, PA: IGI Global. doi:10.4018/978-1-5225-0463-4.ch007

Eneanya, A. N. (2016). Health Policy Implementation and Its Barriers: The Case Study of US Health System. In R. Gholipour & K. Rouzbehani (Eds.), *Social, Economic, and Political Perspectives on Public Health Policy-Making* (pp. 42–63). Hershey, PA: IGI Global. doi:10.4018/978-1-4666-9944-1.ch003

Entico, G. J. (2016). Knowledge Management and the Medical Health Librarians: A Perception Study. In J. Yap, M. Perez, M. Ayson, & G. Entico (Eds.), *Special Library Administration, Standardization and Technological Integration* (pp. 52–77). Hershey, PA: IGI Global. doi:10.4018/978-1-4666-9542-9.ch003

Ferradji, M. A., & Zidani, A. (2016). Collaborative Environment for Remote Clinical Reasoning Learning. *International Journal of E-Health and Medical Communications*, *7*(4), 62–81. doi:10.4018/IJEHMC.2016100104

Fisher, J. (2018). Sociological Perspectives on Improving Medical Diagnosis Emphasizing CAD. In M. Khosrow-Pour, D.B.A. (Ed.), Encyclopedia of Information Science and Technology, Fourth Edition (pp. 1017-1024). Hershey, PA: IGI Global. doi:10.4018/978-1-5225-2255-3.ch088

Flores, C. D., Respício, A., Coelho, H., Bez, M. R., & Fonseca, J. M. (2016). Simulation for Medical Training. In M. Cruz-Cunha, I. Miranda, R. Martinho, & R. Rijo (Eds.), *Encyclopedia of E-Health and Telemedicine* (pp. 827–842). Hershey, PA: IGI Global. doi:10.4018/978-1-4666-9978-6.ch064

Frank, E. M. (2018). Healthcare Education: Integrating Simulation Technologies. In V. Bryan, A. Musgrove, & J. Powers (Eds.), *Handbook of Research on Human Development in the Digital Age* (pp. 163–182). Hershey, PA: IGI Global. doi:10.4018/978-1-5225-2838-8.ch008

Garner, G. (2018). Foundations for Yoga Practice in Rehabilitation. In S. Telles & N. Singh (Eds.), *Research-Based Perspectives on the Psychophysiology of Yoga* (pp. 263–307). Hershey, PA: IGI Global. doi:10.4018/978-1-5225-2788-6.ch015

Gasmelseid, T. M. (2016). Improving Pharmaceutical Care through the Use of Intelligent Pharmacoinformatics. In T. Gasmelseid (Ed.), *Advancing Pharmaceutical Processes and Tools for Improved Health Outcomes* (pp. 167–188). Hershey, PA: IGI Global. doi:10.4018/978-1-5225-0248-7.ch007

Gavurová, B., Kováč, V., & Šoltés, M. (2018). Medical Equipment and Economic Determinants of Its Structure and Regulation in the Slovak Republic. In M. Khosrow-Pour, D.B.A. (Ed.), Encyclopedia of Information Science and Technology, Fourth Edition (pp. 5841-5852). Hershey, PA: IGI Global. doi:10.4018/978-1-5225-2255-3.ch508

Ge, X., Wang, Q., Huang, K., Law, V., & Thomas, D. C. (2017). Designing Simulated Learning Environments and Facilitating Authentic Learning Experiences in Medical Education. In J. Stefaniak (Ed.), *Advancing Medical Education Through Strategic Instructional Design* (pp. 77–100). Hershey, PA: IGI Global. doi:10.4018/978-1-5225-2098-6.ch004

Gewald, H., & Gewald, C. (2018). Inhibitors of Physicians' Use of Mandatory Hospital Information Systems (HIS). *International Journal of Healthcare Information Systems and Informatics, 13*(1), 29–44. doi:10.4018/IJHISI.2018010103

Ghosh, D., & Dinda, S. (2017). Health Infrastructure and Economic Development in India. In R. Das (Ed.), *Social, Health, and Environmental Infrastructures for Economic Growth* (pp. 99–119). Hershey, PA: IGI Global. doi:10.4018/978-1-5225-2364-2.ch006

Ghosh, K., & Sen, K. C. (2017). The Potential of Crowdsourcing in the Health Care Industry. In N. Wickramasinghe (Ed.), *Handbook of Research on Healthcare Administration and Management* (pp. 418–427). Hershey, PA: IGI Global. doi:10.4018/978-1-5225-0920-2.ch024

Ghrab, S., & Saad, I. (2016). Identifying Crucial Know-How and Knowing-That for Medical Decision Support. *International Journal of Decision Support System Technology*, *8*(4), 14–33. doi:10.4018/IJDSST.2016100102

Giokas, K., Tsirmpas, C., Anastasiou, A., Iliopoulou, D., Costarides, V., & Koutsouris, D. (2016). Contemporary Heart Failure Treatment Based on Improved Knowledge and Personalized Care of Comorbidities. In D. Fotiadis (Ed.), *Handbook of Research on Trends in the Diagnosis and Treatment of Chronic Conditions* (pp. 301–314). Hershey, PA: IGI Global. doi:10.4018/978-1-4666-8828-5.ch014

Gopalan, V., Chan, E., & Ho, D. T. (2018). Deliberate Self-Harm and Suicide Ideology in Medical Students. In C. Smith (Ed.), *Exploring the Pressures of Medical Education From a Mental Health and Wellness Perspective* (pp. 122–143). Hershey, PA: IGI Global. doi:10.4018/978-1-5225-2811-1.ch005

Goswami, S., Dey, U., Roy, P., Ashour, A., & Dey, N. (2017). Medical Video Processing: Concept and Applications. In N. Dey, A. Ashour, & P. Patra (Eds.), *Feature Detectors and Motion Detection in Video Processing* (pp. 1–17). Hershey, PA: IGI Global. doi:10.4018/978-1-5225-1025-3.ch001

Goswami, S., Mahanta, K., Goswami, S., Jigdung, T., & Devi, T. P. (2018). Ageing and Cancer: The Epigenetic Basis, Alternative Treatment, and Care. In B. Prasad & S. Akbar (Eds.), *Handbook of Research on Geriatric Health, Treatment, and Care* (pp. 206–235). Hershey, PA: IGI Global. doi:10.4018/978-1-5225-3480-8.ch012

Gouva, M. I. (2017). The Psychological Impact of Medical Error on Patients, Family Members, and Health Professionals. In M. Riga (Ed.), *Impact of Medical Errors and Malpractice on Health Economics, Quality, and Patient Safety* (pp. 171–196). Hershey, PA: IGI Global. doi:10.4018/978-1-5225-2337-6.ch007

Gürcü, M., & Tengilimoğlu, D. (2017). Health Tourism-Based Destination Marketing. In A. Bayraktar & C. Uslay (Eds.), *Strategic Place Branding Methodologies and Theory for Tourist Attraction* (pp. 308–331). Hershey, PA: IGI Global. doi:10.4018/978-1-5225-0579-2.ch015

Gürsel, G. (2016). Mobility in Healthcare: M-Health. In A. Panagopoulos (Ed.), *Handbook of Research on Next Generation Mobile Communication Systems* (pp. 485–511). Hershey, PA: IGI Global. doi:10.4018/978-1-4666-8732-5.ch019

Gürsel, G. (2017). For Better Healthcare Mining Health Data. In S. Bhattacharyya, S. De, I. Pan, & P. Dutta (Eds.), *Intelligent Multidimensional Data Clustering and Analysis* (pp. 135–158). Hershey, PA: IGI Global. doi:10.4018/978-1-5225-1776-4.ch006

Guzman-Lugo, G., Lopez-Martinez, M., Lopez-Ramirez, B., & Avila-Vazquez, D. (2016). City-Driven Approach to Determine Health Services Based on Current User Location and Collaborative Information. *International Journal of Knowledge Society Research*, *7*(1), 53–62. doi:10.4018/IJKSR.2016010104

Gyaase, P. O., Darko-Lartey, R., William, H., & Borkloe, F. (2017). Towards an Integrated Electronic Medical Records System for Quality Healthcare in Ghana: An Exploratory Factor Analysis. *International Journal of Computers in Clinical Practice*, *2*(2), 38–55. doi:10.4018/IJCCP.2017070103

Handayani, P. W., Sandhyaduhita, P. I., Hidayanto, A. N., Pinem, A. A., Fajrina, H. R., Junus, K. M., ... Ayuningtyas, D. (2016). Integrated Hospital Information System Architecture Design in Indonesia. In T. Iyamu & A. Tatnall (Eds.), *Maximizing Healthcare Delivery and Management through Technology Integration* (pp. 207–236). Hershey, PA: IGI Global. doi:10.4018/978-1-4666-9446-0.ch013

Hanel, P. (2017). Is China Catching Up?: Health-Related Applications of Biotechnology. In T. Bas & J. Zhao (Eds.), *Comparative Approaches to Biotechnology Development and Use in Developed and Emerging Nations* (pp. 465–520). Hershey, PA: IGI Global. doi:10.4018/978-1-5225-1040-6.ch016

Harmsen, C. A., & Royle, R. N. (2016). St. Stephen's Hospital Hervey Bay: Study of Developing a Digital Hospital. In J. Moon & M. Galea (Eds.), *Improving Health Management through Clinical Decision Support Systems* (pp. 127–153). Hershey, PA: IGI Global. doi:10.4018/978-1-4666-9432-3.ch006

Harp, D., Shim, R. S., Johnson, J., Harp, J. A., Wilcox, W. C., & Wilcox, J. K. (2016). Race and Gender Inequalities in Medicine and Biomedical Research. In U. Thomas & J. Drake (Eds.), *Critical Research on Sexism and Racism in STEM Fields* (pp. 115–134). Hershey, PA: IGI Global. doi:10.4018/978-1-5225-0174-9.ch006

Hartman, A., & Brown, S. (2017). Synergism through Therapeutic Visual Arts. In V. Bryan & J. Bird (Eds.), *Healthcare Community Synergism between Patients, Practitioners, and Researchers* (pp. 29–48). Hershey, PA: IGI Global. doi:10.4018/978-1-5225-0640-9.ch002

Hazra, J., Chowdhury, A. R., & Dutta, P. (2016). Cluster Based Medical Image Registration Using Optimized Neural Network. In S. Bhattacharyya, P. Banerjee, D. Majumdar, & P. Dutta (Eds.), *Handbook of Research on Advanced Hybrid Intelligent Techniques and Applications* (pp. 551–581). Hershey, PA: IGI Global. doi:10.4018/978-1-4666-9474-3.ch018

Hung, S., Huang, W., Yen, D. C., Chang, S., & Lu, C. (2016). Effect of Information Service Competence and Contextual Factors on the Effectiveness of Strategic Information Systems Planning in Hospitals. *Journal of Global Information Management*, *24*(1), 14–36. doi:10.4018/JGIM.2016010102

Iltchev, P., Śliwczyński, A., Szynkiewicz, P., & Marczak, M. (2016). Mobile Health Applications Assisting Patients with Chronic Diseases: Examples from Asthma Care. In A. Moumtzoglou (Ed.), *M-Health Innovations for Patient-Centered Care* (pp. 170–196). Hershey, PA: IGI Global. doi:10.4018/978-1-4666-9861-1.ch009

Iqbal, S., Ahmad, S., & Willis, I. (2017). Influencing Factors for Adopting Technology Enhanced Learning in the Medical Schools of Punjab, Pakistan. *International Journal of Information and Communication Technology Education*, *13*(3), 27–39. doi:10.4018/IJICTE.2017070103

Jagan, J., Dalkiliç, Y., & Samui, P. (2016). Utilization of SVM, LSSVM and GP for Predicting the Medical Waste Generation. In G. Hua (Ed.), *Smart Cities as a Solution for Reducing Urban Waste and Pollution* (pp. 224–251). Hershey, PA: IGI Global. doi:10.4018/978-1-5225-0302-6.ch008

Jagiello, K., Sosnowska, A., Mikolajczyk, A., & Puzyn, T. (2017). Nanomaterials in Medical Devices: Regulations' Review and Future Perspectives. *Journal of Nanotoxicology and Nanomedicine*, *2*(2), 1–11. doi:10.4018/JNN.2017070101

Jena, T. K. (2018). Skill Training Process in Medicine Through Distance Mode. In U. Pandey & V. Indrakanti (Eds.), *Optimizing Open and Distance Learning in Higher Education Institutions* (pp. 228–243). Hershey, PA: IGI Global. doi:10.4018/978-1-5225-2624-7.ch010

Jesus, Â., & Gomes, M. J. (2016). Web 2.0 Tools in Biomedical and Pharmaceutical Education: Updated Review and Commentary. In T. Gasmelseid (Ed.), *Advancing Pharmaceutical Processes and Tools for Improved Health Outcomes* (pp. 52–78). Hershey, PA: IGI Global. doi:10.4018/978-1-5225-0248-7.ch003

Joseph, V., & Miller, J. M. (2018). Medical Students' Perceived Stigma in Seeking Care: A Cultural Perspective. In C. Smith (Ed.), *Exploring the Pressures of Medical Education From a Mental Health and Wellness Perspective* (pp. 44–67). Hershey, PA: IGI Global. doi:10.4018/978-1-5225-2811-1.ch002

Joyce, B. L., & Swanberg, S. M. (2017). Using Backward Design for Competency-Based Undergraduate Medical Education. In J. Stefaniak (Ed.), *Advancing Medical Education Through Strategic Instructional Design* (pp. 53–76). Hershey, PA: IGI Global. doi:10.4018/978-1-5225-2098-6.ch003

Kaljo, K., & Jacques, L. (2018). Flipping the Medical School Classroom. In M. Khosrow-Pour, D.B.A. (Ed.), Encyclopedia of Information Science and Technology, Fourth Edition (pp. 5800-5809). Hershey, PA: IGI Global. doi:10.4018/978-1-5225-2255-3.ch504

Karon, R. (2016). Utilisation of Health Information Systems for Service Delivery in the Namibian Environment. In T. Iyamu & A. Tatnall (Eds.), *Maximizing Healthcare Delivery and Management through Technology Integration* (pp. 169–183). Hershey, PA: IGI Global. doi:10.4018/978-1-4666-9446-0.ch011

Kasina, H., Bahubalendruni, M. V., & Botcha, R. (2017). Robots in Medicine: Past, Present and Future. *International Journal of Manufacturing, Materials, and Mechanical Engineering*, *7*(4), 44–64. doi:10.4018/IJMMME.2017100104

Katehakis, D. G. (2018). Electronic Medical Record Implementation Challenges for the National Health System in Greece. *International Journal of Reliable and Quality E-Healthcare*, *7*(1), 16–30. doi:10.4018/IJRQEH.2018010102

Katz, A., & Shtub, A. (2016). Design and Build a Wizard of Oz (WOZ) Telemedicine Simulator Platform. In M. Cruz-Cunha, I. Miranda, R. Martinho, & R. Rijo (Eds.), *Encyclopedia of E-Health and Telemedicine* (pp. 128–141). Hershey, PA: IGI Global. doi:10.4018/978-1-4666-9978-6.ch011

Kaur, P. D., & Sharma, P. (2017). Success Dimensions of ICTs in Healthcare. In B. Singh (Ed.), *Computational Tools and Techniques for Biomedical Signal Processing* (pp. 149–173). Hershey, PA: IGI Global. doi:10.4018/978-1-5225-0660-7.ch007

Kaushik, P. (2018). Comorbidity of Medical and Psychiatric Disorders in Geriatric Population: Treatment and Care. In B. Prasad & S. Akbar (Eds.), *Handbook of Research on Geriatric Health, Treatment, and Care* (pp. 448–474). Hershey, PA: IGI Global. doi:10.4018/978-1-5225-3480-8.ch025

Khachane, M. Y. (2017). Organ-Based Medical Image Classification Using Support Vector Machine. *International Journal of Synthetic Emotions*, *8*(1), 18–30. doi:10.4018/IJSE.2017010102

Kirci, P. (2018). Intelligent Techniques for Analysis of Big Data About Healthcare and Medical Records. In N. Shah & M. Mittal (Eds.), *Handbook of Research on Promoting Business Process Improvement Through Inventory Control Techniques* (pp. 559–582). Hershey, PA: IGI Global. doi:10.4018/978-1-5225-3232-3.ch029

Kldiashvili, E. (2016). Cloud Computing as the Useful Resource for Application of the Medical Information System for Quality Assurance Purposes. *International Journal of Computers in Clinical Practice*, *1*(2), 1–23. doi:10.4018/IJCCP.2016070101

Kldiashvili, E. (2018). Cloud Approach for the Medical Information System: MIS on Cloud. In M. Khosrow-Pour (Ed.), *Incorporating Nature-Inspired Paradigms in Computational Applications* (pp. 238–261). Hershey, PA: IGI Global. doi:10.4018/978-1-5225-5020-4.ch008

Kldiashvili, E., Burduli, A., Ghortlishvili, G., & Sheklashvili, I. (2016). Georgian Experience in Telecytology. In M. Cruz-Cunha, I. Miranda, R. Martinho, & R. Rijo (Eds.), *Encyclopedia of E-Health and Telemedicine* (pp. 62–71). Hershey, PA: IGI Global. doi:10.4018/978-1-4666-9978-6.ch006

Ko, H., Mesicek, L., Choi, J., Choi, J., & Hwang, S. (2018). A Study on Secure Contents Strategies for Applications With DRM on Cloud Computing. *International Journal of Cloud Applications and Computing*, *8*(1), 143–153. doi:10.4018/IJCAC.2018010107

Komendziński, T., Dreszer-Drogorób, J., Mikołajewska, E., Mikołajewski, D., & Bałaj, B. (2016). Interdisciplinary Education for Research and Everyday Clinical Practice: Lessons Learned from InteRDoCTor Project. In A. Rosiek & K. Leksowski (Eds.), *Organizational Culture and Ethics in Modern Medicine* (pp. 78–110). Hershey, PA: IGI Global. doi:10.4018/978-1-4666-9658-7.ch004

Komendziński, T., Mikołajewska, E., & Mikołajewski, D. (2018). Cross-Cultural Decision-Making in Healthcare: Theory and Practical Application in Real Clinical Conditions. In A. Rosiek-Kryszewska & K. Leksowski (Eds.), *Healthcare Administration for Patient Safety and Engagement* (pp. 276–298). Hershey, PA: IGI Global. doi:10.4018/978-1-5225-3946-9.ch015

Konecny, L. T. (2018). Medical School Wellness Initiatives. In C. Smith (Ed.), *Exploring the Pressures of Medical Education From a Mental Health and Wellness Perspective* (pp. 209–228). Hershey, PA: IGI Global. doi:10.4018/978-1-5225-2811-1.ch009

Konieczna, A., & Słomkowski, P. (2016). Confrontation of Human Rights in Daily Clinical Situations. In A. Rosiek & K. Leksowski (Eds.), *Organizational Culture and Ethics in Modern Medicine* (pp. 255–281). Hershey, PA: IGI Global. doi:10.4018/978-1-4666-9658-7.ch011

Kromrei, H., Solomonson, W. L., & Juzych, M. S. (2017). Teaching Residents How to Teach. In J. Stefaniak (Ed.), *Advancing Medical Education Through Strategic Instructional Design* (pp. 164–185). Hershey, PA: IGI Global. doi:10.4018/978-1-5225-2098-6.ch008

Kulkarni, S., Savyanavar, A., Kulkarni, P., Stranieri, A., & Ghorpade, V. (2018). Framework for Integration of Medical Image and Text-Based Report Retrieval to Support Radiological Diagnosis. In M. Kolekar & V. Kumar (Eds.), *Biomedical Signal and Image Processing in Patient Care* (pp. 86–122). Hershey, PA: IGI Global. doi:10.4018/978-1-5225-2829-6.ch006

Kumar, A., & Sarkar, B. K. (2018). Performance Analysis of Nature-Inspired Algorithms-Based Bayesian Prediction Models for Medical Data Sets. In U. Singh, A. Tiwari, & R. Singh (Eds.), *Soft-Computing-Based Nonlinear Control Systems Design* (pp. 134–155). Hershey, PA: IGI Global. doi:10.4018/978-1-5225-3531-7.ch007

Kurtz, R. S. (2016). Fortitude: A Study of African Americans in Surgery in New York City. In U. Thomas & J. Drake (Eds.), *Critical Research on Sexism and Racism in STEM Fields* (pp. 153–169). Hershey, PA: IGI Global. doi:10.4018/978-1-5225-0174-9.ch009

Labbadi, W., & Akaichi, J. (2017). Efficient Algorithm for Answering Fuzzy Medical Requests in Pervasive Healthcare Information Systems. *International Journal of Healthcare Information Systems and Informatics, 12*(2), 46–64. doi:10.4018/IJHISI.2017040103

Lagumdzija, A., & Swing, V. K. (2017). Health, Digitalization, and Individual Empowerment. In F. Topor (Ed.), *Handbook of Research on Individualism and Identity in the Globalized Digital Age* (pp. 380–402). Hershey, PA: IGI Global. doi:10.4018/978-1-5225-0522-8.ch017

Lamey, T. W., & Davidson-Shivers, G. V. (2017). Instructional Strategies and Sequencing. In J. Stefaniak (Ed.), *Advancing Medical Education Through Strategic Instructional Design* (pp. 30–52). Hershey, PA: IGI Global. doi:10.4018/978-1-5225-2098-6.ch002

Leon, G. (2017). The Role of Forensic Medicine in Medical Errors. In M. Riga (Ed.), *Impact of Medical Errors and Malpractice on Health Economics, Quality, and Patient Safety* (pp. 144–170). Hershey, PA: IGI Global. doi:10.4018/978-1-5225-2337-6.ch006

Lidia, B., Federica, G., & Maria, V. E. (2016). The Patient-Centered Medicine as the Theoretical Framework for Patient Engagement. In G. Graffigna (Ed.), *Promoting Patient Engagement and Participation for Effective Healthcare Reform* (pp. 25–39). Hershey, PA: IGI Global. doi:10.4018/978-1-4666-9992-2.ch002

Love, L., & McDowelle, D. (2018). Developing a Comprehensive Wellness Program for Medical Students. In C. Smith (Ed.), *Exploring the Pressures of Medical Education From a Mental Health and Wellness Perspective* (pp. 190–208). Hershey, PA: IGI Global. doi:10.4018/978-1-5225-2811-1.ch008

Lovell, K. L. (2017). Development and Evaluation of Neuroscience Computer-Based Modules for Medical Students: Instructional Design Principles and Effectiveness. In J. Stefaniak (Ed.), *Advancing Medical Education Through Strategic Instructional Design* (pp. 262–276). Hershey, PA: IGI Global. doi:10.4018/978-1-5225-2098-6.ch013

Lubin, R., & Hamlin, M. D. (2018). Medical Student Burnout: A Social Cognitive Learning Perspective on Medical Student Mental Health and Wellness. In C. Smith (Ed.), *Exploring the Pressures of Medical Education From a Mental Health and Wellness Perspective* (pp. 92–121). Hershey, PA: IGI Global. doi:10.4018/978-1-5225-2811-1.ch004

Luk, C. Y. (2018). Moving Towards Universal Health Coverage: Challenges for the Present and Future in China. In B. Fong, A. Ng, & P. Yuen (Eds.), *Sustainable Health and Long-Term Care Solutions for an Aging Population* (pp. 19–45). Hershey, PA: IGI Global. doi:10.4018/978-1-5225-2633-9.ch002

Mahat, M., & Pettigrew, A. (2017). The Regulatory Environment of Non-Profit Higher Education and Research Institutions and Its Implications for Managerial Strategy: The Case of Medical Education and Research. In L. West & A. Worthington (Eds.), *Handbook of Research on Emerging Business Models and Managerial Strategies in the Nonprofit Sector* (pp. 336–351). Hershey, PA: IGI Global. doi:10.4018/978-1-5225-2537-0.ch017

Maitra, I. K., & Bandhyopadhyaay, S. K. (2017). Adaptive Edge Detection Method towards Features Extraction from Diverse Medical Imaging Technologies. In S. Bhattacharyya, S. De, I. Pan, & P. Dutta (Eds.), *Intelligent Multidimensional Data Clustering and Analysis* (pp. 159–192). Hershey, PA: IGI Global. doi:10.4018/978-1-5225-1776-4.ch007

Mangu, V. P. (2017). Mobile Health Care: A Technology View. In C. Bhatt & S. Peddoju (Eds.), *Cloud Computing Systems and Applications in Healthcare* (pp. 1–18). Hershey, PA: IGI Global. doi:10.4018/978-1-5225-1002-4.ch001

Manirabona, A., Fourati, L. C., & Boudjit, S. (2017). Investigation on Healthcare Monitoring Systems: Innovative Services and Applications. *International Journal of E-Health and Medical Communications*, *8*(1), 1–18. doi:10.4018/IJEHMC.2017010101

Mannai, M. M., & Karâa, W. B. (2016). Biomedical Image Processing Overview. In W. Karâa & N. Dey (Eds.), *Biomedical Image Analysis and Mining Techniques for Improved Health Outcomes* (pp. 1–12). Hershey, PA: IGI Global. doi:10.4018/978-1-4666-8811-7.ch001

Manzoor, A. (2016). RFID in Health Care-Building Smart Hospitals for Quality Healthcare. *International Journal of User-Driven Healthcare*, *6*(2), 21–45. doi:10.4018/IJUDH.2016070102

Marwan, M., Kartit, A., & Ouahmane, H. (2018). A Framework to Secure Medical Image Storage in Cloud Computing Environment. *Journal of Electronic Commerce in Organizations*, *16*(1), 1–16. doi:10.4018/JECO.2018010101

Masoud, M. P., Nejad, M. K., Darebaghi, H., Chavoshi, M., & Farahani, M. (2018). The Decision Support System and Conventional Method of Telephone Triage by Nurses in Emergency Medical Services: A Comparative Investigation. *International Journal of E-Business Research*, *14*(1), 77–88. doi:10.4018/IJEBR.2018010105

McDonald, W. G., Martin, M., & Salzberg, L. D. (2018). From Medical Student to Medical Resident: Graduate Medical Education and Mental Health in the United States. In C. Smith (Ed.), *Exploring the Pressures of Medical Education From a Mental Health and Wellness Perspective* (pp. 145–169). Hershey, PA: IGI Global. doi:10.4018/978-1-5225-2811-1.ch006

Medhekar, A. (2017). The Role of Social Media for Knowledge Dissemination in Medical Tourism: A Case of India. In R. Chugh (Ed.), *Harnessing Social Media as a Knowledge Management Tool* (pp. 25–54). Hershey, PA: IGI Global. doi:10.4018/978-1-5225-0495-5.ch002

Medhekar, A., & Haq, F. (2018). Urbanization and New Jobs Creation in Healthcare Services in India: Challenges and Opportunities. In U. Benna & I. Benna (Eds.), *Urbanization and Its Impact on Socio-Economic Growth in Developing Regions* (pp. 198–218). Hershey, PA: IGI Global. doi:10.4018/978-1-5225-2659-9.ch010

Mehta, G., Dutta, M. K., & Kim, P. S. (2016). An Efficient and Lossless Cryptosystem for Security in Tele-Ophthalmology Applications Using Chaotic Theory. *International Journal of E-Health and Medical Communications*, *7*(4), 28–47. doi:10.4018/IJEHMC.2016100102

Mehta, P. (2017). Framework of Indian Healthcare System and its Challenges: An Insight. In V. Bryan & J. Bird (Eds.), *Healthcare Community Synergism between Patients, Practitioners, and Researchers* (pp. 247–271). Hershey, PA: IGI Global. doi:10.4018/978-1-5225-0640-9.ch011

Metelmann, B., & Metelmann, C. (2016). M-Health in Prehospital Emergency Medicine: Experiences from the EU funded Project LiveCity. In A. Moumtzoglou (Ed.), *M-Health Innovations for Patient-Centered Care* (pp. 197–212). Hershey, PA: IGI Global. doi:10.4018/978-1-4666-9861-1.ch010

Mi, M. (2017). Informal Learning in Medical Education. In J. Stefaniak (Ed.), *Advancing Medical Education Through Strategic Instructional Design* (pp. 225–244). Hershey, PA: IGI Global. doi:10.4018/978-1-5225-2098-6.ch011

Miglioretti, M., Mariani, F., & Vecchio, L. (2016). Could Patient Engagement Promote a Health System Free From Malpractice Litigation Risk? In G. Graffigna (Ed.), *Promoting Patient Engagement and Participation for Effective Healthcare Reform* (pp. 240–264). Hershey, PA: IGI Global. doi:10.4018/978-1-4666-9992-2.ch012

Misra, S. C., & Bisui, S. (2016). Feasibility of Large Scale Implementation of Personalized Medicine in the Current Scenario. *International Journal of E-Health and Medical Communications*, *7*(2), 30–49. doi:10.4018/IJEHMC.2016040103

Misra, S. C., Bisui, S., & Fantazy, K. (2016). Identifying Critical Changes in Adoption of Personalized Medicine (PM) in Healthcare Management. *International Journal of E-Health and Medical Communications*, *7*(3), 1–15. doi:10.4018/IJEHMC.2016070101

Mohammadian, M., Hatzinakos, D., Spachos, P., & Jentzsh, R. (2016). An Intelligent and Secure Framework for Wireless Information Technology in Healthcare for User and Data Classification in Hospitals. In V. Wang (Ed.), *Handbook of Research on Advancing Health Education through Technology* (pp. 452–479). Hershey, PA: IGI Global. doi:10.4018/978-1-4666-9494-1.ch019

Mokeddem, S., & Atmani, B. (2016). Assessment of Clinical Decision Support Systems for Predicting Coronary Heart Disease. *International Journal of Operations Research and Information Systems*, *7*(3), 57–73. doi:10.4018/IJORIS.2016070104

Mokrzycka, A., & Kowalska-Bobko, I. (2016). Public Health Legislation and Patient's Rights: Health2020 Strategy, European Perspective. In A. Rosiek & K. Leksowski (Eds.), *Organizational Culture and Ethics in Modern Medicine* (pp. 298–322). Hershey, PA: IGI Global. doi:10.4018/978-1-4666-9658-7.ch013

Moon, J. D., & Galea, M. P. (2016). Overview of Clinical Decision Support Systems in Healthcare. In J. Moon & M. Galea (Eds.), *Improving Health Management through Clinical Decision Support Systems* (pp. 1–27). Hershey, PA: IGI Global. doi:10.4018/978-1-4666-9432-3.ch001

Mosadeghrad, A. M., & Woldemichael, A. (2017). Application of Quality Management in Promoting Patient Safety and Preventing Medical Errors. In M. Riga (Ed.), *Impact of Medical Errors and Malpractice on Health Economics, Quality, and Patient Safety* (pp. 91–112). Hershey, PA: IGI Global. doi:10.4018/978-1-5225-2337-6.ch004

Moumtzoglou, A. (2017). Digital Medicine: The Quality Standpoint. In A. Moumtzoglou (Ed.), *Design, Development, and Integration of Reliable Electronic Healthcare Platforms* (pp. 179–195). Hershey, PA: IGI Global. doi:10.4018/978-1-5225-1724-5.ch011

Moumtzoglou, A., & Pouliakis, A. (2018). Population Health Management and the Science of Individuality. *International Journal of Reliable and Quality E-Healthcare, 7*(2), 1–26. doi:10.4018/IJRQEH.2018040101

Mpofu, C. (2016). International Medical Experiences Outbound New Zealand: An Economic and Medical Workforce Strategy. In D. Velliaris & D. Coleman-George (Eds.), *Handbook of Research on Study Abroad Programs and Outbound Mobility* (pp. 446–469). Hershey, PA: IGI Global. doi:10.4018/978-1-5225-0169-5.ch018

Mukhtar, W. F., & Abuelyaman, E. S. (2017). Opportunities and Challenges of Big Data in Healthcare. In N. Wickramasinghe (Ed.), *Handbook of Research on Healthcare Administration and Management* (pp. 47–58). Hershey, PA: IGI Global. doi:10.4018/978-1-5225-0920-2.ch004

Munugala, S., Brar, G. K., Syed, A., Mohammad, A., & Halgamuge, M. N. (2018). The Much Needed Security and Data Reforms of Cloud Computing in Medical Data Storage. In M. Lytras & P. Papadopoulou (Eds.), *Applying Big Data Analytics in Bioinformatics and Medicine* (pp. 99–113). Hershey, PA: IGI Global. doi:10.4018/978-1-5225-2607-0.ch005

Narasimhamurthy, A. (2016). An Overview of Machine Learning in Medical Image Analysis: Trends in Health Informatics. In N. Dey & A. Ashour (Eds.), *Classification and Clustering in Biomedical Signal Processing* (pp. 23–45). Hershey, PA: IGI Global. doi:10.4018/978-1-5225-0140-4.ch002

Ngara, R. (2017). Multiple Voices, Multiple Paths: Towards Dialogue between Western and Indigenous Medical Knowledge Systems. In P. Ngulube (Ed.), *Handbook of Research on Theoretical Perspectives on Indigenous Knowledge Systems in Developing Countries* (pp. 332–358). Hershey, PA: IGI Global. doi:10.4018/978-1-5225-0833-5.ch015

O'Connor, Y., & Heavin, C. (2018). Defining and Characterising the Landscape of eHealth. In M. Khosrow-Pour, D.B.A. (Ed.), Encyclopedia of Information Science and Technology, Fourth Edition (pp. 5864-5875). Hershey, PA: IGI Global. doi:10.4018/978-1-5225-2255-3.ch510

Ochonogor, W. C., & Okite-Amughoro, F. A. (2018). Building an Effective Digital Library in a University Teaching Hospital (UTH) in Nigeria. In A. Tella & T. Kwanya (Eds.), *Handbook of Research on Managing Intellectual Property in Digital Libraries* (pp. 184–204). Hershey, PA: IGI Global. doi:10.4018/978-1-5225-3093-0.ch010

Olaniran, B. A. (2016). ICTs, E-health, and Multidisciplinary Healthcare Teams: Promises and Challenges. *International Journal of Privacy and Health Information Management*, *4*(2), 62–75. doi:10.4018/IJPHIM.2016070105

Olaniran, B. A. (2016). ICT Use and Multidisciplinary Healthcare Teams in the Age of e-Health. *International Journal of Reliable and Quality E-Healthcare*, *5*(1), 18–31. doi:10.4018/IJRQEH.2016010102

Olivares, S. L., Cruz, A. G., Cabrera, M. V., Regalado, A. I., & García, J. E. (2017). An Assessment Study of Quality Model for Medical Schools in Mexico. In S. Mukerji & P. Tripathi (Eds.), *Handbook of Research on Administration, Policy, and Leadership in Higher Education* (pp. 404–439). Hershey, PA: IGI Global. doi:10.4018/978-1-5225-0672-0.ch016

Omidoyin, E. O., Opeke, R. O., & Osagbemi, G. K. (2016). Utilization Pattern and Privacy Issues in the use of Health Records for Research Practice by Doctors: Selected Nigerian Teaching Hospitals as Case Study. *International Journal of Privacy and Health Information Management*, *4*(1), 1–11. doi:10.4018/IJPHIM.2016010101

Omoruyi, E. A., & Omidele, F. (2018). Resident Physician and Medical Academic Faculty Burnout: A Review of Current Literature. In C. Smith (Ed.), *Exploring the Pressures of Medical Education From a Mental Health and Wellness Perspective* (pp. 171–189). Hershey, PA: IGI Global. doi:10.4018/978-1-5225-2811-1.ch007

Osop, H., & Sahama, T. (2016). Data-Driven and Practice-Based Evidence: Design and Development of Efficient and Effective Clinical Decision Support System. In J. Moon & M. Galea (Eds.), *Improving Health Management through Clinical Decision Support Systems* (pp. 295–328). Hershey, PA: IGI Global. doi:10.4018/978-1-4666-9432-3.ch014

Ossowski, R., & Izdebski, P. (2016). Ethical Aspects of Talking to a Patient. In A. Rosiek & K. Leksowski (Eds.), *Organizational Culture and Ethics in Modern Medicine* (pp. 203–235). Hershey, PA: IGI Global. doi:10.4018/978-1-4666-9658-7.ch009

Pandian, P. S. (2016). An Overview of Telemedicine Technologies for Healthcare Applications. *International Journal of Biomedical and Clinical Engineering*, *5*(2), 29–52. doi:10.4018/IJBCE.2016070103

Papadopoulou, P., Lytras, M., & Marouli, C. (2018). Bioinformatics as Applied to Medicine: Challenges Faced Moving from Big Data to Smart Data to Wise Data. In M. Lytras & P. Papadopoulou (Eds.), *Applying Big Data Analytics in Bioinformatics and Medicine* (pp. 1–25). Hershey, PA: IGI Global. doi:10.4018/978-1-5225-2607-0.ch001

Paraskou, A., & George, B. P. (2018). An Overview of Reproductive Tourism. In *Legal and Economic Considerations Surrounding Reproductive Tourism: Emerging Research and Opportunities* (pp. 1–17). Hershey, PA: IGI Global. doi:10.4018/978-1-5225-2694-0.ch001

Park, S., & Moon, J. (2016). Strategic Approach towards Clinical Information Security. In J. Moon & M. Galea (Eds.), *Improving Health Management through Clinical Decision Support Systems* (pp. 329–359). Hershey, PA: IGI Global. doi:10.4018/978-1-4666-9432-3.ch015

Pereira, D., Castro, A., Gomes, P., Areias, J. C., Reis, Z. S., Coimbra, M. T., & Cruz-Correia, R. (2016). Digital Auscultation: Challenges and Perspectives. In M. Cruz-Cunha, I. Miranda, R. Martinho, & R. Rijo (Eds.), *Encyclopedia of E-Health and Telemedicine* (pp. 910–927). Hershey, PA: IGI Global. doi:10.4018/978-1-4666-9978-6.ch070

Peters, R. A., & Cruz, M. (2016). The States as Generators of Incremental Change in American Health Care Policy: 1935 to 1965. In R. Gholipour & K. Rouzbehani (Eds.), *Social, Economic, and Political Perspectives on Public Health Policy-Making* (pp. 86–114). Hershey, PA: IGI Global. doi:10.4018/978-1-4666-9944-1.ch005

Phuritsabam, B., & Devi, A. B. (2017). Information Seeking Behavior of Medical Scientists at Jawaharlal Nehru Institute of Medical Science: A Study. In S. Ram (Ed.), *Library and Information Services for Bioinformatics Education and Research* (pp. 177–187). Hershey, PA: IGI Global. doi:10.4018/978-1-5225-1871-6.ch010

Pieczka, B. (2018). Management of Risk and Adverse Events in Medical Entities. In A. Rosiek-Kryszewska & K. Leksowski (Eds.), *Healthcare Administration for Patient Safety and Engagement* (pp. 31–46). Hershey, PA: IGI Global. doi:10.4018/978-1-5225-3946-9.ch003

Poduval, J. (2016). Curriculum Development. In *Optimizing Medicine Residency Training Programs* (pp. 45–102). Hershey, PA: IGI Global. doi:10.4018/978-1-4666-9527-6.ch003

Poduval, J. (2016). Ethics and Professionalism. In *Optimizing Medicine Residency Training Programs* (pp. 103–133). Hershey, PA: IGI Global. doi:10.4018/978-1-4666-9527-6.ch004

Poduval, J. (2016). Management Skills and Leadership. In *Optimizing Medicine Residency Training Programs* (pp. 182–205). Hershey, PA: IGI Global. doi:10.4018/978-1-4666-9527-6.ch008

Poduval, J. (2016). Medicine Residency Training. In *Optimizing Medicine Residency Training Programs* (pp. 1–27). Hershey, PA: IGI Global. doi:10.4018/978-1-4666-9527-6.ch001

Poduval, J. (2016). Personal Issues. In *Optimizing Medicine Residency Training Programs* (pp. 206–221). Hershey, PA: IGI Global. doi:10.4018/978-1-4666-9527-6.ch009

Poduval, J. (2017). Medical Errors: Impact on Health Care Quality. In M. Riga (Ed.), *Impact of Medical Errors and Malpractice on Health Economics, Quality, and Patient Safety* (pp. 33–60). Hershey, PA: IGI Global. doi:10.4018/978-1-5225-2337-6.ch002

Politis, D., Stagiopoulos, P., Aidona, S., Kyriafinis, G., & Constantinidis, I. (2018). Autonomous Learning and Skill Accreditation: A Paradigm for Medical Studies. In A. Kumar (Ed.), *Optimizing Student Engagement in Online Learning Environments* (pp. 266–296). Hershey, PA: IGI Global. doi:10.4018/978-1-5225-3634-5.ch012

Pomares-Quimbaya, A., Gonzalez, R. A., Quintero, S., Muñoz, O. M., Bohórquez, W. R., García, O. M., & Londoño, D. (2016). A Review of Existing Applications and Techniques for Narrative Text Analysis in Electronic Medical Records. In M. Cruz-Cunha, I. Miranda, R. Martinho, & R. Rijo (Eds.), *Encyclopedia of E-Health and Telemedicine* (pp. 796–811). Hershey, PA: IGI Global. doi:10.4018/978-1-4666-9978-6.ch062

Pomares-Quimbaya, A., González, R. A., Sierra, A., Daza, J. C., Muñoz, O., García, A., ... Bohórquez, W. R. (2017). ICT for Enabling the Quality Evaluation of Health Care Services: A Case Study in a General Hospital. In A. Moumtzoglou (Ed.), *Design, Development, and Integration of Reliable Electronic Healthcare Platforms* (pp. 196–210). Hershey, PA: IGI Global. doi:10.4018/978-1-5225-1724-5.ch012

Pouliakis, A., Margari, N., Karakitsou, E., Archondakis, S., & Karakitsos, P. (2018). Emerging Technologies Serving Cytopathology: Big Data, the Cloud, and Mobile Computing. In I. El Naqa (Ed.), *Emerging Developments and Practices in Oncology* (pp. 114–152). Hershey, PA: IGI Global. doi:10.4018/978-1-5225-3085-5.ch005

Queirós, A., Silva, A. G., Ferreira, A., Caravau, H., Cerqueira, M., & Rocha, N. P. (2016). Assessing Mobile Applications Considered Medical Devices. In M. Cruz-Cunha, I. Miranda, R. Martinho, & R. Rijo (Eds.), *Encyclopedia of E-Health and Telemedicine* (pp. 111–127). Hershey, PA: IGI Global. doi:10.4018/978-1-4666-9978-6.ch010

Raffaeli, L., Spinsante, S., & Gambi, E. (2016). Integrated Smart TV-Based Personal e-Health System. *International Journal of E-Health and Medical Communications*, *7*(1), 48–64. doi:10.4018/IJEHMC.2016010103

Rai, A., Kothari, R., & Singh, D. P. (2017). Assessment of Available Technologies for Hospital Waste Management: A Need for Society. In R. Singh, A. Singh, & V. Srivastava (Eds.), *Environmental Issues Surrounding Human Overpopulation* (pp. 172–188). Hershey, PA: IGI Global. doi:10.4018/978-1-5225-1683-5.ch010

Ramamoorthy, S., & Sivasubramaniam, R. (2018). Image Processing Including Medical Liver Imaging: Medical Image Processing from Big Data Perspective, Ultrasound Liver Images, Challenges. In M. Lytras & P. Papadopoulou (Eds.), *Applying Big Data Analytics in Bioinformatics and Medicine* (pp. 380–392). Hershey, PA: IGI Global. doi:10.4018/978-1-5225-2607-0.ch016

Rathor, G. P., & Gupta, S. K. (2017). Improving Multimodality Image Fusion through Integrate AFL and Wavelet Transform. In V. Tiwari, B. Tiwari, R. Thakur, & S. Gupta (Eds.), *Pattern and Data Analysis in Healthcare Settings* (pp. 143–157). Hershey, PA: IGI Global. doi:10.4018/978-1-5225-0536-5.ch008

Rawat, D. B., & Bhattacharya, S. (2016). Wireless Body Area Network for Healthcare Applications. In N. Meghanathan (Ed.), *Advanced Methods for Complex Network Analysis* (pp. 343–358). Hershey, PA: IGI Global. doi:10.4018/978-1-4666-9964-9.ch014

Rea, P. M. (2016). Advances in Anatomical and Medical Visualisation. In M. Pinheiro & D. Simões (Eds.), *Handbook of Research on Engaging Digital Natives in Higher Education Settings* (pp. 244–264). Hershey, PA: IGI Global. doi:10.4018/978-1-5225-0039-1.ch011

Rexhepi, H., & Persson, A. (2017). Challenges to Implementing IT Support for Evidence Based Practice Among Nurses and Assistant Nurses: A Qualitative Study. *Journal of Electronic Commerce in Organizations*, *15*(2), 61–76. doi:10.4018/JECO.2017040105

Reychav, I., & Azuri, J. (2016). Including Elderly Patients in Decision Making via Electronic Health Literacy. In M. Cruz-Cunha, I. Miranda, R. Martinho, & R. Rijo (Eds.), *Encyclopedia of E-Health and Telemedicine* (pp. 241–249). Hershey, PA: IGI Global. doi:10.4018/978-1-4666-9978-6.ch020

Richards, D., & Caldwell, P. H. (2016). Gamification to Improve Adherence to Clinical Treatment Advice: Improving Adherence to Clinical Treatment. In D. Novák, B. Tulu, & H. Brendryen (Eds.), *Handbook of Research on Holistic Perspectives in Gamification for Clinical Practice* (pp. 47–77). Hershey, PA: IGI Global. doi:10.4018/978-1-4666-9522-1.ch004

Rissman, B. (2016). Medical Conditions Associated with NLD. In B. Rissman (Ed.), *Medical and Educational Perspectives on Nonverbal Learning Disability in Children and Young Adults* (pp. 27–66). Hershey, PA: IGI Global. doi:10.4018/978-1-4666-9539-9.ch002

Rosiek, A. (2018). The Assessment of Actions of the Environment and the Impact of Preventive Medicine for Public Health in Poland. In A. Rosiek-Kryszewska & K. Leksowski (Eds.), *Healthcare Administration for Patient Safety and Engagement* (pp. 106–119). Hershey, PA: IGI Global. doi:10.4018/978-1-5225-3946-9.ch006

Rosiek, A., Leksowski, K., Goch, A., Rosiek-Kryszewska, A., & Leksowski, Ł. (2016). Medical Treatment and Difficult Ethical Decisions in Interdisciplinary Hospital Teams. In A. Rosiek & K. Leksowski (Eds.), *Organizational Culture and Ethics in Modern Medicine* (pp. 121–153). Hershey, PA: IGI Global. doi:10.4018/978-1-4666-9658-7.ch006

Rosiek, A., & Rosiek-Kryszewska, A. (2018). Managed Healthcare: Doctor Life Satisfaction and Its Impact on the Process of Communicating With the Patient. In A. Rosiek-Kryszewska & K. Leksowski (Eds.), *Healthcare Administration for Patient Safety and Engagement* (pp. 244–261). Hershey, PA: IGI Global. doi:10.4018/978-1-5225-3946-9.ch013

Rosiek-Kryszewska, A., Leksowski, Ł., Rosiek, A., Leksowski, K., & Goch, A. (2016). Clinical Communication in the Aspect of Development of New Technologies and E-Health in the Doctor-Patient Relationship. In A. Rosiek & K. Leksowski (Eds.), *Organizational Culture and Ethics in Modern Medicine* (pp. 18–51). Hershey, PA: IGI Global. doi:10.4018/978-1-4666-9658-7.ch002

Rosiek-Kryszewska, A., & Rosiek, A. (2018). The Involvement of the Patient and his Perspective Evaluation of the Quality of Healthcare. In A. Rosiek-Kryszewska & K. Leksowski (Eds.), *Healthcare Administration for Patient Safety and Engagement* (pp. 121–144). Hershey, PA: IGI Global. doi:10.4018/978-1-5225-3946-9.ch007

Rosiek-Kryszewska, A., & Rosiek, A. (2018). The Impact of Management and Leadership Roles in Building Competitive Healthcare Units. In A. Rosiek-Kryszewska & K. Leksowski (Eds.), *Healthcare Administration for Patient Safety and Engagement* (pp. 13–30). Hershey, PA: IGI Global. doi:10.4018/978-1-5225-3946-9.ch002

Roşu, S. M., Păvăloiu, I. B., Dragoi, G., Apostol, C. G., & Munteanu, D. (2016). Telemedicine Based on LMDS in the Urban/Metropolitan Area: A Romanian Case Study. In M. Cruz-Cunha, I. Miranda, R. Martinho, & R. Rijo (Eds.), *Encyclopedia of E-Health and Telemedicine* (pp. 96–109). Hershey, PA: IGI Global. doi:10.4018/978-1-4666-9978-6.ch009

Rouzbehani, K. (2017). Health Policy Implementation: Moving Beyond Its Barriers in United States. In N. Wickramasinghe (Ed.), *Handbook of Research on Healthcare Administration and Management* (pp. 541–552). Hershey, PA: IGI Global. doi:10.4018/978-1-5225-0920-2.ch032

Ruiz, I. M., Cohen, D. S., & Marco, Á. M. (2016). ISO/IEEE11073 Family of Standards: Trends and Applications on E-Health Monitoring. In M. Cruz-Cunha, I. Miranda, R. Martinho, & R. Rijo (Eds.), *Encyclopedia of E-Health and Telemedicine* (pp. 646–660). Hershey, PA: IGI Global. doi:10.4018/978-1-4666-9978-6.ch050

Sam, S. (2017). Mobile Phones and Expanding Human Capabilities in Plural Health Systems. In K. Moahi, K. Bwalya, & P. Sebina (Eds.), *Health Information Systems and the Advancement of Medical Practice in Developing Countries* (pp. 93–114). Hershey, PA: IGI Global. doi:10.4018/978-1-5225-2262-1.ch006

Sankaranarayanan, S., & Ganesan, S. (2016). Applications of Intelligent Agents in Health Sector-A Review. *International Journal of E-Health and Medical Communications*, *7*(1), 1–30. doi:10.4018/IJEHMC.2016010101

Santos-Trigo, M., Suaste, E., & Figuerola, P. (2018). Technology Design and Routes for Tool Appropriation in Medical Practices. In M. Khosrow-Pour, D.B.A. (Ed.), Encyclopedia of Information Science and Technology, Fourth Edition (pp. 3794-3804). Hershey, PA: IGI Global. doi:10.4018/978-1-5225-2255-3.ch329

Sarivougioukas, J., Vagelatos, A., Parsopoulos, K. E., & Lagaris, I. E. (2018). Home UbiHealth. In M. Khosrow-Pour, D.B.A. (Ed.), Encyclopedia of Information Science and Technology, Fourth Edition (pp. 7765-7774). Hershey, PA: IGI Global. doi:10.4018/978-1-5225-2255-3.ch675

Sarkar, B. K. (2017). Big Data and Healthcare Data: A Survey. *International Journal of Knowledge-Based Organizations*, *7*(4), 50–77. doi:10.4018/IJKBO.2017100104

Saxena, K., & Banodha, U. (2017). An Essence of the SOA on Healthcare. In R. Bhadoria, N. Chaudhari, G. Tomar, & S. Singh (Eds.), *Exploring Enterprise Service Bus in the Service-Oriented Architecture Paradigm* (pp. 283–304). Hershey, PA: IGI Global. doi:10.4018/978-1-5225-2157-0.ch018

Schmeida, M., & McNeal, R. (2016). Consulting Online Healthcare Information: E-Caregivers as Knowledgeable Decision Makers. *International Journal of Computers in Clinical Practice*, *1*(1), 42–52. doi:10.4018/IJCCP.2016010104

Sen, K., & Ghosh, K. (2018). Incorporating Global Medical Knowledge to Solve Healthcare Problems: A Framework for a Crowdsourcing System. *International Journal of Healthcare Information Systems and Informatics*, *13*(1), 1–14. doi:10.4018/IJHISI.2018010101

Shakdher, A., & Pandey, K. (2017). REDAlert+: Medical/Fire Emergency and Warning System using Android Devices. *International Journal of E-Health and Medical Communications*, *8*(1), 37–51. doi:10.4018/IJEHMC.2017010103

Shekarian, E., Abdul-Rashid, S. H., & Olugu, E. U. (2017). An Integrated Fuzzy VIKOR Method for Performance Management in Healthcare. In M. Tavana, K. Szabat, & K. Puranam (Eds.), *Organizational Productivity and Performance Measurements Using Predictive Modeling and Analytics* (pp. 40–61). Hershey, PA: IGI Global. doi:10.4018/978-1-5225-0654-6.ch003

Shi, J., Erdem, E., & Liu, H. (2016). Expanding Role of Telephone Systems in Healthcare: Developments and Opportunities. In A. Dwivedi (Ed.), *Reshaping Medical Practice and Care with Health Information Systems* (pp. 87–131). Hershey, PA: IGI Global. doi:10.4018/978-1-4666-9870-3.ch004

Shijina, V., & John, S. J. (2017). Multiple Relations and its Application in Medical Diagnosis. *International Journal of Fuzzy System Applications*, *6*(4), 47–62. doi:10.4018/IJFSA.2017100104

Shipley, N., & Chakraborty, J. (2018). Big Data and mHealth: Increasing the Usability of Healthcare Through the Customization of Pinterest – Literary Perspective. In J. Machado, A. Abelha, M. Santos, & F. Portela (Eds.), *Next-Generation Mobile and Pervasive Healthcare Solutions* (pp. 46–66). Hershey, PA: IGI Global. doi:10.4018/978-1-5225-2851-7.ch004

Singh, A., & Dutta, M. K. (2017). A Reversible Data Hiding Scheme for Efficient Management of Tele-Ophthalmological Data. *International Journal of E-Health and Medical Communications*, *8*(3), 38–54. doi:10.4018/IJEHMC.2017070103

Sivaji, A., Radjo, H. K., Amin, M., & Abu Hashim, M. A. (2016). Design of a Hospital Interactive Wayfinding System: Designing for Malaysian Users. In N. Mohamed, T. Mantoro, M. Ayu, & M. Mahmud (Eds.), *Critical Socio-Technical Issues Surrounding Mobile Computing* (pp. 88–123). Hershey, PA: IGI Global. doi:10.4018/978-1-4666-9438-5.ch005

Skourti, P. K., & Pavlakis, A. (2017). The Second Victim Phenomenon: The Way Out. In M. Riga (Ed.), *Impact of Medical Errors and Malpractice on Health Economics, Quality, and Patient Safety* (pp. 197–222). Hershey, PA: IGI Global. doi:10.4018/978-1-5225-2337-6.ch008

Smith, C. R. (2018). Medical Students' Quest Towards the Long White Coat: Impact on Mental Health and Well-Being. In C. Smith (Ed.), *Exploring the Pressures of Medical Education From a Mental Health and Wellness Perspective* (pp. 1–42). Hershey, PA: IGI Global. doi:10.4018/978-1-5225-2811-1.ch001

Smith, S. I., & Dandignac, M. (2018). Perfectionism: Addressing Lofty Expectations in Medical School. In C. Smith (Ed.), *Exploring the Pressures of Medical Education From a Mental Health and Wellness Perspective* (pp. 68–91). Hershey, PA: IGI Global. doi:10.4018/978-1-5225-2811-1.ch003

Sobrinho, Á. A., Dias da Silva, L., Perkusich, A., Cunha, P., Pinheiro, M. E., & Melo de Medeiros, L. (2016). Towards Medical Systems to Aid the Detection and Treatment of Chronic Diseases. In D. Fotiadis (Ed.), *Handbook of Research on Trends in the Diagnosis and Treatment of Chronic Conditions* (pp. 50–69). Hershey, PA: IGI Global. doi:10.4018/978-1-4666-8828-5.ch003

Soczywko, J., & Rutkowska, D. (2018). The Patient/Provider Relationship in Emergency Medicine: Organization, Communication, and Understanding. In A. Rosiek-Kryszewska & K. Leksowski (Eds.), *Healthcare Administration for Patient Safety and Engagement* (pp. 74–105). Hershey, PA: IGI Global. doi:10.4018/978-1-5225-3946-9.ch005

Sołtysik-Piorunkiewicz, A., Furmankiewicz, M., & Ziuziański, P. (2016). Web Healthcare Applications in Poland: Trends, Standards, Barriers and Possibilities of Implementation and Usage of E-Health Systems. In I. Deliyannis, P. Kostagiolas, & C. Banou (Eds.), *Experimental Multimedia Systems for Interactivity and Strategic Innovation* (pp. 258–283). Hershey, PA: IGI Global. doi:10.4018/978-1-4666-8659-5.ch013

Soni, P. (2018). Implications of HIPAA and Subsequent Regulations on Information Technology. In M. Gupta, R. Sharman, J. Walp, & P. Mulgund (Eds.), *Information Technology Risk Management and Compliance in Modern Organizations* (pp. 71–98). Hershey, PA: IGI Global. doi:10.4018/978-1-5225-2604-9.ch004

Spinelli, R., & Benevolo, C. (2016). From Healthcare Services to E-Health Applications: A Delivery System-Based Taxonomy. In A. Dwivedi (Ed.), *Reshaping Medical Practice and Care with Health Information Systems* (pp. 205–245). Hershey, PA: IGI Global. doi:10.4018/978-1-4666-9870-3.ch007

Srivastava, A., & Aggarwal, A. K. (2018). Medical Image Fusion in Spatial and Transform Domain: A Comparative Analysis. In M. Anwar, A. Khosla, & R. Kapoor (Eds.), *Handbook of Research on Advanced Concepts in Real-Time Image and Video Processing* (pp. 281–300). Hershey, PA: IGI Global. doi:10.4018/978-1-5225-2848-7.ch011

Srivastava, S. K., & Roy, S. N. (2018). Recommendation System: A Potential Tool for Achieving Pervasive Health Care. In J. Machado, A. Abelha, M. Santos, & F. Portela (Eds.), *Next-Generation Mobile and Pervasive Healthcare Solutions* (pp. 111–127). Hershey, PA: IGI Global. doi:10.4018/978-1-5225-2851-7.ch008

Stancu, A. (2016). Correlations and Patterns of Food and Health Consumer Expenditure. In A. Jean-Vasile (Ed.), *Food Science, Production, and Engineering in Contemporary Economies* (pp. 44–101). Hershey, PA: IGI Global. doi:10.4018/978-1-5225-0341-5.ch003

Stanimirovic, D. (2017). Digitalization of Death Certification Model: Transformation Issues and Implementation Concerns. In S. Saeed, Y. Bamarouf, T. Ramayah, & S. Iqbal (Eds.), *Design Solutions for User-Centric Information Systems* (pp. 22–43). Hershey, PA: IGI Global. doi:10.4018/978-1-5225-1944-7.ch002

Stavros, A., Vavoulidis, E., & Nasioutziki, M. (2016). The Use of Mobile Health Applications for Quality Control and Accreditational Purposes in a Cytopathology Laboratory. In A. Moumtzoglou (Ed.), *M-Health Innovations for Patient-Centered Care* (pp. 262–283). Hershey, PA: IGI Global. doi:10.4018/978-1-4666-9861-1.ch013

Sukkird, V., & Shirahada, K. (2018). E-Health Service Model for Asian Developing Countries: A Case of Emergency Medical Service for Elderly People in Thailand. In M. Khosrow-Pour (Ed.), *Optimizing Current Practices in E-Services and Mobile Applications* (pp. 214–232). Hershey, PA: IGI Global. doi:10.4018/978-1-5225-5026-6.ch011

Sygit, B., & Wąsik, D. (2016). Patients' Rights and Medical Personnel Duties in the Field of Hospital Care. In A. Rosiek & K. Leksowski (Eds.), *Organizational Culture and Ethics in Modern Medicine* (pp. 282–297). Hershey, PA: IGI Global. doi:10.4018/978-1-4666-9658-7.ch012

Sygit, B., & Wąsik, D. (2016). The Idea of Human Rights in Conditions of Hospital Treatment. In A. Rosiek & K. Leksowski (Eds.), *Organizational Culture and Ethics in Modern Medicine* (pp. 236–254). Hershey, PA: IGI Global. doi:10.4018/978-1-4666-9658-7.ch010

Talbot, T. B. (2017). Making Lifelike Medical Games in the Age of Virtual Reality: An Update on "Playing Games with Biology" from 2013. In B. Dubbels (Ed.), *Transforming Gaming and Computer Simulation Technologies across Industries* (pp. 103–119). Hershey, PA: IGI Global. doi:10.4018/978-1-5225-1817-4.ch006

Tamposis, I., Pouliakis, A., Fezoulidis, I., & Karakitsos, P. (2016). Mobile Platforms Supporting Health Professionals: Need, Technical Requirements, and Applications. In A. Moumtzoglou (Ed.), *M-Health Innovations for Patient-Centered Care* (pp. 91–114). Hershey, PA: IGI Global. doi:10.4018/978-1-4666-9861-1.ch005

Tiago, M. T., Tiago, F., Amaral, F. E., & Silva, S. (2016). Healthy 3.0: Healthcare Digital Dimensions. In A. Dwivedi (Ed.), *Reshaping Medical Practice and Care with Health Information Systems* (pp. 287–322). Hershey, PA: IGI Global. doi:10.4018/978-1-4666-9870-3.ch010

Tripathy, B. (2016). Application of Rough Set Based Models in Medical Diagnosis. In S. Dash & B. Subudhi (Eds.), *Handbook of Research on Computational Intelligence Applications in Bioinformatics* (pp. 144–168). Hershey, PA: IGI Global. doi:10.4018/978-1-5225-0427-6.ch008

Turcu, C. E., & Turcu, C. O. (2017). Social Internet of Things in Healthcare: From Things to Social Things in Internet of Things. In C. Reis & M. Maximiano (Eds.), *Internet of Things and Advanced Application in Healthcare* (pp. 266–295). Hershey, PA: IGI Global. doi:10.4018/978-1-5225-1820-4.ch010

Unwin, D. W., Sanzogni, L., & Sandhu, K. (2017). Developing and Measuring the Business Case for Health Information Technology. In K. Moahi, K. Bwalya, & P. Sebina (Eds.), *Health Information Systems and the Advancement of Medical Practice in Developing Countries* (pp. 262–290). Hershey, PA: IGI Global. doi:10.4018/978-1-5225-2262-1.ch015

Urooj, S., & Singh, S. P. (2016). Wavelet Transform-Based Soft Computational Techniques and Applications in Medical Imaging. In P. Saxena, D. Singh, & M. Pant (Eds.), *Problem Solving and Uncertainty Modeling through Optimization and Soft Computing Applications* (pp. 339–363). Hershey, PA: IGI Global. doi:10.4018/978-1-4666-9885-7.ch016

Vasant, P. (2018). A General Medical Diagnosis System Formed by Artificial Neural Networks and Swarm Intelligence Techniques. In U. Kose, G. Guraksin, & O. Deperlioglu (Eds.), *Nature-Inspired Intelligent Techniques for Solving Biomedical Engineering Problems* (pp. 130–145). Hershey, PA: IGI Global. doi:10.4018/978-1-5225-4769-3.ch006

Waegemann, C. P. (2016). mHealth: History, Analysis, and Implementation. In A. Moumtzoglou (Ed.), M-Health Innovations for Patient-Centered Care (pp. 1-19). Hershey, PA: IGI Global. doi:10.4018/978-1-4666-9861-1.ch001

Watfa, M. K., Majeed, H., & Salahuddin, T. (2016). Computer Based E-Healthcare Clinical Systems: A Comprehensive Survey. *International Journal of Privacy and Health Information Management*, *4*(1), 50–69. doi:10.4018/IJPHIM.2016010104

Wietholter, J. P., Coetzee, R., Nardella, B., Kincaid, S. E., & Slain, D. (2016). International Healthcare Experiences: Caring While Learning and Learning While Caring. In D. Velliaris & D. Coleman-George (Eds.), *Handbook of Research on Study Abroad Programs and Outbound Mobility* (pp. 470–496). Hershey, PA: IGI Global. doi:10.4018/978-1-5225-0169-5.ch019

Witzke, K., & Specht, O. (2017). M-Health Telemedicine and Telepresence in Oral and Maxillofacial Surgery: An Innovative Prehospital Healthcare Concept in Structurally Weak Areas. *International Journal of Reliable and Quality E-Healthcare*, *6*(4), 37–48. doi:10.4018/IJRQEH.2017100105

Wójcik, A., & Chojnacki, M. (2016). Behavior and Ethical Problems in the Functioning of the Operating Theater (Case Study). In A. Rosiek & K. Leksowski (Eds.), *Organizational Culture and Ethics in Modern Medicine* (pp. 154–179). Hershey, PA: IGI Global. doi:10.4018/978-1-4666-9658-7.ch007

Wolk, K., & Marasek, K. P. (2016). Translation of Medical Texts using Neural Networks. *International Journal of Reliable and Quality E-Healthcare*, *5*(4), 51–66. doi:10.4018/IJRQEH.2016100104

Wong, A. K., & Lo, M. F. (2018). Using Pervasive Computing for Sustainable Healthcare in an Aging Population. In B. Fong, A. Ng, & P. Yuen (Eds.), *Sustainable Health and Long-Term Care Solutions for an Aging Population* (pp. 187–202). Hershey, PA: IGI Global. doi:10.4018/978-1-5225-2633-9.ch010

Wu, W., Martin, B. C., & Ni, C. (2017). A Systematic Review of Competency-Based Education Effort in the Health Professions: Seeking Order Out of Chaos. In K. Rasmussen, P. Northrup, & R. Colson (Eds.), *Handbook of Research on Competency-Based Education in University Settings* (pp. 352–378). Hershey, PA: IGI Global. doi:10.4018/978-1-5225-0932-5.ch018

Yadav, N., Aliasgari, M., & Poellabauer, C. (2016). Mobile Healthcare in an Increasingly Connected Developing World. *International Journal of Privacy and Health Information Management*, *4*(2), 76–97. doi:10.4018/IJPHIM.2016070106

Yadav, S., Ekbal, A., Saha, S., Pathak, P. S., & Bhattacharyya, P. (2017). Patient Data De-Identification: A Conditional Random-Field-Based Supervised Approach. In S. Saha, A. Mandal, A. Narasimhamurthy, S. V, & S. Sangam (Eds.), Handbook of Research on Applied Cybernetics and Systems Science (pp. 234-253). Hershey, PA: IGI Global. doi:10.4018/978-1-5225-2498-4.ch011

Yu, B., Wijesekera, D., & Costa, P. C. (2017). Informed Consent in Healthcare: A Study Case of Genetic Services. In A. Moumtzoglou (Ed.), *Design, Development, and Integration of Reliable Electronic Healthcare Platforms* (pp. 211–242). Hershey, PA: IGI Global. doi:10.4018/978-1-5225-1724-5.ch013

Yu, B., Wijesekera, D., & Costa, P. C. (2017). Informed Consent in Electronic Medical Record Systems. In I. Management Association (Ed.), Healthcare Ethics and Training: Concepts, Methodologies, Tools, and Applications (pp. 1029-1049). Hershey, PA: IGI Global. doi:10.4018/978-1-5225-2237-9.ch049

Yu, M., Li, J., & Wang, W. (2017). Creative Life Experience among Students in Medical Education. In C. Zhou (Ed.), *Handbook of Research on Creative Problem-Solving Skill Development in Higher Education* (pp. 158–184). Hershey, PA: IGI Global. doi:10.4018/978-1-5225-0643-0.ch008

Zarour, K. (2017). Towards a Telehomecare in Algeria: Case of Diabetes Measurement and Remote Monitoring. *International Journal of E-Health and Medical Communications*, *8*(4), 61–80. doi:10.4018/IJEHMC.2017100104

Zavyalova, Y. V., Korzun, D. G., Meigal, A. Y., & Borodin, A. V. (2017). Towards the Development of Smart Spaces-Based Socio-Cyber-Medicine Systems. *International Journal of Embedded and Real-Time Communication Systems*, *8*(1), 45–63. doi:10.4018/IJERTCS.2017010104

Zeinali, A. A. (2018). Word Formation Study in Developing Naming Guidelines in the Translation of English Medical Terms Into Persian. In M. Khosrow-Pour, D.B.A. (Ed.), Encyclopedia of Information Science and Technology, Fourth Edition (pp. 5136-5147). Hershey, PA: IGI Global. doi:10.4018/978-1-5225-2255-3.ch446

Ziminski, T. B., Demurjian, S. A., Sanzi, E., & Agresta, T. (2016). Toward Integrating Healthcare Data and Systems: A Study of Architectural Alternatives. In T. Iyamu & A. Tatnall (Eds.), *Maximizing Healthcare Delivery and Management through Technology Integration* (pp. 270–304). Hershey, PA: IGI Global. doi:10.4018/978-1-4666-9446-0.ch016

Ziminski, T. B., Demurjian, S. A., Sanzi, E., Baihan, M., & Agresta, T. (2016). An Architectural Solution for Health Information Exchange. *International Journal of User-Driven Healthcare*, *6*(1), 65–103. doi:10.4018/IJUDH.2016010104

Zineldin, M., & Vasicheva, V. (2018). Reducing Medical Errors and Increasing Patient Safety: TRM and 5 Q's Approaches for Better Quality of Life. In *Technological Tools for Value-Based Sustainable Relationships in Health: Emerging Research and Opportunities* (pp. 87–115). Hershey, PA: IGI Global. doi:10.4018/978-1-5225-4091-5.ch005

About the Contributors

Thomas Heinrich Musiolik was born in Strzelce Opolskie (Poland) and grew up in Berlin. He studied International Business and International Management (Marketing and Communication) at the universities of Breda (Netherlands) and Berlin (Germany). He is currently a doctoral student at the Berlin University of the Arts. Thomas Heinrich Musiolik is Editor-in-Chief of the Journal of Future Robot Life and Chair of the Conference on Future Applications of AI, Sensors, and Robotics in Society. He is Lecturer for Digital Brand Management, Digital Experience, Multisensory Experience and Online Communication at German, Swiss, Austrian, South American and Polish universities. He is also expert for the European Commission and reviewer for scientific publishers and journals (for example, Marketing Review St. Gallen) and author of several books and articles in journals specializing in Marketing & Communication. Musiolik is also a scientific ambassador of Brain City Berlin. Since 2011, he has been investigating the functions of the brain and the influence of digital media. The goal of his work is to understand the customer needs and to map these findings in a dynamic model and to integrate them into the digital space, as a fully automated interface. The result would be automated and perfect experiences. He is also researching the societal changes that are emerging in the context of digitization. The aim of his work is to better understand the digitization and its effects on the human brain and make it usable as an benefit for the society. Personally and as a scientist he stands for clear decisions, infectious ideas and the permanent questioning of the status quo.

* * *

Jesmond Attard is a Visiting Senior Lecturer at the Faculty of Health Sciences and Research Support Officer at the Faculty of Engineering, University of Malta. He is a qualified Orthotist/Prosthetist, and is the Chief Scientific Officer (Orthotics & Prosthetics) with the Department of Health, Malta.

Andrew Cachia is an experienced software developer specialized in innovative technologies including Artificial Intelligence, Virtual Reality, Blockchain and FinTech. He has completed an MSc in Artificial Intelligence as well as a BSc in IT (Computing for Finance).

Vanessa Camilleri is an academic at the Department of Artificial Intelligence, Faculty of ICT, University of Malta. Her expertise is in the area of Human Computer Interactions, with a specialisation in Virtual Worlds and Serious Games. Her areas of interest include Virtual Reality applications for developing emotional intelligence values. Her previous experience in the area of education and pedagogy, as well as educational technologies and use of games for learning have contributed to her overall academic profile. Her main publications are in the areas of online learning and the use of innovative and emerging technologies for learning. She also has worked on a number of EU funded projects in the areas of game-based learning. More recently she has started working on developing virtual reality experiences for teaching and learning purposes related to various aspects of emotional intelligence.

Cornelia Eicher studied business in Cambridge, England and Basel, Switzerland (M.Sc. International Management) and Public Health in Berlin, Germany (MPH). Her doctoral thesis pursued the topic of assistive and robotic health technologies and devices for vulnerable patient groups (Dr. rer. medic.). Since 2017 Dr. Eicher has been doing research in the Geriatrics Research Group of the Charité - Universitätsmedizin Berlin within different R&D projects related to technologies for the ageing population and people in need of support.

Paulann Grech is a senior lecturer with the Department of Mental Health, University of Malta. In addition to lecturing, she is involved in research projects related to critical psychiatry, service user involvement and approaches to understanding and managing mental distress. Dr.Grech is the chairperson of the NGO Hearing Voices Malta, which is the Maltese branch of the Hearing Voices Network. She is also a committee member of the Life Resources Foundation and sits on the board of directors of the European Centre of Excellence (CoE) for Research in Continuing Professional Development. Dr. Grech is a mental health activist and is a co-organiser of three ongoing campaigns, namely #StopStigma, #myreality and #togetherwithonevoice. In this role, she regularly co-organises awareness events and participates in others as an invited speaker, focusing on different mental health aspects. As a writer, Dr.Grech is particularly interested in observing and blogging about life from a mental health perspective via her thrice weekly mini-articles on: https://www.facebook.com/paulann.grech. She has just published a book called Coping with Coronus: Self-help notes for a Pandemic.

Jan Kalina is a researcher in the fields of machine learning and data analysis with experience with medical informatics. He studied mathematical statistics at the Faculty of Mathematics and Physics of the Charles University in Prague and then obtained his Ph.D. from the University of Duisburg-Essen in 2007. He works at the Czech Academy of Sciences, Institute of Computer Science. He served as the head of Department of Medical Informatics in 2013-2017 and is currently the deputy head of the Department of Machine Learning since 2018.

Robert Klebbe does research and his doctorate degree in the Geriatrics Research Group of the Charité - Universitätsmedizin Berlin. He is a professional geriatric nurse and studied Sociology of Technology (B.A./M.A.) at the Technical University of Berlin. His research focuses on human-technology interaction of older adults in the context of innovative, digital health technologies as well as on the sociology of technology and health. His current research focuses on human-robot interaction in the care of older adults and people with neuromuscular diseases.

Alexei Sammut joined the Department of Mental Health, University of Malta in 2016. Previously Alexei had a career in the public sector as a Mental Health Nurse. He holds both general and mental health nursing qualifications and has worked in a variety of mental health settings, including acute, learning disabilities and old age psychiatry. Alexei Sammut has completed his Doctorate in Philosophy at Kingston University and St Georges University of London under the supervision of Professor Mary Chambers, Mr Robert Grant and Dr Josianne Scerri, with his thesis Maltese Nurses' and Midwives' Attitudes Mental Illness: A National Comparative Study. Alexei is the coordinator of the Bachelor of Science Mental Health Nursing Part Time programme. He has presented in several conferences. Apart from his teaching load he acts as a dissertation supervisor. Alexei acts as a reviewer for several local and international journals. Dr Sammut is an elected board member of Horatio, European Psychiatric Nurses, representing psychiatric and mental health nurses across Europe.

Josianne Scerri completed her undergraduate studies at the University of Malta. She continued her postgraduate studies obtaining a Master's in Education, and then read for her Doctorate at the University of Nottingham. Her Doctoral research was a prospective study examining the illness perceptions and emotional adjustment of patients with chronic illnesses and their carers. At present Josianne is Head, Department of Mental Health, Faculty of Health Sciences, University of Malta. She is also an Honorary Research Fellow at Kingston University and St George's University of London. Josianne is also an Associate member of the Person-centred Practice Research International Community of Practice and a member of the European Centre of Excellence (CoE) for Research in Continuing Professional Development. She presently is also a member of the University Research and Ethics committee and an Associate Editor of the Malta Journal of Health Sciences. As a keynote speaker at both local and international conferences, she has addressed issues relating to the experiences of patients and carers, as well as means of empowerment with health professionals, patients, carers and the academic community. In addition to her regular lecturing load and the conducting of her own research, she supervises students undertaking dissertations from undergraduate to doctoral level.

Nicole Tobišková is a first-year PhD student at University West in Trollhättan, Sweden. She received a bachelor's degree in Computer Science from Czech Technical University in Prague and a master's degree in Human-Computer Interaction from Umeå University in Sweden. Her current research focus lies on the intersection of Artificial Intelligence - driven Human-Computer Interaction and Production Technology.

Satvik Tripathi (born Jan 04, 2004 in Lucknow, India) is an incoming freshman at the College of Computing & Informatics, Drexel University, and an active researcher in the field of AI in Medicine. His main areas of concentration are Artificial Intelligence, Neuroscience, Radiology, and Mathematics. He recently attended Stanford Pre-Collegiate Summer Institute to study Artificial Intelligence course. He is currently working as a Research Intern at Neosoma. Alongside, he is also serving as the Treasurer at Drexel AI and the Student Officer at the Medical Intelligence Society. He authored his first book chapter at the age of 15, and due to his expertise in the field, he has been serving as a Reviewer at IGI Global Publication. He is well experienced with neuroradiological imaging and developing as well as implementing Deep Learning techniques for clinical use. His main research interests include Computer Vision, Neurosymbolic AI, Pattern Recognition, Generative Adversarial Networks, and Neuro-inspired Machine Learning.

Index

M

N

O

P

R

S

T

U

www.ingramcontent.com/pod-product-compliance
Lightning Source LLC
LaVergne TN
LVHW081520300926
849161LV00006B/1231

9781799878889